(You Can Be....)

WELL AT ANY AGE

Your Definitive Guide To
Vibrant Health & Longevity

For information address Institute of Nutritional Science
9528 Miramar Road #180, San Diego, CA 92126
USA

10 9 8 7 6 5 4 3 2 1

First Edition

Library of Congress Cataloging-in-Publication Data

Whiting, K Steven

You Can Be... Well At Any Age: Your Definitive Guide to Vibrant Health & Longevity/
K Steven Whiting

Includes bibliographical references and index.

1. Dietary Supplements
2. Prevention/ Reversal of Chronic Disease
3. Longevity

Library of Congress Control Number: 00-134230

ISBN 0-9701302-0-1

This book does not intend to diagnose disease nor to provide specific medical advice. Its intention is solely to inform and to educate. The author intends that readers will use the information presented in this book in cooperation with the advice of a qualified health professional trained in such field.

About the Author...

Dr. Whiting is an Orthomolecular Nutritionist. His degrees include a Masters in psychology as well as a Doctorate in biochemistry. While his degrees were earned outside the United States, his more than 27 years of experience in the field of human nutrition make his approach both relevant and insightful.

His many years in the nutrition industry include extensive research into such chronic conditions as heart disease, arthritis, diabetes, osteoporosis and prostate problems, to name a few. The result of this research has lead to the development of nutritional protocols for the prevention, management and reversal of these conditions.

Studies he has conducted have led to a totally new system of weight management based on 'body typing', wherein how a person's body handles foods is evaluated *before* they are put on a weight management program that's customized for them.

Recently, he has focused his attention on the human immune system. His subsequent research into deep viral infections has led to the use of oxygen therapy as well as other all-natural potent immune boosters for the management of immune-compromised conditions. Further, his work with AIDS and cancer patients using meditation, biofeedback and visualization has received worldwide attention.

Dr. Whiting has served as both consultant and staff member to many of the leading alternative & complimentary hospitals in Europe and Latin America, where he has had the opportunity of testing his concepts on those individuals who were most in need. This resulted in the development of nutritional support protocols for a variety of chronic health challenges. Through his international affiliations, he remains current on the very latest progressive applications of nutrition for a wide variety of chronic degenerative disorders, for which orthodox medicine has offered little hope.

In 1991, he founded the international organization, The Institute of Nutritional Science Ltd. with offices in London, England, Den Haag, The Netherlands and in San Diego, California. The purpose of the Institute is to gather and conduct research on how natural supplements can prevent and manage disease conditions. The Institute publishes a monthly Journal, available by subscription, dispensing this information in an easy to understand user-friendly fashion. Further, The Institute provides ongoing education in the field of nutrition and preventive health via their books, audio tapes and special reports. The Institute also offers certificate-training programs, through their Holland office, for those individuals wishing to further pursue their knowledge and training in the field of clinical nutrition.

He is the author of numerous self-help booklets on nutrition and progressive health, as well as the author of a textbook entitled **Gaining and Maintaining Total Health**. His book **SelfHealth, Your Complete Guide to Optimal Wellness,** which was published in 1996, rapidly became a best seller. This present work, **You Can Be... Well At Any Age: Your Definitive Guide to Vibrant Health & Longevity**, is the most comprehensive work of it's kind, containing over 250 protocols for a wide variety of human health challenges.

Author, lecturer, teacher, product formulator and consultant, Dr. Whiting is dedicated to educating others in helping themselves towards a more healthful existence through a better understanding of the nutritional needs of the body. His application of nutritional principles and mental therapeutics has enabled thousands of individuals to realize a return to vibrant health. Through these combined efforts, Dr. Whiting and The Institute of Nutritional Science are committed to empowering the individual with the very latest nutritional information in the hopes that this will serve to enhance both the quality and quantity of life for everyone in the years ahead.

Acknowledgements

I would like to thank my staff at The Institute of Nutritional Science for their endless hours of time in the preparation and proof reading of this work. I would also like to extend a special thank you to Roy Muecke for his editorial talents in making this book more readable and user friendly. To all the graphic artists, typesetters, and printers, your talents are reflected herein.

To Robert de la Bije, who has taken on the task of the foreign language editions, many thanks for making this information available to the people in other countries. Also, thanks go to the countless number of people around the world who have supported my work both financially and philosophically.

"When you sell a man a book,
you don't sell him 12 ounces of
paper and ink and glue-
you sell him a whole new life."

- Christopher Morley

Table of Contents

Table of Contents

Introduction

Humanity is poised on the edge of a new century. What an exciting time! It seems that everyone is looking forward to the millennium, each for their own reasons. For most, it is the anticipation of what the ensuing years hold in the way of scientific and social progress. If the past century alone is any indication, the changes in the next 100 years will be anyone's guess.

As we enter both a new century and a new millennium, sadly, we carry much old baggage with us. The latter half of the last century saw the control over much infectious disease through the advent of the antibiotic during World War II. While infectious diseases are once again on the slight rise due to antibiotic abuse, they do not represent even a fraction of the threat of decades past.

The lessening threat of infectious disease has been replaced by a much larger and ominous threat, namely that of chronic degenerative disease. Chronic diseases are identified as, generally, non-contagious in nature, and once acquired, remain with us for a very long time, if not the rest of our lives. Diseases such as heart disease, cancer, arthritis, diabetes, toxic overload conditions such as fibromyalgia, prostate problems and autoimmune disorders are so common that everyone knows someone who has at least one of these problems. In fact, just 60 years ago, one in six people (17%) had a chronic disease. Today that figure has jumped to one in two (50%)! As more and more of us reach age 50 and beyond, chronic disease will affect two out of every three people (67%).

Allopathic, or "conventional medicine", is poorly equipped, at best, for handling these chronic conditions. Through its reactive nature, medical treatment, over a prolonged period of time, frequently produces more problems for the patient than it alleviates. Focus on prevention and reversal of these chronic conditions will be essential if we are to ensure any degree of quality of life for the millions and millions of people who have entered the last one-third of their lives.

Science has learned a great deal in the last two decades about how and why we age. Even though we have barely scratched the surface, the information at hand offers keys to enhancing both the quality and quantity of life ahead.

Even though the average life span has increased precious little since the turn of the last century, we are equipped to make a considerable change in statistics - if we put into practice the knowledge at hand. In fact, if we can manage to avoid some of the more obvious pitfalls (obesity, stress, immune system compromise, toxic overload, etc), which contribute to premature aging and death, we have the potential to make the last third of our lives some of the best years of all.

For many, retirement means having the time to enjoy all the many hobbies and other activities that we have always had to put off due to demands of job and family. Sadly, when many of us reach those 'golden years', they are tarnished with doctor visits, therapies, side effects from numerous drugs, surgical procedures, prolonged hospital stays and deterioration of both mind and body. All too often, we find ourselves more restricted than we were when we had to work and raise the family. The golden years become discolored and it is no wonder that depression is the most common ongoing complaint of elderly people.

It doesn't have to be that way, however. A United States Congressional investigation, prior to the passage of the Dietary Supplement Health and Education Act (DSHEA), revealed that more than 90 percent of all chronic diseases could be either prevented or greatly improved if people would exercise and take the proper dietary supplements. Thousands and thousands of clinical studies into the application of specific dietary supplements repeatedly prove this finding. Today there are both safe and effective methods of preventing and even reversing many of the top robbers of the quality and quantity of life. Diseases such as heart disease, diabetes, arthritis, prostate problems and even cancer can be prevented, improved and even reversed, not through drugs and surgery, but through exercise, proper diet and the appropriated use of nutritional supplements.

By providing the body with a Full Spectrum of vitamins, minerals, fatty acids, amino acids, phytonutrients (from plants), and heavy hitting antioxidants, we can both slow down the aging process and ward off most of the diseases of maturity. We have come to realize that there is more to optimal nutrition than randomly taking some vitamins and minerals. We now know that ratio is equally as important as potency, if not more so. We also know that nutrients work at their best when they are all present at the same time. This concept of totality establishes and nourishes the internal harmonics of the living body, giving us our best possible chance at quality longevity.

Through understanding the importance of maintaining chemical balance in our bodies and providing all the raw materials we need, on a daily basis, we can create an environment wherein the body can establish and maintain internal synergy.

By learning how to both choose and prepare foods in a healthy way, we can avoid the pitfalls of the Standard American Diet (SAD). This particular diet has likely contributed more to the loss of "quality of life" than all other causes, including substance abuse, combined.

Instead of trying to drug, cut, burn, and otherwise poison sick people well, we now know that there are better ways. Complimentary protocols for most of today's common health concerns are not only well researched, but have been proven to be highly effective in helping many people dramatically improve the quality of their lives. As a result, society is now demanding that "alternative medicine" options be made more widely available. These demands will eventually force the conventional medical professionals and the pharmaceutical industry to make many changes.

The vast conglomerate, known as the 'baby boomers', has governed the politics, economy, and social trends of an entire civilization. Their force, as a unit, has dictated the way both products and services are marketed.

There were over 76 million people born in the United States alone during the years from 1946 to 1964. If we follow this mass of people, we can see clearly what has taken place. In 1940 there were 270 million jars of baby food sold. By 1953 that number had jumped to 1.5 billion! In 1960, a small company called The Gap, posted revenues of $600,000 in sales of blue jeans. By 1976, as the baby boomers became teenagers and young adults, their revenue soared to 99 million! In 1982 the home gym and fitness equipment industry generated about $75 million in sales. By 1985, as many 'boomers' reached middle age, the industry boasted a whopping $1 billion in revenue!

The morale of this story is that this vast generation can afford to have whatever interests them. Today their interests lie in preventing and reversing the ravages of time and aging. The next decade will witness the greatest increase in the use of dietary supplements and health foods in history. Further, it will drive the medical industry into preventive, complimentary forms of medicine because their patients will demand it.

For now, where do you get all the answers to these essential, yet complicated, questions? My friends, you hold those answers in your hands.

My goal in writing this book was to provide a handbook for gleaning the very best out of life ahead. Ninety percent of everything we know about longevity and nutrition we learned in the last 20 years. This rapid influx of information has caused a virtual overload to the point where most people are just plain confused.

What you now hold in your hands is a guidebook to help you apply what we know to your best possible advantage. The best news of all is that it doesn't have to be complicated, in fact it isn't. You don't have to radically change your lifestyle to benefit from current knowledge in longevity. The principles outlined in this book are attainable and doable by every single person, regardless of age or present physical condition.

One of the most common questions we receive at the Institute is, ' Is it too late for me"? The answer is simple: still life - still hope. As long as you are still breathing, you can benefit, and benefit profoundly, from the program outlined herein.

The key to all of these potential benefits lies in a

cooperation between you and me. I will provide you with the programs, specific programs that will address your own individual needs. You must take responsibility for your future and apply the protocols accordingly. Together we can change the future, your future. The time is now.

Part 1: Facing the Problem

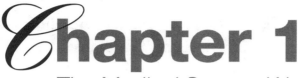

Chapter 1
The Medical System Worldwide

While this book is primarily designed to put forth a plan for health and longevity through the use of methods other than conventional allopathic medicine, I think it would be both interesting and beneficial to understand where we have come from regarding our "mind set" towards health. Certainly as recently as twenty years ago, virtually the only option in health care available on any widespread basis was either conventional medicine or perhaps, chiropractic. Even though there is still widespread opposition to alternative healing modalities, at least there are choices available today. In fact, for the first time in recorded history, in 1998, more people sought the counsel, therapies, and advice of alternative health care practitioners than those of conventional medical doctors.

Why has there been such staunch opposition to anything that is outside the scope of conventional medicine? To answer this question, we have to take a look at both the philosophy of modern medicine as well as the politics of the institution.

Hypocrites (460-377 BC), known as the father of medicine, defined health as the balance between the various components of person's nature, environment, and ways of life. The Hippocratic oath requires that the physician remember, under all circumstances, that he or she should "Of first, do no harm". Hypocrites stated "It is more important to know what sort of person has a disease than to know what sort of disease a person has". At the turn of the last century, this philosophy was revived by physician William Osler. Today, we are relearning the connection between the mind and the body, and that one cannot expect to cut, burn, and poison sick people well.

The emphasis upon understanding the patient vanished somewhere in the 1960's. As conventional medicine grew larger, it became cold and impersonal. No longer was the family physician available for house calls. Through large insurance muscle, doctors lost their flexibility and were forced to pool resources, forming medical groups consisting of many physicians. This meant that not only did the Doctor no longer make house calls, you may not even see the same Doctor when you come back to the same office.

The de-humanizing of the medical profession was a product of insurance companies, the success of pharmaceuticals such as the antibiotics that made Doctors feel invincible, the advent of super high technology, and at least to some extent, the shear numbers of patients.

By 1985, the health care expenditure in the United

States alone had reached $360 billion, nearly a billion dollars every day! For this, we boast the greatest diagnostic system in the history of medicine. Increasingly sophisticated devices, designed to diagnose disease, potential disease, and even possible disease, remove the physician farther and farther from his patients. There are more than 11 billion of these sophisticated medical tests being performed every year in the United States alone.

Not only are these medial tests out of control but the treatments have become high tech, costly and inhumane as well. Radiation devices for cancer treatment, specialized equipment for kidney dialysis, artificial body parts and elaborate intensive care units to care for people experiencing these treatments have driven the cost of maintaining the deteriorating human body almost unattainable.

Medical costs in the United States alone account for over 11 percent of the nation's gross national product. At approximately one trillion dollars, it equates to over $3,000 for every U.S. citizen. Other so-called 'civilized nations' are not far behind us. In the United Kingdom each and every citizen is spending over $450.00 annually on healthcare. In Japan it's $500.00, in France, $800.00, and in Germany nearly $1000.00! How did we get into this mess?

Any economist will tell you that when a service industry attains monopoly status, quality of goods and services will deteriorate while costs will continue to rise. In fact, we are careful to ensure that vital goods and services are not subject to a monopoly situation through many complicated business laws. Yet the most important industry, the health care system, has operated in a near total monopoly for decades.

After the successful advent of the antibiotic in the 1940's, conventional medical practitioners rose to a God-like status, at least in their own minds. Pharmaceutical companies, riding on the success of specific key drugs, grew into one of the most financially powerful conglomerates in the world. Today, we have a situation in which the drug companies are so powerful that they actually dictate policy in medicine through their large financial contributions to such political organizations as the American Medical Association. They fund many medical journals through their high priced advertising. It is estimated that the pharmaceutical industry spends in excess of two billion dollars every year in order to solicit their drugs to physicians. In a past issue of Fortune Magazine, it was uncovered that while the pharmaceutical industry claims to spend 15 percent of its sales on research and development, they spent over twice that much on advertisements appearing in medical journals, alone! Much of the rest of their staggering advertising budget is spent on the army of drug salespeople who personally visit physicians with literature, gifts, and incentives.

A Harvard University study has shown that physicians will routinely pick up erroneous information from these 'salespeople', which is in direct contradiction to the actual clinical studies involving the drugs that they are selling. According to Milton Silverman of the University of California at San Francisco, "In medical school, we teach students to prescribe on the basis of scientific evidence.... Five years after medical school, they are not prescribing as they were taught. They are brainwashed by detail men."

These drugs are so prolifically prescribed, that it is now believed that during any given 24 hour period, as many as 50 to 80 percent of all adults in the United States swallow a medically prescribed drug.

According to the Bureau of Statistics and published in U.S. News and World Report back in January of 1995, "Up to 2 million people are hospitalized each year as a result of significant side effects from prescription medications." The side effects must have indeed been significant if it drove the patient to the hospital. Worse, much worse, according to the same reliable source, as many as 140,000 of those people die as a result of the side effects or reactions related to consuming those various prescription drugs!

If you factor the figure of 140,00 deaths into all the other causes of death such as heart disease, cancer etc., at 140,000 deaths, it makes prescription drugs the fifth leading cause of death worldwide!

If this atrocity were to occur in virtually any other area of professionalism, the public would have long ago demanded review and revision. So how can this occur, year after year, and no one says a word? The answer, although complicated, goes back to the fact that allopathic medicine holds or at least has held the monopoly over health care worldwide for many decades. This has allowed them, and their counterparts such as the pharmaceutical industry, to amass such financial power that to question them seems almost impossible.

Fortunately this monopoly is breaking down. During the last 20 years, conventional medicine has lost much of the public confidence it once held due to repeated failures in properly addressing both the prevention and treatment of leading causes of disease and premature death.

The medical industry's last shining hour was the development of the antibiotic prior to 1950. Since that time very little in the way of disease eradication has been developed. Today, while infectious diseases have been reduced substantially, they have been replaced by a group of diseases called chronic degenerative diseases, which are proving to respond poorly to the standard medical model. In fact, it is estimated that at least 70 percent of all medical costs are generated by the mismanagement of these chronic conditions.

Heart disease is still the number one cause of death in spite of such invasive and expensive procedures as angioplasty and the bypass operation. Cancer, the most feared disease of the Twentieth Century, not only remains at number two as we enter the new millennium, but will likely overtake heart disease as the leading cause of death within the next decade. Other diseases such as diabetes, which has gone from relative obscurity at the turn of the last century, now sits at number three in the new millennium ahead. Arthritis, while not directly responsible for high numbers of fatalities, robs more people of the quality of their retirement years than at any other time in human history. Chronic prostate inflammation and complications from menopause continue to add to the burdens of aging. Burdens by the way, which are not being effectively addressed by our present system of medical care.

As we proceed into the new century, more and more people worldwide will cross over the 50 year old mark. In fact, in another 10 years, we will have more people alive over the age of 50 than at any time in recorded history. This vast population is the very target for chronic degenerative disease and not only has medicine failed in its management of these conditions, they have failed to properly educate the public in proven ways to prevent the occurrence of these diseases in the first place.

This dilemma has been caused by a failure to modify the standard medical model of diagnosis and treatment as well as a realization that these very chronic conditions are what continue to support the entire medical industry. If heart disease, cancer, arthritis and diabetes were to be suddenly eradicated from our lives, the medical industry would collapse into bankruptcy overnight. There is little hope of this occurring as long as conventional medicine continues to treat chronic diseases with the old "Standard Medical Model".

The Standard Medical Model

Whenever you, or anyone else for that matter, visit a medical doctor, you will be treated according to the 'standard medical model.' This is the way doctors have all been trained to view their patients. In fact, they are brainwashed from the first day of medical school up until their day of graduation that all patients are addressed and managed in exactly the same way. Further, they are advised that if they always follow this medical model and something should go wrong, organizations such as The American Medical Association and others will be there to back them up and protect them. However, should they deviate from this medical model, well, they will be on their own.... Alone.

What is this standard medical model? It is a system of patient management that developed primarily out of the success with antibiotics. When you apply it to infectious diseases or emergency situations, the medical model can be a lifesaver. However, when this same line of thinking is applied to chronic degenerative disease, the results are dismal at best and a total failure most of the time. Let's take a closer look at what has gone wrong.

The standard medical model is as follows...

1. Diagnose Disease
2. Prescribe Drugs
3. Perform Surgery

When we apply this concept to an emergency procedure for example, it works well. Let's say that you have just been hit by a car and your leg is broken in several places. You will be very glad indeed, that there is an emergency room nearby where trained doctors can diagnose the extent of your damage, perform surgery, set bones, apply casts, and prescribe medications to prevent infection, inflammation, and pain. All will likely be well and a full recovery would be expected. Now, what happens in the case of a chronic disease?

Let's take arthritis, for example, and apply the medical model to the management of this disease. First of all the doctor will perform an examination and perhaps run some tests. After which a diagnosis of arthritis is handed down. Next, the doctor will prescribe drugs such as pain-killers and anti-inflammatories. Since none of these chemicals actually addresses the cause of arthritis, the disease will continue to progress with time. This will necessitate the use of stronger and stronger drugs. At some point in time, the physician will make the determination that the side effects of the drug therapy are worse than the apparent benefit and will suggest that they move to stage three of the medical model and perform some surgery. In the case of arthritis, it might likely be joint replacement.

It should be seen by this example that none of the treatments or procedures outlined above did anything for the actual arthritis. Even the replacement of the joint with a plastic counterpart does not signify the end, since over time, other joints will be affected and the process and the discomfort will continue.

If you apply the standard medical model to any chronic disease condition, you will end up at the same point of no results. This is why chronic disease is the leading cause of suffering and death in our society. Until medicine is willing to look at the cause of these diseases, they will continue to rob more and more people of both the quality and quantity of their lives ahead.

As more and more of us pass the age 50 mark, we become increasingly more vulnerable to chronic disease. Since these diseases are a result of the biochemical breakdown of the living human chemistry, our chances of developing one or more of these conditions increases dramatically after the age of 45 or 50 and continues to increase with every year thereafter.

The majority of the casualties of the medical system are due to side effects of drugs, chronic disease not addressed, surgical procedures improperly performed, and the excessive use of testing procedures. These casualties occur most often in the elderly.

It is not uncommon for many older people to be taking 15 or more prescription drugs at any given time. The side effects of drug therapy increases exponentially with the increase in the number of drugs taken. Among the older population, the use of non-steroidal anti-inflammatory drugs (NSAIDs) for arthritis, common aches and pains, and other conditions can be linked to many complications.Serious digestive problems can lead the list according to a study conducted at Emory University. The over the counter pain killers were found to cause gastroesophageal reflux disease, resulting in chronic acid injury and imbalance. The clinical study found that 35% of patients over 65 years of age showed significant damage as a result of regular use of NSAIDs.

You might think that this would discourage the practice of routinely prescribing these drugs to older people. To the contrary, a report published in the Annuals of Internal Medicine showed that doctors are not only prescribing these drugs more than in the past but that they are frequently prescribing them unnecessarily. Another study, conducted in Canada, revealed that NSAIDs were being prescribed unnecessarily as often as 41 percent of the time!

Older members of the population continue to suffer the most at the hands of medicine "gone awry". According to a study conducted in Jerusalem and presented to the American Geriatrics Society in Atlanta, Georgia in May of 1997, elderly people may not benefit from the flu shot. Yet, in spite of this study, and other credible evidence substantiating its findings, older people remain the primary recipients of the flu shot. The study's coordinator, Haim Dannenberg of the Hadassah University Hospital revealed that the subjects who had been given repeated flu shots had lower antibody levels than those who had not been vaccinated! This phenomena seemed to increase with age, the older participants fairing less well.

In spite of the overwhelming evidence for misuse

of drug therapy on older people, pharmaceutical companies continue to target the older population in the bulk of their advertising and promotion.

There are currently over 45 million people in the United States and Europe who are presently over 65. That is a marketing dream, and one that has not been overlooked by the drug companies. At any given time, there are over 200 drugs being developed or in trials specifically for senior citizens. While the industry is proud of this 'contribution', it doesn't seem to acknowledge that few, if any, of these drugs have actually been shown to cure any disease or disorder. Further, according to Harvard University, at least 40 percent of all older people are routinely given prescriptions for drugs they have no business taking.

What about all those high tech tests? The use of diagnostic testing on older people has increased by more than 300 percent over the last seven years alone. Researchers at the Veterans Affairs Medical Center and the Dartmouth Medical School warned that there is significant risk to over-diagnosing. Many of the diagnostic procedures are, themselves, not without risk or side effects. The worst outcome, according to these findings, was the fact the over-diagnosing often created a patient where there was none before.

Is It the Doctor's Fault?

With all of these overwhelming concerns regarding the conventional medical system, is it any wonder that millions and millions of people the world over are not only looking elsewhere for health care, but are routinely following programs other than allopathic medicine. With this mass exodus from conventional thinking we must ask ourselves, "is it the fault of the Doctors?"

I attended university classes with men and women whose goal was to become a physician. For the most part these were all very dedicated and sincere individuals. In fact, in my over 27 years in the health and nutrition industry, I cannot remember meeting a single medical doctor who said, "I can hardly wait to get my license so that I can go out and kill people!" Everyone starts out with the most noble of intents, with the common goal of hoping to relieve some small part of human suffering. What goes wrong?

The physician is no longer in charge of his or her own practice. They are brainwashed by drug companies, threatened by organizations such as the AMA who are supposed to be protecting them, and overworked by an unmanageable patient workload. Is it any wonder that not one physician in 100 reads their medical journals. They simply don't have time.

In the meantime, we have to begin to learn to take responsibility for our own health care. We all need to learn how to determine when it's time to see a physician. More importantly, we must also learn how to determine whether it is in our best interests to listen to his advice exclusively, or to also seek information about some of the less invasive options available elsewhere.

This book is all about those options. As we have already established, chronic, non-infectious diseases are the main cause of ill health as we age; they also are the poorest managed forms of health problems.

It is estimated that anyone born from today forward will have a better than 90 percent chance of living to age 100 and past. At what price? Today, the average life span is in the mid seventies, yet for many millions of people, the last 20 or 30 years of that life span is without any appreciable quality attached to it.

Instead of our retirement years being filled with the joy and activities that free time can provide, we are all congregating at doctors' offices, therapy centers, pharmacies to get the latest wonder drug, experiencing the side effects of those wonder drugs, and undergoing surgical procedures.

Quantity of life must be intrinsically linked to quality or the results are of little value. I could not agree more with the future thinkers that ages of over 100 years are well within our grasp, but the quality factor must also be equally addressed.

The quality of life a person may expect in the 'golden years' may be directly traced back to how they lived their life in the past as well as the genetics they were born with. While we can do little to change our genetic characteristics, we surely can positively affect the quality of our future years.

The human body is the most complicated chemical laboratory ever invented by anyone. In all our great scientific achievement, we have barely begun to delve into its complexity. Yet, that vast chemical universe within us is almost totally self-sufficient. If we give it some quality food, pure water, and about 120 or so nutrients, it can and will take care of us very nicely. Chronic disease is the result of a human biochemistry long out of balance. Treating the effects or symptoms of these conditions will do little to enhance the quality or quantity of anyone's life. Only when we come to the understanding of what this body of ours needs and then how to provide for those needs, will we be in a position to positively affect both quality and quantity of life ahead. The guideposts to that journey begin by turning this page.

Chapter 2
What We Know About Aging

Remember back when you were in your teens and twenty's? Remember how invincible you thought you were? It's true, we were, compared to today! The things we used to take for granted, such as eating all manner of junk and still digesting it are gone. Now we must be careful of everything we eat and anti-acids are part of too many meals.

It's this thing called aging. We all acknowledge that it is inevitable; most of us certainly don't look forward to it and very few people understand what aging is. Without at least a basic knowledge of the aging process, it becomes difficult to 'face the enemy'. In this case, the enemy is truly within, deep in the heart of our own biochemistry.

In the last chapter, I left you with the concept that quality of life is as important, if not more so, than shear quantity alone. When we discuss aging, we are concerned with both the quality and quantity of the years ahead. So often you hear older people speak negatively of life extension. They cannot understand the benefits of living an extra decade if it is to be filled with the same aches & pains and limitations of the previous ten years. And right they are. Any program that addresses aging must address the preservation of an active, meaningful life as well.

First of all, any discussion concerning aging and longevity must be prefaced with the statement that no one yet has all the answers to the aging problem. What we do know, however, can make a profound difference in the future life of a middle-aged individual.

While great strides have been made in understanding the free radical and its relationship to the premature aging of living tissue, it cannot be overlooked, the role our state of mind plays in the longevity equation. Without the right attitude towards both longevity and life itself, you will find the mere biochemical substances will leave you feeling flat and unfulfilled. It is important that you understand the many negatives society perpetuates relative to aging and especially the quality of the aging life. If you buy into these concepts, you will have lost before you have begun. Many ancient philosophies have stated the concept of 'as you think, so are you.' This applies in countless direct ways, in the maintenance of this home we call the human body.

In a society that seeks excuses rather than solutions, we routinely hear such negative concepts as 'nothing can be done about aging', or 'if most doctors don't know about life extension, it can't be real.' What about the excuse 'life extension is difficult, complicated and expensive', or 'life extension might be a reality for my grandchildren but it's too late for me'. As long as we maintain these attitudes, we will fail. Just because we don't know 'everything' about aging, we have no excuse not to use what we do know.

Just because the general public, sadly, does not know about or understand the concept of aging doesn't mean you can't. What is this process called aging? It is the time in biochemical activity where more healthy body cells die than the body is able to replace. Aging is a natural progressive deterioration of numerous biochemical and cellular functions, which have been interfered with by the introduction of such biochemical altering factors as free radicals, toxins and stress.

Have you ever wondered why some people seem to age faster than others? While there are many possible factors, an understanding of the aging process may shed some light on this question. The rate of aging in any individual directly depends upon the relationship between the "destruction and repair" of living cells, tissues, and organ systems. The yin and yang of destruction and repair occurs literally from the moment of conception. As we progress through life, we have the opportunity to avoid much of the destruction which takes place. But as we age, the destruction/repair ratio declines against us. The more destruction that is not repaired, the less we are able to resist new destruction around the corner. This is why the older we get, the faster we age. But by providing cellular protection, we can slow down the destruction rate and by giving the body the right raw materials, we can increase the repair rate. The end result will be both a slowing of actual aging, and more importantly, a slowing of the ravages of aging.

Just because heart disease, cancer and diabetes are the top three leading causes of death, doesn't mean that you have to develop one of them and die from it as well. We all to frequently look at the odds against us without also looking at the factors that produce those odds. Yes, in order to reduce the risk, self-responsibility and positive action are necessary. It doesn't mean that path has to be complicated, expensive or boring. Did you know that by just a few small life style changes and additions, you could reduce your risk of diseases, including the "big three" just referred to, by more than 70 percent? That's right, science now has the ability to stack the deck in your favor, but you must actively participate in that exercise. There is no magic pill, no single magic potion that can guarantee you safe immunity from chronic disease, but there is a program, outlined in this book, that can come very, very close.

Factors That Contribute To Premature Aging

The jury is still out on many factors affecting the aging process of the human body. Many researchers are still at odds over the degree of influence that certain specific aging factors have in the aging person.

However, there are many solid, indisputable facts which scientists and researchers agree upon; these factors affect both the length and quality of remaining life at any given stage. Effective control of these factors is now within our grasp.

In essence, anything that affects a cell's ability to feed, cleanse, and repair itself causes aging. This list is long and wide indeed, but for the sake of immediate understanding we can group these many factors into a few categories.

Free Radicals

The free radical may be likened to a chemical buzz bomb. It is a molecule with an imbalance in the number of electrons, making it highly reactive. Seeking to balance itself, once in the body, it will attach itself to almost any cell structure, stealing the material needed to stabilize itself. In the process living tissue is damaged, sometimes permanently through an alteration or mutation of the cells genetic material. Free radicals are formed in the body naturally, as a byproduct of life metabolism. Within the body lies the means to neutralize this naturally occurring free radical activity, mostly through the production of hydrogen peroxide. The problem begins when free radical production and activity exceeds the body's ability to neutralize it. This can occur in the presence of toxins from the environment, including smoke and engine exhaust, and in the presence of other factors including radiation, pharmaceuticals, unmanaged stress, by-products of adulterated or chemically altered foods, and poor digestion.

Under these circumstances, free radical proliferation can rapidly lead to cross linkage of cell structures and permanent DNA damage. These mutations are forever replicated each time the damaged cell divides and replaces itself.

Our environment is so polluted that today we are exposed to more toxic, free radical inducing substances than at any time in the past. In fact, it is estimated that the average person living today is exposed to 1000 more specific free radical inducing chemicals in one 24 hour period than their grandparents experienced in their entire lifetime! With this onslaught, the body cannot hope to manage the juggling act.

Not surprisingly, the chronic, degenerative diseases that threaten the quality and quantity of our lives are the results of this uncontrolled free radical activity in the body. Conditions such as heart disease, peripheral vascular disease, coronary artery disease, cancer, diabetes, arthritis, Alzheimer's disease, Parkinson's disease, auto-immune diseases, allergies and degenerative eye diseases such as glaucoma, cataracts, and macular degeneration, to name a few, are all the result of wild free radical damage.

Chronic and Infectious Disease

The disease process and the presence of disease itself is a source of explosive free radical production. In the case of infectious disease, white blood cell proliferation produces, as a by-product, intense chemical "free- radical" activity. These levels can rise to enormous heights during an acute infection. For this reason extra free radical protection is always advised during an acute infectious illness such as a cold, flu or other bacteria or virus pathology.

Chronic disease, like infectious disease, produces free radicals but at a much slower rate due to the absence of high white blood cell activity. The problem with chronic disease is that it is present twenty-four hours a day, seven days a week for long periods of time, sometimes years. This provides a constant source of free radical production and activity since the presence of chronic disease already indicates an altered biochemistry. The waste products produced at the cellular level, within the body as a result of the presence of chronic degenerative disease serves as the catalyst for steady and continual free radical formation. It is essential therefore, to provide adequate free radical inhibition to compensate for anyone who already has a chronic disease.

Stress

Another major area of free radical formation within the body is caused by the biochemical changes that take place during periods of unmanageable stress.

Stress, in and of itself, is not bad. The excess stress over and above the body's ability to neutralize and the emotional stress that is not effectively managed can cause a profound biochemical change in the internal environment of the human body.

An example of physical stress may be seen in many athletes. We often think of top athletes in any field as the epitome of health and fitness. They may be physically fit, but chances are they are aging faster than most people do and are filled with free radical activity caused by the physical stress of excess exercise. When we exercise, especially to the extreme, we break down body tissues in higher amounts than the body is able to repair and replace. This battle, which most athletes fight, is called "recovery time". When a muscle is exercised, it grows only because it has been broken down by the exercise first. As it rebuilds, it becomes bigger and stronger than before. While this is a normal and healthy process, the by-product of this catabolism (destructive metabolism) is the intense creation of free radicals.

Another example of physical free radical formation may be seen in people who spend a great deal of time outdoors. The radiation from the sun causes cross linkage and free radical damage to the sub-dermal layers of the skin. This produces wrinkling and that leather-like look associated with weathered aging.

While these examples affect a small percentage of the population, a much larger segment is similarly adversely affected by internal, emotional stress, which is not properly managed. This can reek havoc with the internal biochemistry of the body, producing free radicals as well as an environment wherein the body is poorly able to recover. If more of us understood the tremendous upheaval that is caused from mismanaged emotional stress, perhaps we would pay closer attention to moderating it in our lives.

Major Free Radicals Present in the Human Body

There are four major "free radical" groups present in the body. Following is a brief description of each, including protocols which have proven to be effective in combating them. You will likely hear these terms bantered around anyway.

Superoxide (02-). This is the most common free radical found in the body. It is really an oxygen molecule with an extra electron. This free radical attacks the cell membranes (the coverings around each individual cell), the mitochondria of the cell (responsible for energy production), and the chromosomes (carries the genetic code). The vast presence of the superoxide radical may account for the high percentage of people who are constantly tired and fatigued since it alters the mitochondria's ability to produce energy. This free radial is neutralized by a substance known as superoxide dismutase (SOD). In the past, we used to give SOD orally in attempts to fight the superoxide radical. Today we know that there are much more effective ways of producing superoxide dismutase and in fact, that which is taken orally is mostly destroyed in the digestive tract anyway. The following protocol for free radical protection discusses substances, which allow the body to manufacture superoxide dismutase internally.

Hydrogen Peroxide (H202). Another by-product of superoxide scavenging is produced at the cellular level in the presence of toxic substances. It should not be confused with food grade hydrogen peroxide taken in supplemental form. Hydrogen peroxide is only dangerous when it forms inside the cells. Extra-cellular hydrogen peroxide disassociates and almost instantly forms stable oxygen for use by the body cells. The most common site for hydrogen peroxide "free radical" damage is at the DNA template. There, the genetic mutations can frequently lead to cancer and other genetic diseases. This free radical is destroyed by glutathione peroxidase or catalase.

Hydroxyl Radical (H0). This is the most toxic free radical of the group and it is produced when intercellular hydrogen peroxide is not completely broken down and converted to water. It can steal hydrogen atoms, which subsequently break down living tissues. This occurs in chain reactions and can affect millions of molecules at once. This free radical is destroyed or neutralized by methionine and most importantly, grape seed extract.

Singlet Oxygen (102). Singlet oxygen is produced primarily by radiation damage to stable oxygen. Over exposure to the sun, medical x-rays and other sources of radiation can accelerate the formation of this nasty free radical. Singlet oxygen specifically attacks joints and connective tissues; it is directly involved in such chronic conditions as arthritis and fibromyalgia. It also plays havoc with the eye tissue causing cataracts and retinal damage such as macular degeneration. This free radical is destroyed, or more appropriately, scavenged by the carotenoids. Lycopene is the most powerful singlet oxygen scavenger we presently know of.

Another reason why free radical damage is so severe and extensive today is that the industrialized diet provides few, if any, of the substances needed by the body to fight off these renegade buzz bombs. These vital substances are called antioxidants. When taken in adequate amounts and ratios combinations, they provide complete protection against free radicals. They do this by preventing formation of new free radicals, destroying existing free radicals and providing "free radical" scavenging services.

The Antioxidant Family

In discussing specific antioxidants and their application to your health and longevity, it might be helpful to discuss, briefly, how antioxidants protect you.

First of all, antioxidants, as the name implies, prevent oxidants or free radicals from forming. They also stop specific minerals from oxidation internally. Minerals, which belong to the 'metals' group of nutrients, have the ability and potential of 'rusting' within the body. This 'rusting', depresses the immune system and we all know what happens after that.

Certain specific antioxidants, through their free radical scavenging potential, intercept oxidants that have already been formed and prevent their chain reaction from continuing. This is much like the row of dominos, once one has fallen; the rest will follow unless something prevents the reaction.

Lastly, antioxidants, in combination, have the ability to actually eliminate molecules or cells that have been severely damaged. This means that antioxidants not only wage the war against oxidative particles and the damage they cause, but they can clean up the mess afterwards!

The most important antioxidants are vitamin C, vitamin E, carotenoids, zinc, selenium, N-acetyl cysteine, CoQ10, milk thistle, lycopene, quercetin, bilberry, alpha lipoic acid and the proanthocyanidins. We will be discussing these along with other supportive antioxidants, so that you may understand the wide reaching benefits that may be derived from incorporating the right combination of them into your daily nutritional program.

It is important to understand that the time-tested concept of totality applies to the use of antioxidants no differently than it does to the use of other nutrients such as vitamins and minerals. The total effectiveness of antioxidants taken together in the right combinations is far greater than the sum of the individual parts. In other words, antioxidants work better together than they do individually.

We can divide the antioxidants into two groups, those that are commonly recognized and those that are new, potent and aggressive in their actions. Group one makes up what we consider to be the minimal baseline of antioxidant protection for every human being, regardless of age or physical condition. Group two represents the 'heavy hitters' and when taken in the right combinations, can provide cellular protection from free radicals at levels we could only imagine even five years ago.

Let's take a look at some of these important nutrients from each group and discuss their individual action within the body.

Group One: The Foundation Antioxidants.

Vitamin A. As an antioxidant, vitamin A performs several important functions. The most important role of this nutrient is in its ability to protect and repair mucous membrane tissue from free radicals caused by smoking, chemicals and other pollutants. Since free radicals explosively multiply in the presence of all pollutants, and the mucous membrane tissues are our first line of defense, it is very important that we protect these tissues and maintain their integrity. Further, while vitamin A is doing this all-important job, it is also working to boost our immune system, a real benefit to us all.

Another concern is damage from various forms of radiation. Studies continually show that both animals and humans, who are ingesting adequate amounts of vitamin A, suffer far less DNA mutation when exposed to radiation.

It is now thought that a common colon condition, called colitis, is caused by free radical damage to the mucous membrane of the intestines. This being the case, vitamin A is vital in all disorders of both chronic and acute intestinal inflammations.

There is some evidence that vitamin A exercises anti-cancer effects as well. This would be especially true for those areas where mucous membrane tissue may be found. One study, involving over 300 people who underwent surgery for lung cancer, found that the group who took very high amounts of vitamin A had far fewer new tumors than people who did not use the vitamin.

All of vitamin A's many benefits have caused me to often say that it is my favorite vitamin.

Beta Carotene. This best known member of the carotenoid family is converted to vitamin A by the liver. While this is the primary reason why most people take beta-carotene, it is also a powerful antioxidant in its own right. Beta-carotene helps prevent lipid oxidation, an important factor in atherosclerosis. In addition to beta-carotene, there are many other far more powerful carotenoids which we will be discussing in group two.

Folic Acid and Pantothenic Acid. These two B-complex nutrients in particular, exercise powerful antioxidant properties under specific conditions. In any case, single B-complex nutrients should never be taken in the absence of the others. To do so causes a rapid and potentially serious deficiency condition.

Vitamin C. This is probably the most commonly known nutrient of all and certainly, next to vitamin E, the best known antioxidant. Vitamin C's many roles as a free radical fighter are well documented. When free radicals strike a cell, one of the most vulnerable sites are the mitochondria, the energy producing centers of the cell. When adequate vitamin C is present in both the intra and extra cellular fluids, it can neutralize free radicals before they can penetrate the cell membrane and really do some serious damage. Other specific sites within the body which are protected by vitamin C include the pancreas, the lungs and the prostate gland, preventing cross linkage of these tissues. This greatly reduces the risk of cancer in these sites. Further, vitamin C, along with glutathione (see group two), prevents damage to eye tissue, preventing the formation of cataracts.

Vitamin C is a coordinator as it were, working together with many other antioxidants In fact, vitamin E will work much better when there is adequate vitamin C present at the same time.

Citrus Bioflavonoids. A member of the vitamin C family, the citrus bioflavonoids are the best known of a much larger group of flavonoids, many of which have been discovered very recently. More about those in our discussion of group two. For now, suffice it to say that citrus bioflavonoids are an absolute must for any Full Spectrum nutritional product. This particular group of bioflavonoids is responsible for capillary integrity. This means that if you want to avoid varicose veins, broken capillaries and capillary leaking (bruising), you had better be sure to get some citrus bioflavonoids on a daily basis. Ever wonder why people who tend to consume too much alcohol have all those broken red capillaries on their face? The alcohol causes free radical "cross linkage" of the cells of the capillaries and they subsequently rupture.

Vitamin E. This nutrient has long been associated with heart health. In fact it helps to control and prevent this number one killer of all so-called 'civilized' nations. Ok, so we all know this, but how does vitamin E do it?

The nutrient exercises a powerful antioxidant effect on the fats of the body, including your LDL, or 'bad cholesterol'. LDL cholesterol and other fats only stick to the artery wall when free radical damage has altered the surface of the artery wall and altered the LDL cholesterol at the same time. By preventing both situations from occurring, vitamin E can virtually halt the progression of this top killer.

Further, vitamin E actually helps to lower overall cholesterol and triglycerides in the bloodstream. Vitamin E is a natural blood thinner and helps to prevent fats, naturally occurring in the blood, from sticking together.

Other areas where vitamin E performs antioxidant and healing effects include some forms of cancer, neurological disorders, lung diseases, immune insufficiency, and menopausal symptoms.

Selenium. This amazing mineral has many functions within the body. We will confine our discussion here to its antioxidant potential, which primarily revolves around the body's need for selenium, together with glutathione, for the production of an enzyme called glutathione peroxidase. This enzyme halts the oxidation of fats, so like vitamin E, it is important in good cardiovascular health. Further along these lines, glutathione peroxidase is essential for the conversion of single amino acids into more complex protein structures. One example that comes to mind is within the eye tissue. When eye tissue naturally breaks down and is not sufficiently repaired or replaced, cataracts can form. This deterioration of the protein structure of the lens of the eye can be halted by the presence of glutathione peroxidase.

Selenium has anti-cancer factors as well. Studies have shown that proper dosages of selenium can reduce lung cancer by as much as 46 percent, esophageal cancers by 67 percent, colon cancer by 62 percent and last yet most impressive, prostate cancer by 72 percent!

Sulfur. There seems to be much misinformation surrounding this important mineral. Sulfur is found in very high amounts within almost all tissues and it is one of the seven major minerals in the body. Many of you may have heard of the numerous health benefits attributed to garlic and garlic extracts. This is due to the high organic sulfur content of this plant.

Sulfur may be safely consumed if from an organic source, as may be found from mineral products derived exclusively from plants. Further, foods like eggs, grains, and some fruits and vegetables all provide high amounts of organic sulfur.

Zinc. Just as vitamin A is my favorite vitamin, zinc has to be my favorite mineral. It has so many functions within the human body that a book could be written on this one nutrient alone. Zinc is the basis of hundreds of enzymes, required by your body for literally thousands of functions. Many of these enzymes are also antioxidants in their own right, one example being superoxide dismutase (SOD). Still, other enzymes created with zinc as a basis are responsible for the production of both DNA and RNA.

Zinc is essential to the proper functioning of the immune response, precisely why it is included in many cough and cold formulations. Zinc levels naturally decline in the body with age, which is why older people, in general, have less of an immune response. This may be remedied through chelated zinc supplementation. This valuable mineral should be part of a Full Spectrum approach to good health.

Zinc is important for healthy sexual activity in males, since semen contains the highest concentration of zinc found anywhere in the body. Zinc is also vital to diabetics, especially the Type I, Juvenile Onset, because zinc is a primary constituent of the hormone insulin, and since they produce very little insulin, zinc can frequently enhance this production.

Symptoms of zinc deficiency include poor appetite, slow healing of wounds, white spots on fingernails, lethargy and loss of sex drive in males.

This preceding list of nutrients comprises what I consider to be the baseline antioxidants. These should all be found in any good Full Spectrum dietary supplement. In fact, you should never take these nutrients alone or even in combination with each other unless all the other essential nutrients are present as well. We must not forget that nutrients are like members of a large orchestra. In order for them to make beautiful music, they must all be present and working together at the same time. You will find out much more about these and all the other essential nutrients in the upcoming chapters on vitamins and minerals.

Group Two: The Heavy Hitters for Complete Cell Protection.

Just when the protective antioxidants, provided in foods from nature, could no longer sufficiently protect us from the tens of thousands of man-made free radical sources, science has been able to isolate and concentrate powerful free radical fighters heretofore hidden deep within nature's realm. These 'super antioxidants' may very well prove to be the weapon we all need to fight off chronic diseases, premature aging, and disability. By adding the right combination of many of these latest antioxidant substances, you too can beat the ravages of aging and forestall the many factors that compromise the quality of life as we age.

Lycopene. Who would have guessed that pasta sauces, ketchup and other tomato products could actually reduce your risk of getting certain types of cancers? Within these foods is a substance called lycopene, a member of the carotenoid family. Like beta-carotene, lycopene is an antioxidant with one small exception; lycopene is ten times more powerful in protecting against cancer!

Much of the current research regarding lycopene and cancer revolves around prostate cancer. It has long been observed that this dreaded cancer occurs with much less frequency in the southern Mediterranean countries such as Italy and Greece. In these countries, cooked tomatoes are a dietary staple.

For some reason, which we cannot totally explain, when tomatoes are cooked, the process concentrates the percentage of lycopene, making it one of the few nutrients known which is not damaged by heating.

In a physiological sense, lycopene is the most prevalent carotenoid in the human body. One of the most concentrated sites may be found in the male prostate. It is believed that, through the presence of lycopene, the human body is able to defend itself from specific cancer causing free radicals.

Other types of cancer that may be prevented through the presence of lycopene in adequate amounts include breast, lung and endometrial.

One of the reasons even people who consume large

amounts of tomato products might be deficient in ly-copene is that, like all carotenoids, it can only be ab-sorbed in the presence of some fat. Therefore, the super low fat diet craze has created a situation where the incredible benefits of all carotenoids may be greatly diminished due to lack of absorption.

Other benefits from lycopene include prevention of heart disease. A recent study conducted in Israel, demonstrated that lycopene greatly increases the resistance of LDL cholesterol to oxidation. This is important because LDL cholesterol is only harmful when free radical oxygen alters the fat structure, oxidizing or literally rusting the fat.

We cannot produce lycopene within our bodies, which means that we must ingest it from foods and supplements. People who are at specific high risk such as smokers, drinkers and those with a high-risk cancer profile, should be cognizant of getting adequate lycopene daily.

Once again, like all balance within the human body, lycopene seems to work much better when combined with other antioxidants. In fact, one study, which used beta-carotene alone, failed in demonstrating an anti-cancer benefit. When researchers combined the beta-carotene with lycopene and tocopherols, the results were amazing.

Quercetin. According to Robert C Atkins, in his book, Dr. Atkins' Vita-Nutrient Solution, quercetin deserves the title of 'King of the Flavonoids'. This is because of its ability to affect so many areas of human health.

Quercetin is a 'secret weapon' when it comes to allergies. Millions of people suffer from a variety of allergies. Those with airborne allergies have the worst time, since they cannot escape the cause of their irritation.

Together with citrus bioflavonoids, clinical studies have shown that quercetin is better than most of the leading anti-histamines in regulating the allergic response. Still other studies are showing consistently that quercetin has the ability to block the production of a specific enzyme that neutralizes cortisone, the body's most powerful natural anti-inflammatory. At the Institute, we have tested, and are now using quercetin with great success in many, heretofore, unmanageable allergy sufferers.

As with all the 'heavy hitter' antioxidants, quercetin has many applications in the body. It protects us against heart disease, the number one cause of death in America and many other countries. Some studies indicate that quercetin's action upon the cardiovascular system may be equal to, or even greater than, that of natural vitamin E. In study after study, a high intake of this nutrient has shown a direct correlation between levels of quercetin and lower risks of cardiovascular disease and stroke.

Quercetin has another amazing ability. It can accelerate the production of specific enzymes that destroy potential carcinogens before they can do their final evil deed and convert healthy cells into cancerous ones.

In foods quercetin may be found in garlic, onions, cayenne pepper and green tea. This is one reason why these foods have had the reputation of being extra healthy. The problem is that most people do not eat a sufficient amount of these foods to ingest enough protective quercetin. Supplementation is a logical solution to this problem.

Bilberry. Unless you have dealt with eye problems in the past, you may never have heard of bilberry. It is a distant relative to the blueberry and the cranberry.

The main benefit derived from bilberry is its ability to improve circulation and blood vessel health. This seems to apply specifically, although not exclusively, to the eye tissues. The United States military used bilberry extract back in World War II to improve the night vision of soldiers, especially air pilots. This practice is still in use to this day.

Research relative to blood vessel integrity and eyesight is quite extensive. Studies conducted in Italy have shown that bilberry can improve circulation to the eyes thereby mitigating such conditions as diabetes-caused glaucoma, day blindness, near sightedness and cataract formation. One such study showed that bilberry, along with vitamin E, stopped cataract formation in 97 percent of the people who took it.

Another condition, which has eluded many other

methods of treatment, is macular degeneration. This problem is becoming more and more prevalent due to free radical damage to the eye tissues from smoke and other pollutants in the air. Bilberry comes to the rescue once again not only because it increases blood flow and hence oxygen to the eye tissue, but it also prevents oxidative damage to the eye.

The specific flavonoids in bilberry, which are called anthocyanosides, not only provide eye tissue support but help to limit calcium deposits and blood clots inside of the arteries. Because of the direct benefit exercised upon the vascular system, bilberry is also very useful in such conditions as leg swelling, varicose veins and even postpartum hemorrhoids.

Lastly, bilberry helps diminish inflammation, a helpful effect in such conditions as arthritis and other inflammatory disorders.

Since bilberry is helpful in improving circulation, it is very good for wound healing. Wounds heal faster and with less infection. Bilberry works together with collagen to rebuild damaged tissues.

Grape Seed Extract. This powerful antioxidant and anti-inflammatory is a member of the specific flavonoid group called the proanthocyanidins.

While grape seed extract demonstrates specific benefits of its own, its primary contribution to an antioxidant compound would have to be its ability to work together with other antioxidants, enhancing their potential.

There has been a debate for some time over which

members of this group are better than others. The truth is that all proanthocyanidins, including cranberries, pine bark, or grape seeds contribute equally. The only difference might be the concentration. Here at the Institute, we use grape seed extract, since it is about 10 to 15 percent higher in proanthocyanidin potency than pine bark.

The earliest indication that something in the grape might be of benefit to human health came from the French. Researchers often pondered as to how the French, who consume very rich, high fatty foods, could have such a low incidence of heart disease. In fact there is very little problem with elevated, imbalanced cholesterol anywhere in France. What was special about the French, or their diet, which precluded them from the epidemic of heart disease problems now prevalent in many other areas of the world? Red wine!

Now, I realize that many people will question why we are promoting an alcoholic beverage as healthy. Sorry folks, the facts stand as they are. Obviously, if you have a biochemical problem with alcohol, you must avoid even red wine. Otherwise, two glasses of red wine per day lowers the risk of heart disease by as much as 10 times more than aspirin! These findings have been confirmed and documented in at least seven major clinical studies.

People often ask if grape juice will produce the same effect. The answer is yes but not nearly to the same degree. The small amount of alcohol in the wine greatly increases the extraction of the proanthocyanidins from the grape. Further, the alcohol helps to calm the system and relax the arteries. In just one of the many studies on the benefits of red wine published in the Journal of Epidemiology, researches found that after studying 24,000 middle-aged men, there was a 35 percent reduction in cardiovascular disease and a 24 percent reduction in cancer, when two to three glasses of red wine were ingested on a daily basis.

What about white wine you say? There are certainly antioxidants present in white wine but not as many as found in the red varieties. Why is this important? Well, proanthocyanidins are up to fifty times more potent than vitamin E in their free radical scavenging ability.

Some of the specific benefits, which may be derived from grape seed extract, include...

- It has the ability to cross the blood-brain barrier so it can scavenge free radicals from within brain tissue.
- It is highly synergistic with other antioxidants, such as vitamins A, C, and E, enhancing their effectiveness.
- Assists in the prevention of histamine formation, an important factor for allergy sufferers.
- Grape Seed extract protects us against radiation from all sources, including the sun, from pesticides in foods and water, and heavy metal poisoning, all of which produce free radicals in the body with great fortitude.

One final word on grape seed extract and red wine. Moderation is the key here. While all the studies have shown a profound benefit from two to three glasses of wine per day, in every case, more was not better. As alcohol consumption went up, the benefits decreased proportionately. If you cannot moderate your consumption, take your grape seed extract by supplementation.

Coenzyme Q10. This amazing nutrient is really not a vitamin, a mineral or even an amino acid, yet it is absolutely essential that we have an adequate supply in order to live safely in our toxic world. Our bodies can make it in certain amounts, but frequently not sufficient to counter all the abusive substances in our environment.

One of the first observed beneficial effects of ubiquinone (Co-Q10), was its ability to produce energy. Through this enhanced energy, individual cells of the body were able to live longer. Today we know that ubiquinone has many other abilities and can protect our body from many very destructive free radicals. Further, it is a natural immune enhancer.

Some of the specific areas where Co-Q10 has proven helpful include chronic conditions such as heart disease, diabetes, high blood pressure, obesity, and even cancer.

The many benefits of Co-Q10 are only available to us if we get the right amount of the nutrient needed. It is the feeling of many nutritionists that this level can only be sustained in the body through the use of supplements.

Since Co-Q10 is tied into energy production, it would stand to reason that it would be most helpful to the heart. No other organ expends so much energy as our heart, which only rests between its beats. There are at least sixty studies, which support the direct benefits of Co-Q10 on such cardiovascular conditions as cardiomyopathy, arrhythmia, coronary artery disease, congestive heart failure, mitral valve prolapse and high blood pressure.

One study showed that when potential heart transplant patients were given sufficient Co-Q10, they no longer needed the surgery!

In another study, Co-Q10 was given to many thousands of people suffering from congestive heart failure. The results were far more successful than any of the pharmaceutical approaches currently in use. An amazing 75 percent obtained dramatic improvements in pulmonary function, heart palpitations and edema, all with virtually no side effects.

Since we know that almost all drugs only mask the effects of a disease or disorder, often replacing those symptoms with side effects from the drug itself, Co-Q10 is an ideal substance for all cardiovascular concerns. It has no side effects and it has consistently proven to be of greater benefit than any pharmaceutical.

It is not uncommon for people with various heart diseases to have at least 25 percent less Co-Q10 than their healthy counterparts. According to Robert C Atkins, a holistic cardiologist, when Co-Q10 levels fall to 25 percent of normal, the heart will stop beating!

Other areas where this wonderful substance comes to our continued rescue is with diabetes. Co-Q10 has been found to help reduce blood sugar while protecting the heart and vascular system from the ravages of the disease.

Studies have shown that Co-Q10 can reverse most periodontal disease, the number one cause of tooth loss in people over fifty years of age.

Very recent studies over the last two years have indicated that Co-Q10 can help slow the progression of Parkinson's disease. This is a condition wherein the sufferer looses precious dopamine in the brain. Co-Q10 was found to greatly slow this loss down.

While this marvelous nutrient can do so much for our well being, absorbing it is not always that easy. Once again, it is a substance that must be taken with some fat. This is another instance where the low fat fanaticism that has swept the country has caused more harm than good. This is especially true with heart disease. We were told to cut all the fat out of our diets and heart disease got worse! One reason is that the super low fat diets prevented the uptake of many of the most powerful heart protecting substances, including Co-Q10.

Milk Thistle. Without a doubt, the most effective of all the herbal detoxifiers has to be Silybum marianum, or milk thistle. This being the case, the organ that would logically benefit most from such a potential must be the liver. All the toxins in the body end up in the liver to be processed before excretion. It has been said that the liver is the chemical laboratory of the body, carrying on thousands of functions at any given moment. When the liver becomes over burdened with toxic build up, it cannot do its job effectively. Silymarin, the active component in the herb, has an amazing ability to protect the liver from oxidative damage as well as boosting its detoxification abilities.

So powerful is milk thistle, that in one study it cut the death rate from cirrhosis by a full 50 percent. Anyone suffering from any form of hepatitis MUST consider milk thistle as part of their treatment and management program.

The liver depends upon one specific substance in order to fulfill much of its duties. That is glutathione. This substance protects the liver from harm while serving as a base for many enzymes needed to protect other cellular structures. One example is the relationship between glutathione and cataracts. As the protein structure of the lens of the eye breaks down, new cells cannot be formed without the presence of an enzyme called glutathione peroxidase. This enzyme is made from glutathione. In fact, glutathione's importance has been recognized by scientists for over 20 years but the problem has been in raising glutathione levels in the body.

Supplements of glutathione are not well absorbed and much of what is ingested orally, is destroyed or broken down in the digestive system. Glutathione supplements are still quite popular but, sadly, are of little benefit to the body.

Milk Thistle, along with our next magic antioxidant N-Acetyl Cysteine, actually produce glutathione in the liver, raising the levels of this vital substance tremendously.

Milk Thistle must be included in any Full Spectrum antioxidant program for it is one of the few nutrients that can serve both as an antioxidant and a free radical scavenger. This makes it of double benefit to us.

Another substance that is manufactured in the body with the help of milk thistle is superoxide dismutase (SOD). This is another popular antioxidant/ enzyme substance, because it controls the superoxide free radical. Again, the problem has always been the delivery system. We would include superoxide dismutase because we knew it was good for us, but we also knew that much of what was ingested orally was also broken down by the digestive process. Even enteric-coated products provided little help. Now we have a way to assist the body in making superoxide dismutase in virtually all the quantities necessary and milk thistle is one of the important ingredients in that chemical process.

N-Acetyl Cysteine. The most miraculous substance we have saved for last. Of all the antioxidants, common and rare, this special form of the amino acid Cysteine is the most powerful, exhibiting more antioxidant potential than virtually all the other known antioxidants combined! We predict that this nutrient will become one of the biggest buzzwords in the field of nutrition over the months and years to come. More and more benefits are being attributed to this amazing substance through clinical studies unfolding almost daily.

If it's so good, why hasn't anybody heard about it? Well, they have. They're just not talking too loudly because it works so well that it could conceivably make many forms of treatment for chronic diseases obsolete.

If you were to visit almost any hospital emergency room across the country, you would find they stock N-Acetyl Cysteine (NAC) and use it as an antidote for many kinds of poisoning. The most common usage is against acetaminophen poisoning, which occurs regularly due to constant over-consumption. (acetaminophen is the NSAID found in Tylenol® and other over the counter painkillers) Excess acetaminophen depletes the liver of glutathione to the point of liver failure. Large doses of NAC can so rapidly restore the glutathione levels that it can detoxify an acetaminophen overdose in a matter of a few hours.

NAC has been used medically to break down lung-clogging mucus in cases of chronic bronchitis and other respiratory disorders since the 1960's.

There are several key functions of NAC already identified, with likely, many more to follow as the nutrient is continually studied. Its primary function, along with milk thistle, is to raise the glutathione levels within the liver, protecting it from the many toxins it has to detoxify and render harmless.

It is well known that glutathione levels are much lower in people with cancer, linking a depletion of that nutrient to the immune system's inability to recognize the foreign cells.

Considering NAC's tremendous antioxidant power, it would stand to reason that it would be helpful in every chronic degenerative disease since free radical damage, causing an altered biochemistry, is responsible for virtually all chronic conditions. Recent studies however, show that it is also a powerful weapon against acute infectious attacks such as colds and flu.

In a study conducted at the Institute of Hygiene and Preventive Medicine at the University of Genoa, Italy, Dr. Silvio De Flora administered NAC or a placebo to over 250 subjects.

The conclusion was that while the NAC did not appear to prevent infection from cold or flu pathogens, only 25 percent of the NAC group developed any significant symptoms while 79 percent of the placebo group had severe flu symptoms. This means that NAC can reduce the symptoms from colds and flu by a whopping two-thirds!

There are other viruses, such as rhinovirus and the Coxsackie virus, that seasonally plague us. The researchers found that NAC was also very effective in dealing with these bugs as well. It seems that NAC is not virus or bacteria specific like many other immune products on the market. Therefore, NAC can provide a broad-spectrum of protection to ease or even eliminate the annoying symptoms of viral and bacterial related infections. This is especially good news for those in high-risk situations, such as persons with immune compromised disorders and the elderly.

In fact, overall, NAC reduced or prevented virtually all the annoying side effects of fall and winter ailments such as headache, 'achiness', nasal discharge, cough and sore throat. This pattern of improvement was observed over and over again in study after study.

NAC is a real lifesaver for those with breathing problems. In fact, conventional medicine uses NAC in many of its inhalants to ward off asthma attacks. Other related conditions in which NAC can help include adult respiratory distress syndrome, and chronic obstructive pulmonary disease (COPD).

NAC is also a potent heart supplement. Better than any pharmaceutical method, it eliminates the dangers of lipoprotein(a), which is a by-product of cholesterol metabolism. The presence of lipoprotein(a) has just recently been recognized as a powerful but independent risk factor for heart disease.

NAC lowers high blood pressure due to the relaxing effect it exercises upon the blood vessels while increasing blood flow to the extremities of the body. Researchers in Australia have demonstrated that if enough NAC is administered just after a heart attack, much more of the heart muscle remains undamaged.

Those suffering from inflammatory bowel conditions, such as irritable bowel syndrome, colitis, diverticulitis, etc., should be aware of the benefits of NAC. As the levels of glutathione rise in the body, these conditions seem to diminish accordingly.

Those experiencing hair loss will be interested in knowing that NAC may be of special value to them. By now, most people are aware of the dangers of the low or non-fat diets, which have been so popular over the past 20 years. One problem connected with them has been that they produce a deficiency of sulfur in the body. One of the consequences of a sulfur deficiency, especially in women, is hair loss. NAC just happens to be one of the best sulfur-containing substances known.

Evidence to show that NAC exercises a profound effect upon the immune system comes from several studies of patients infected with the human immunodeficiency virus (HIV). One particular study, conducted at Stanford University, determined that patients with HIV infections and acquired immunodeficiency syndrome (AIDS) had low levels of glutathione. These studies also determined that the declining glutathione levels were actually a better indication of life expectancy in these patients than was a decrease in CD4 immune cells. The study tracked the health of over 200 AIDS patients for three years. Some of the participants received mega doses of NAC while others received a placebo for six-week intervals. Those taking NAC had increased blood levels of glutathione. After this phase of the study was complete, the researchers gave all willing participants NAC supplements for six months.

During this time, it was shown that those taking the NAC were more than twice as likely to survive for two years than the subjects who elected not to take the NAC.

All things considered, NAC is the most vital antioxidant for the new millennium. We will continue to poison our environment, consume diets consisting of dead lifeless foods, subject ourselves to ever-increasing radiation from electronic devices, high frequency signals, and even the sun itself, through the breakdown of the ozone layer. This being the case, NAC is the only single antioxidant that addresses every major chronic disease in our society! It may further be said that N-Acetyl Cysteine is the universal antioxidant for it activates and increases the potential of all the other antioxidants.

Alpha Lipoic Acid This is an extraordinary antioxidant in that it addresses so much of the free radical issue, quenching a wide range of free radicals. This antioxidant also has the ability to raise glutathione levels, an important factor of many antioxidants. Additionally, lipoic acid helps to conserve and recycle other important nutrients and antioxidants. Lipoic acid has been shown to be beneficial in cases of diabetes, especially type II, adult onset diabetes. As we mentioned earlier, diabetes, like most chronic degenerative diseases, is caused by free radical damage. Through this protecting mechanism, lipoic acid increased insulin sensitivity and thus enhances glucose uptake.

These powerful ingredients, any one of which could change the course of human cell life, together are an unstoppable combination, providing an unparalleled dual level of protection to all living systems.

Like other, more familiar nutrients such as vitamins, minerals and amino acids, antioxidants and free radical scavengers are best taken in combination with each other. The total value is much greater than the mere sum of the parts involved.

According to Dr Michael Murray, "extensive research shows that a combination of antioxidants provides greater protection than does taking a high dose of any single antioxidant. Mixtures of antioxidant nutrients appear to work together harmoniously to produce the phenomenon known as synergy, where the whole is greater than the sum of the parts. In other words, when it comes to the benefits of antioxidants, one plus one equals three."

Maximizing Your Antioxidant Benefits

Your need for antioxidants can vary widely from day to day, depending upon your involvement with free radical forming factors. For example, on one day everything may be going along fairly normally, then the next day you find yourself under inordinate amounts of stress and tension at work. After work you go out and have a few drinks to unwind, increasing your alcohol consumption above your normal level. Your antioxidant requirements for those two days will be quite different.

Studies conducted here, at The Institute of Nutritional Science, have shown a wide variance of antioxidant needs, depending upon lifestyle changes, from one day to another. For this reason, establishing a dose range to ensure optimal free radical protection takes a bit of work.

We will offer two basic protocols. The first is what the 'average' person, living with 'average' free radical factors should follow. The second will be for those who are generally exposed to higher levels of free radical forming factors.

If you are predominately in one group over the other, then you will be following that protocol most of the time. If you should occasionally slide from one group to another, you can temporarily alter your intake of nutrients accordingly.

Foundation Protocol

The following represents the minimum antioxidant and free radical scavenging protection that everyone should have on a daily basis.

Vitamin A	10,000 IU
Beta Carotene	10,000 IU
Folic Acid	400 mcg
Pantothenic Acid	200 mg
Vitamin C	1,000 mg
Citrus Bioflavonoids	200 mg
Vitamin E (d-alpha tocopherol)	400 IU

```
Selenium ........................ 100 mcg
Sulfur ............................ 100 mcg
Zinc .............................. 20 mg
N-Acetyl Cysteine ....... 100-200 mg
Silybum marianum ........ 50-100 mg
Quercetin ...................... 50 mg
Co-enzyme Q10 ............. 10-20 mg
Lycopene (extract).......... 25-50 mg
Grape Seed Extract ........ 20-30 mg
```

Higher Risk Protocol

Those individuals who are exposed to higher free radical producing factors such as smoking, excess alcohol consumption, pesticides, food additives, auto exhaust, cigarette smoke, radiation, impure water, toxic metals, industrial chemicals, excessive pharmaceuticals or stress, should consider the following potencies to ensure that adequate cellular protection has been achieved.

```
Vitamin A........................ 10,000 IU
Beta Carotene ................. 10,000 IU
Folic Acid....................... 600 mcg
Pantothenic Acid .............. 800 mg
Vitamin C ...................... 2,000 mg
Citrus Bioflavonoids .......... 400 mg
Vitamin E (d-alpha tocopherol) .. 400 IU
```

Selenium	200 mcg
Sulfur	100 mcg
Zinc	40 mg
N-Acetyl Cysteine	200-400 mg
Silybum marianum	200-300 mg
Quercetin	100 mg
Co-enzyme Q10	20-50 mg
Lycopene (extract)	50-100 mg
Grape Seed Extract	50-100 mg

This protocol will protect most individuals from many of the ravages of free radical proliferation in the body. But like all nutrients and human need, it can vary, sometimes greatly, depending upon circumstances. Persons suffering from chronic disease often need much, much higher doses of antioxidants because the disease process itself is actually producing incredibly high amounts of free radicals. Dosages for these individuals must be adjusted accordingly.

Take the Guess Work Out

The most accurate way to determine your antioxidant/free radical scavenging nutrient needs is through a diagnostic test. The Institute of Nutritional Science is offering a diagnostic urine test for free radicals, which may be self-administered in the comfort of your own home.

The test period is for four weeks, during which time you will need to take your antioxidants in varying doses. Depending upon the results of the test, we will know whether to raise or lower your antioxidant intake. Once we establish a baseline intake, you can easily up the dose during periods wherein you are exposed to greater free radical forming factors.

We live in a time where ignoring the problems caused by impure food, contaminated water, and a polluted environment can be very dangerous indeed. By burying our head in the proverbial sand, we only expose our backside to greater and greater threats from free radical proliferation!

This need not be the case. The knowledge and the road to its proper application is available to every man, woman and child alive today. To not take advantage of it is just as surely suicide as pointing the weapon to your head. The only difference is that it's a much slower process.

Other Popular Anti-Aging Ingredients

There are several other substances, discovered by science and made available by the nutrition industry, which can contribute to slowing and improving the aging process. Since these substances can have a downside for some, we do not necessarily recommend them for everyone. We will discuss each one individually and offer our findings. We certainly encourage your experimentation with these substances, providing you do not fall into one of the restricted categories and that your health care provider monitors your progress.

DHEA

Dehydroepiandrosterone (DHEA) has been labeled the 'mother hormone', because the body uses this base material in the manufacture of several important hormone systems. Through this activity, we might say that DHEA is the 'excitement' hormone. To highlight a few of its functions, it stimulates brain activity, muscle growth, and immune function. DHEA has been used in athletic circles for some time because of its ability to not only increase muscle mass but to preserve existing muscle from catabolism as well.

DHEA is produced naturally by the body's adrenal glands. This production begins to decrease slowly at about age 35 and rapidly decreases after the age of 50. In fact if you are over fifty, you likely have only 20 to 25 percent of the DHEA you had when you were in your mid-twenties.

Other potential benefits of taking DHEA in supplement form include its positive effect on diabetes. Because DHEA can help reduce overall body fat, it can improve insulin sensitivity. Further, since DHEA is also an antioxidant, it helps prevent the lipid peroxidation and free radical damage seen in surges of high blood sugar. The majority of the ravages of diabetes such as blindness, circulatory problems, kidney problems and impotence are a result of free radical damage to these tissues, generated by the bouncing between high levels of blood sugar and insulin.

If DHEA is so important, why haven't I included it the preceding "base-line" antioxidant protocol? Well, a closer look at this potentially powerful hormone precursor leads us to be cautious with regard to its application in certain people.

Since DHEA is a relatively new discovery, there have been no long-term studies regarding prolonged use. Because of its action on both estrogens and androgens, DHEA would not be good for postmenopausal women, or for men who are at high risk for prostate cancer.

If you wish to add DHEA to your total program here are some general guidelines:

1. Do not take it at all if you are under age 30.
2. Do not take more than 25 mg per day without a blood test and medical supervision.
3. Do not take DHEA if you have, or are at risk for, prostate cancer.
4. Do not take DHEA if you are menopausal or postmenopausal.

Much of the data from the clinical studies we do have indicate that DHEA is both safe and effective for the majority of people. However, since this book is written for a large section of the population, we must consider all possible readers.

One final note on DHEA and that is don't be fooled by promoters of Mexican yam as a source for

DHEA. Mexican yam DOES NOT raise levels of DHEA in the human body. The herb may have other benefits, but this is not one of them. Save your money and if you decide to use it, use pure DHEA.

Melatonin

Melatonin is another substance in the hormone/hormone precursor category. While we certainly know more about Melatonin than DHEA, still it may not be universally beneficial for everyone. Further, since you need relatively little Melatonin, the risk for overdose is a real possibility.

Just what is Melatonin and how can it help us? Melatonin is related to melanin, the skin pigment and serotonin, a neurotransmitter found in the brain, responsible for generating happy, upbeat feelings. Melatonin is an antioxidant, in fact it is, by volume, the most powerful antioxidant ever discovered!

The most common use for Melatonin is in sleep disorders and for combating jet lag. Since I travel a great deal by air, I can personally attest to the benefits of using Melatonin upon arrival in distant time zones. It really makes a profound difference in reducing the amount of time to recover from the time shift. Further, Melatonin acts as a specific antioxidant against electromagnetic radiation. This is likely why it improves or prevents jet lag. This tired, out of sorts feeling that can come with long airplane travel is believed to be caused, at least in part, by overexposure to radiation at higher altitudes.

Other studies show that Melatonin may be helpful in boosting the immune system. One study showed that Melatonin actually helped to grow back a damaged thymus gland. Since this amazing substance is such a powerful antioxidant, it has a rightful place as an anti-cancer factor as well.

Lastly, since Melatonin stimulates testosterone and estrogen, it may both improve and extend the quality and quantity of your sex life.

While Melatonin seems to be generally safe, there are some concerns that have kept me from including it for everyone on a daily basis. For example, Melatonin should be taken only at night, shortly before bed. It can rapidly raise serotonin levels in the body and it induces sleep and sets sleep cycles. This can make it impractical to include it in a multi-antioxidant formula.

You should not take Melatonin without the approval and supervision of a qualified health care practitioner if...

1. You are taking any medication to boost serotonin levels, lower blood pressure, or increase hormones. Further do not take if you are on birth control pills or thyroid medications.
2. Do not take if you have cancer, hormonal disease, depression, or autoimmune disorders.
3. Do not take if you are nursing or pregnant.

4. Melatonin should not be taken by anyone under the age of 25.

If you choose to take Melatonin you can either do so on an "as needed" basis, such as for jet lag or time zone adjustment, or you may choose to take a smaller amount regularly. A safe dose of Melatonin would be somewhere between 1 and 3 milligrams per day. Doses higher than 3 milligrams should definitely not be taken without the express supervision of a knowledgeable professional.

Human Growth Hormone

Another naturally occurring hormone found in healthy young people is human growth hormone (hGH). This hormone is produced in the pituitary gland in the brain. In theory, supplementing with hGH, especially as we age, may prove beneficial. However, the risks of misuse are also considerable.

The first thing we must clear up is that no matter what you hear or read, human growth hormone is not available from anyone over the counter. It is a highly regulated substance and requires both a doctor's prescription and close monitoring throughout administration. The products sold in health food stores DO NOT contain hGH no matter how cleverly their promotional materials may be worded. Buyer beware!

Therapy with human growth hormone is currently very expensive, in excess of 18,000 dollars per year. Since the side effects from abuse of hGH are extensive and potentially devastating, be sure that your physician is knowledgeable in the use of hGH before you embark on a program.

The science of life extension is still young. Undoubtedly we will see tremendous advancements in this arena over the next decade alone. In the meantime however, don't wait for the next news, utilize what we already know. It is never too late to improve the quality of your life ahead.

Lastly, remember that most of what we label age-related health problems have little or nothing to do with aging at all. Decades of cigarette smoking, excessive abuse of alcohol, poor diet and lack of exercise do far more to destroy the quality of later life than natural aging. Through some simple lifestyle changes and making use of the longevity knowledge we have available, we can truly add more years to our life and more life to our years.

In the next chapter, we will discuss some of these many pitfalls such as obesity, stress, immune suppression and lack of exercise. We will be showing you how simple it really is to greatly eliminate these proven risks from your life.

Chapter 3
Avoiding Pitfalls on the "Road of Life"

In planning for the quality and quantity of our life ahead, we must recognize and learn to minimize certain pitfalls that can interfere with even the best health-promoting program. These include such obvious deterrents to longevity as cigarette smoking, unmanageable stress, and obesity. In other words a good exercise program, healthy diet and dietary supplements will work a lot less effectively if you are simultaneously abusing yourself in other ways.

If you were to listen to many health writers, they would have you believe that you must give up everything that is pleasant in your life in order to achieve good health. The point raised by this thinking is, "if this is true, do I really want to live an extra 10 years with all the pleasures of life removed?" Fortunately, all of our research indicates that you do not need to live the life of a monk, denying yourself virtually every pleasure in order to reap the rewards of a healthy life. When we look at life, we find just as many people who have attained healthy longevity and maintained negative habits as those who abstained from seemingly everything. The key here is moderation, often referred to as the longest four-letter word in the English language! We humans love extremes, one month we are eating junk food and smoking 2 packs a day, the next day we swear it all off and eat nothing but tofu. A study of the human body has revealed to me that stress is the cardinal cause of all illness. Extremes, in either direction, produce stress. That being said, there still remain a few factors that have been proven so overwhelmingly to cause havoc within the body that they should be at least controlled.

Let's take a look at some of these obvious and avoidable factors that can negatively impact our goal of maintaining a healthy life.

Cigarette Smoking

We'll get the obvious out of the way first. It is estimated that 500 million people, worldwide, will die as a result of cigarettes in the coming years. There is such overwhelming evidence proving that cigarette smoking causes a multitude of diseases. It is difficult to imagine that millions of people still engage in this suicidal habit. On the other hand, that is what the tobacco industry had in mind for us all along. In fact, at one time, there were nearly 100 chemical additives put into cigarette tobacco, many of these additives suspiciously resembled very addictive substances. While the tobacco industry has never been forced to release the full list of these chemicals, we know that something must be in the cigarette to produce such an overwhelming addiction. Yes, I know we have been told that nicotine is the culprit, but that just doesn't quite add up. Nicotine is now available in a variety of forms, gum, tablets, and most popular the patches. Yet the success rate in using these aids to quit is very dismal. If nicotine were the problem, their success rate should be over 90 percent!

Here at our Institute we have helped hundreds of people either quite cigarette smoking, or at least improve their odds of survival if they choose to continue. Wanting to quite, really wanting to quit, is the first requisite. We must recognize that there are many people who, knowingly or subconsciously do not want to stop smoking. For these people no program will help them. But if you are smoking cigarettes and really wish to quit, consider the following options.

Firstly, it is important to switch to a cigarette that does not contain any chemical additives. At the time of this writing, I know of only two companies who widely market additive free cigarettes. They are American Spirit of New Mexico and the other is Nat Sherman of New York. Both companies have ensured us that their cigarettes do not contain chemical additives. Those who begin smoking chemical free cigarettes may perhaps find them unsatisfying and will likely feel some withdrawal symptoms. This only proves that it is not the nicotine that's the problem because these cigarettes contain just as much nicotine as all the rest. Stick with these 'clean cigarettes' until you can smoke them comfortably.

Once you have reached this stage, you should begin to reduce the number of cigarettes you smoke daily, until you are able to quit entirely. You will find that cutting back on an additive free cigarette will be far easier than you think, especially if you have tried to quit before. There are some specific nutrients that help protect the body from the ravages of cigarette smoke and you may wish to take these in addition to your regular supplementation program.

Insurance for Smokers

Choline	2,000 mg
Selenium	200 mcg
Extra B-Complex	50 mg
Cysteine HCl	1,000 mg
Vitamin C	3,000 mg
Tyrosine	500 mg

Remember, as with all of our targeted nutrient recommendations, the preceding formula should be taken together with a multi-nutrient formula which provides the Full Spectrum of known human nutritional needs (see the chapter on nutrients for a complete listing).

Currently in progress at the Institute is work on a formulation for smokers and those exposed to "second-hand smoke". The formula will include not only the preceding nutrient factors, but will contain other natural substances which have also proven to be beneficial in smoking cessation programs. While providing antioxidant and free radical scavenging protection, the formula will assist the smoker in quitting by reducing cravings. If you are interested in this formulation, I suggest that you contact my office for updated information on this project.

Hyper-Toxicity

There have always been toxins in our environment. From the first time people sat huddled around a campfire for warmth, we have been exposed to toxins from burning organic matter. As we have tried to stress throughout this book, the body possesses an amazing ability to adapt and compensate for changes, even negative changes, in our environment, but there is a limit to that adaptability potential. In the last 25 years, we have dumped tens of thousands of potentially toxic substances into the environment. Since most of these are man-made compounds, we do not possess the genetic knowledge or experience to metabolize or safely break them down. This overload is so depressing our immune system that it is nearly at the point of failure. In fact, we are seeing many 'new disorders' and 'designer conditions' that are certainly linked to this excess toxicity. Further, many immune related diseases that have been with us for longer periods of time are becoming epidemic in their occurrence.

Conditions such as fibromyalgia, chronic fatigue syndrome and other problems are rising rapidly. The cause of many of these disorders has eluded scientists for years. It is my feeling that they are a by-product of toxic overload upon the living chemical system of the body. Our work with fibromyalgia patients has proven that, when you properly detoxify these people, their symptoms lessen and fade away. Further, clinical evidence shows that vitamin C, in very large doses, often produces dramatic results. This further supports the hyper-toxicity concept because vitamin C is both a diuretic and a powerful antioxidant.

Cancer, an immune deficient disease, has become so epidemic, it will exceed heart disease as the leading cause of death within 5 years. No other single factor has changed so dramatically in the last one hundred years to account for this increase other than diet and the number and levels of toxins in the environment.

It may be argued that if toxins are indeed causing these problems, why isn't everyone getting it. Statistics show that we are well on our way! Since there is such a concept as biochemical individuality, some of us have greater resistance than others. This is the reason why some get the flu in winter and others don't.

In managing hyper-toxicity, our emphasis must be placed upon the importance of antioxidants, since they are consumed in high amounts during the breakdown of foreign substances in the body. Further, adjunct support for the specific tissues or organ systems involved should also be considered (protocols for specific conditions may be found in the chapter entitled "The Natureceutical Pharmacopia").

Lack of Exercise

Everyone knows that exercise is a good thing, but few of us actually follow through and do it. If you were to ask a broad section of the population about the importance of exercise, they would almost universally agree that it is an essential factor for good health. Why then, don't we do it? It is easy to answer this question simply by saying that most people are lazy or choose the easy way out. Since that is likely the case for many, a better understanding of why we are lazy may help us to overcome the stigma attached to it.

There are many reasons, in fact, why people don't exercise regularly. For example, as we grow older, we are just too busy. Our younger years were filled with both the energy and the opportunity to consume that energy via our favorite sport or activity. As we mature, responsibilities increase with financial obligation and family demands. Statistics show that the major problem people face is lack of time management skills, which lead to a majority of stress in life. With the inability to properly manage one's time, exercise is one of the last things to be considered and one of the first items to be crossed off an already too hectic schedule.

Health clubs are frequently an effective alternative to a completely self-motivated home program. In choosing a health club, what should you look for?

1. Choose a club that has well trained instructors, qualified to work with your particular age group.

2. Be sure, if you travel, that it has branches in the places you go.
3. Check the hours of operation and be sure they fit your schedule.
4. Does it offer a variety of exercise options, weight training, aerobics equipment and classes, swimming pool, etc.?
5. Does it offer supportive therapies such as massage, if you are interested?

Once you have chosen a club, it is important to attend regularly. In order to achieve any significant benefit from exercise, one must do it consistently. The body responds to exercise ten times more effectively if you do it on a consistent basis. Health clubs go through a variety of hoops to try and keep their members motivated to come in. They know that if you stop coming to their club, you will likely not renew your membership. In the end, however, it is you that must provide the motivation and discipline to be consistent with exercise.

If you haven't done any exercise for some time, be sure you start slowly and that your program is geared for both your age and your physical abilities. You should plan to exercise on at least three days per week for at least 30 minutes at a time.

A list of do's and don'ts follows:

The "Do's" Include:

1. Be consistent with your exercise program.
2. Do warm up, especially if you haven't exercised in a while.
3. Do cool down by exercising only lightly during the last five minutes of each session.
4. Do combine weight resistance and aerobic exercise. One cannot replace the other; each is equally important.
5. When doing aerobic exercise, a safe rule is to raise your pulse rate to 220 beats per minute minus your age.
6. Do undergo a physical exam prior to starting an exercise program if you are over 40 years of age and have not exercised during the past year.
7. Do supplement your diet with Full Spectrum nutrition as outlined in this book. Remember that exercise creates a greater demand for nutrients, not less.

The "Don'ts" Include:

1. Don't exercise intensely within one hour of a heavy meal.
2. Don't exercise if you have a cold, flu, or other respiratory condition.
3. Don't progress too fast; go at your pace, not someone else's.

4. Don't sit or lie down immediately after exercise. Keep moving, walking around for at least 10 minutes.
5. Don't waste valuable time with passive exercise equipment such as rollers, vibrators, etc. They don't improve your health.
6. Don't follow an exercise program that produces fatigue or discomfort. Be sure it's right for you.
7. Don't use rubber suits, belts or hot tubs to try and lose weight. These gimmicks only dehydrate the body.

The best way to ensure your compliance with the exercise schedule you have set is to make an appointment with yourself. If you are working, set your health club appointments for 4 to 8 weeks ahead. That way, you will not be booking that time with something else. Treat these appointments just as you would any other 'business' commitment. If you are retired, getting an appointment book and doing the same thing is frequently helpful. I have met many a retired person who is so busy they can't seem to find time for anything either!

A note about soreness, when you begin a new exercise program, it is normal and expected that you will experience some muscle stiffness and soreness. If this persists beyond two weeks, consult your exercise instructor for modifications in either your exercises or the amount of weight you are using. In order to greatly reduce soreness from exercise of any kind, you should increase your intake of vitamin C. This nutrient prevents the formation and buildup of lactic acid in the muscle fibers, the cause of the soreness. You should benefit substantially from the addition of 2 to 3 grams (2 to 3 thousand milligrams) per day.

In closing this section on exercise, we need to briefly discuss the subject of rest. Exercising actually tears down muscle tissue. When you rest, your body rebuilds and repairs that muscle tissue. When the muscle is repaired by the body, it becomes bigger and a little stronger than before. This is the main reason rest is just as important to your health and physical fitness as is the actual exercise. The benefits of exercise materialize during periods of rest. For this reason, it is not recommended that you exercise every day. Take a day off between exercise sessions or do less demanding activities on those days.

Weight Management

Obesity is epidemic in most industrialized nations. In the United States it is estimated that one in three people is overweight! As we age, carrying more than 20 % over your ideal bodyweight increasingly raises the liability. Certainly, after the age of 35, if you are excessively overweight, you should consider taking aggressive steps to correct this situation.

Obesity is practically a national epidemic in America. We are told that it's due to constantly over eating. Most all diet programs, certainly those given by dieticians and medical doctors, focus on a reduction of calories to the point where, in theory, more calories are burned than consumed.

If this were universally the case, then a 1500 calorie diet should produce a safe and steady weight loss in virtually every one on that diet; even a sedentary individual burns about 2000 calories per day. Any doctor or dietician will tell you, however, that they must use diets providing as little as 1000 calories or less per day in many cases. They will further tell you that some of their patients actually gain weight on a 1000-calorie diet. Their explanation however, is that 'they must be cheating.'

In carefully controlled studies conducted here at The Institute of Nutritional Science, we have found that it is possible for many people to lose weight poorly, or not at all, on a calorie-restricted diet.

What we must come to realize, if we ever hope to resolve this problem of obesity, is that there are many factors which cause the body to accumulate and carry excessive weight. Only one of them is excess calorie consumption.

About 75 percent of the people who are overweight by 25 pounds or more are probably not eating too much food; they are, likely, eating the wrong kinds of food for their metabolism and body chemistry.

There is a name for this condition. Identified more than 25 years ago, hyperinsulinemia, or excess insulin production, has only recently been given a more generalized acceptance.

Insulin, is a powerful hormone, responsible for regulating glucose in the blood stream. The proper level of glucose is essential for body function. Too much glucose, and you have multiple side effects and a disorder called diabetes. Too little glucose, and you have a different set of side effects and a disorder called hypoglycemia. Insulin first converts excess sugar from the diet into glycogen (the storage sugar) and then into triglycerides which are stored as body fat. When blood sugar falls too low, glycogen is converted back into available blood glucose.

Many diets in industrialized nations provide sugar or sugar forming foods in gross excess of what the human body was genetically programmed to manage. It is this over-consumption of refined carbohydrates and sugars that eventually exhausts the insulin and insulin receptor mechanisms of the body. This leads to either hypoglycemia or diabetes.

Adult onset diabetes or type II diabetes is the most rampant epidemic in the world today. It is caused virtually completely by dietary abuse. At the turn of the last century, the average American consumed about 10 to 12 pounds of sugar per year. Diabetes, at that time, was number 100 in the sequence of frequency of diseases. It was so rare that only specialists in larger cities understood the condition. Today, a mere 100 years later, the average American consumes about 200 pounds or more of sugar, or sugar forming foods, annually. Diabetes today is always in the top ten diseases and it is estimated that it will exceed heart disease as a cause of death within the next ten years.

The low carbohydrate type diets that first became popular in the 1970's with Dr. Robert C. Atkins, have been duplicated, with a few variations, over and over again. Their popularity remains such that even many mainstream 'calorie concept' diet centers are now offering the 'low carbo alternative.' Dr. Atkins was a pioneer and a brave genius. His work freed many hundreds of thousands of people from the shackles of "yo-yo dieting" and "semi-starvation dieting" because of the low calorie consumption diets.

Like the low calorie diet, not everyone responds to a low carbohydrate, higher protein program either. The key is determining what your metabolic typing is. In other words, how your body chemically processes foods. If we could determine this, with some degree of accuracy, it would be much easier to choose the type of diet and eating plan to best fit your chemistry.

Research into this concept of body typing has been going on at The Institute of Nutritional Science for more than 10 years. During that time we have been able to isolate seven specific, distinct and different classifications of "body chemistries". Members of certain groups respond favorably to slightly different types of weight management programs.

Response is a pivotal factor in the success of any weight management program. Dieting is not fun under the best of circumstances. We all want to eat our favorite foods. Therefore, we are constantly on the lookout for that "magic bullet", which will allow us to do that, and still loose weight or maintain an ideal weight. The first step in solving the weight management problem is to accept the fact that there is no "magic bullet", period.

That having been said, what is the next best thing? Finding an eating program that works with your particular body chemistry rather than against it.

Why do you suppose those people we mentioned earlier did not loose weight on that 1000 calorie diet? Were they all cheating? That's doubtful.

The answer to this question surfaces when we look at hyperinsulinemia as a cause for obesity. Excess insulin converts glucose into triglycerides, often before it has the opportunity to serve as a source of energy. By the way, this explains why many severely overweight people virtually have no energy at all, making the exercise that they need an insurmountable obstacle. The low calorie diets consistently recommended by dietitians, doctors, and many weight loss center chains are frequently high in sugar or sugar forming foods and low in protein and fat. Since they are counting calories only, the diet emphasizes lower calorie carbohydrate foods. For variety, they turn to sweet, refined carbohydrates. It is not unusual for the standard 1000 or 1200 calorie diet to be made up of as much as 60 percent or more refined carbohydrates. All of these turn to triglycerides in the presence of excess insulin in the hyperinsulinemic individual. Now we can better see why many people do not fare well on low calorie diets.

If you're still not convinced that carbohydrates and not fat can make you fat, consider these facts...

1. In the last 25 years fat consumption is down by a whopping 40 percent, yet the number of overweight people has continued to rise at an alarming rate.
2. During the last 25 years the number of obese people has risen from one in five to one in three.
3. During the last 25 years the consumption of refined grain products, which convert to sugar rapidly in the body, has risen by 60 percent.
4. During the last 25 years the consumption of soft drinks increased by 25 percent and the amount of concentrated fruit juices increased in children by over 300 percent!
5. During the last 25 years, the amount of sugar consumed by the average person has gone up from about 140 pounds per year to over 200 pounds.

It can clearly be seen that the old concept of 'a calorie is a calorie', no longer is valid for the majority of those engaged in the "Battle of the Bulge" (note: for those suffering from either hypoglycemia or especially diabetes, it is essential that you learn to restrict and control your consumption of sugar-forming foods. See the section on diabetes for further guidelines).

How can we determine the manner in which our own body handles food? How can we obtain the edge that comes from knowing what type of diet program would produce the best, safest and longest lasting results?

There are some simple tests, developed by the staff here at The Institute of Nutritional Science, which are amazingly accurate in determining your metabolic typing. While there are several tests available to clients visiting The Institute personally, the following two tests will tell you quite accurately, whether you tend to be calorie sensitive (eat too much food) or carbohydrate intolerant (eat too many sugar forming foods).

Directions: The following two tests consist of yes or no type statements. As you take each test, check off the statements which apply to you.

Test For Excess Calorie Consumption

1. You had a normal body weight when younger, but slowly gained weight after age 30.
2. You are presently overweight, but by less than 25 pounds.
3. You have a normal appetite - you get hungry at mealtimes.
4. You have few, if any, real food cravings.
5. You have maintained the same basic eating habits all your life.

6. You eat three meals a day - you rarely skip a meal.
7. You have gained a certain amount of extra body weight, but the gaining seems to have tapered off and you are not continuing to gain more and more weight.

Test For Excess Carbohydrate Consumption

1. You are more than 25 pounds overweight.
2. You have had a tendency to be overweight all your adult life.
3. You have been overweight since you were a child.
4. You often have a poor appetite and often skip meals.
5. You prefer not to eat in the morning.
6. You have food cravings that temporarily go away when starchy or sugary foods are eaten.
7. There are foods that you feel you absolutely could not do without.

Scoring: Add up the number of checks separately in each of the two tests. If you had more yes answers to test one, you are likely calorie sensitive and need to restrict your caloric intake. If you answered yes to more statements in test two, you are very likely carbohydrate intolerant and need to restrict the amount of carbohydrates you consume.

By these two simple tests alone you may now know more about the way your own body processes food than the majority of dieters. With this information you can begin to tailor your diet accordingly, either cutting down on calories or eliminating a large percentage of your carbohydrate intake and replace it with protein foods and green vegetables.

For those interested in the full program of weight management and lifestyle as offered by The Institute, you may contact one of our offices or call the main office and ask for The Institute's new book on weight management.

Lifestyle Findings

Results of how better lifestyle factors can positively affect both the quality and quantity of life have been compared in studies conducted since the early 1970's. A summary of these factors from all the studies follows...

Smoking: The least risk was obviously found in people who did not smoke. The next category, were those living with second hand smoke. The third risk group were those that smoked less than a pack a day and the highest risk group were those smoking two or more packs per day.

Alcohol: People who drank two cocktails, or even better, two glasses of red wine per day, had the greatest longevity, followed by those who consumed no alcohol at all. The group with the highest mortality were those regularly consuming an excess of two cocktails daily.

Weight: The group who maintained their ideal weight and the group who were a few percentage points over their ideal weight had about the same mortality risk. Those consistently 20 percent or more over their ideal weight had the greatest risk factor.

Exercise: This seemed to be a very important risk factor in all the studies conducted. Those who exercised regularly, three or four times per week, had a mortality rate only about half as high as those who never exercised do.

Rest: Men who sleep between seven and eight hours a night were better off than men who slept less or more. The best duration of sleep for women was found to be about seven hours or a little less.

Diet: Those who ate erratically, or those who maintained extreme eating habits, had the highest risk. Those eating diets consisting of more than 30 percent processed foods were equally at high risk. Those eating a consistently good diet of the same number of meals per day were at the least risk.

It may be seen by these summaries that moderation is crucial to living a longer and healthier life. Time and time again, it is the extremes of too much or too little which cause us the most problems. With very little modification of your lifestyle, you can greatly enhance the positive elements in your life. And, with very small changes, you can substantially minimize potentially negative life-affecting factors. It is my hope that this information will help you avoid many stumbling blocks and pitfalls as you continue your journey through life.

Chapter 4
Chronic Disease: The Scourge of the New Century

During World War II, medical science developed its most shining star, the antibiotic. Through its use, literally millions of lives were saved from acute bacterial disease. So much so, that infectious disease had begun to take a back seat. People gave much less credence to these acute conditions because they knew there was a 'cure' just a doctor's visit away.

Today, infectious disorders are on the rise once again. This is primarily due to two factors. Firstly, our immune systems are so compromised through high levels of toxic pollutants in our environment. Secondly, the antibiotic has been so over-prescribed, that the bugs are rapidly becoming resistant to the most powerful combinations. This downfall, as it were, of antibiotics came about because they worked so well. It was so easy to administer a ten-day series of a particular antibiotic and the problem, large or small, disappeared. When a patient was ailing because of an infected ingrown toenail, instead of sending that patient home with a box of Epsom salts, doctors prescribed a powerful antibiotic - because they could. Today, it is not uncommon for a small child to have had 8 to 10 rounds of antibiotic therapy before having reached school age. This abuse has led us to a precarious position wherein when we need these powerful substances, they will fail us.

Through substances such as antibiotics and procedures such as improved cleanliness, infectious disease has indeed taken that back seat. Sadly though, they have been replaced by a group of diseases, which, in many ways, are far worse than those they have replaced.

We are talking about chronic degenerative diseases. By definition, a chronic disease is, unlike an acute condition, one that will be around for long periods of time. A degenerative illness continues to worsen over time, frequently becoming a life-long problem for the victim.

A group of chronic degenerative diseases consistently make the top-ten list of causes of debilitation and death. Non-infectious in nature, they include conditions such as heart disease, cancer, diabetes, arthritis, osteoporosis, prostate problems, and many others. A non-infectious disease is one that cannot be passed from one person to another. However, once these diseases enter your life, they are often with you forever.

This epidemic of chronic disease manifestation dwarfs infectious diseases to the point where two out of every three people over the age of 40 suffer from one or more of them.

The tragedy of this situation is obvious. The golden years of your life, those after retirement, should be your reward for a lifetime of work. Finally, we likely have a few dollars in the bank and many of our day to day responsibilities generated by job and family are over. This is the ideal time for us to really enjoy life, to travel or to pursue the hobbies and interests that we have had to put off for so long due to time constraints.

Sounds good doesn't it? Sadly, this is not going to be the case for the majority of us who reach that age. Instead of vacations, hobbies, sports, and other pleasures, our days will likely be filled with doctor visits, trips to the pharmacy to fill prescriptions, compromised health from side effect of drugs, surgical procedures, convalescent therapy, rehabilitation, loss of energy, depression & mood swings, and of course the final insult to the living body, premature death.

Every day, many thousands of "baby-boomers" turn 50. This phenomenon will continue for at least another decade. As more people than ever before in human history pass into the last one-third of their lives, these chronic degenerative diseases will continue to rise.

If we take a closer look at some of these common chronic diseases, the rate of prevalence is both frightening and staggering.

Heart disease has been the leading cause of death in most industrialized nations for several decades. While deaths from heart disease are down considerably from

25 years ago, the actual number of people who have heart disease has never been greater. Procedures, such as angioplasty and the coronary by-pass operation, have temporarily saved lives. However, these procedures have done NOTHING to prevent or reverse the disease. This is supported by the fact that every 30 seconds, 24 hours a day, month after month, year after year, somebody dies of cardiovascular disease. Further, it is estimated that 57 million Americans currently live with some form of cardiovascular disease. Does this sound as though conventional medical science has this problem under control? I think not.

Cancer is, at the time of this writing, the second leading cause of death worldwide. If the incidence of cancer continues its rise at the present rate, it will exceed heart disease as the leading cause of death within the next five years.

Conventional medical methods for fighting and managing this disease have had a dismal response. According to the American Cancer Society, medical science is no closer to conquering cancer today than it was 50 years ago. Estimates place the incidence of cancer frequency at one in three adults over the age of 40. Conventional medical methodologies, such as radiation and chemotherapy, often unleash such devastation upon the immune system that it should not be surprising that the incidence of cancer reoccurrence is so high. We have not yet accepted the fact that you cannot poison a sick person well.

Another disease, in fact the most epidemic condition of modern times, is so rampant that there are over 2200 new cases diagnosed every single day. This disease, a mere hundred years ago, was so obscure that a sufferer had to oftentimes travel hundreds of miles to find a doctor who might even recognize it. This disease is called diabetes.

As of 1998, there were over 16 million diabetics in the United States alone. In other industrialized nations, such as the United Kingdom, diabetes is on the rapid rise. As more and more countries adopt the "junk food" eating habits of Americans, their populace experience a similar increase of this disease.

One of the worst characteristics of diabetes is that it frequently doesn't have the decency to kill you quickly. Diabetes affects nearly every part of the body, slowly destroying it step by step. Complications of diabetes include blindness, kidney disease, nerve disease, circulatory problems, amputations, heart disease and stroke, to name a few. Because the disease eats you up one piece at a time, I have frequently referred to diabetes as the non-infectious leprosy of the 20th Century. Sadly we are marching into the 21st Century with no end in sight for diabetes and most other chronic diseases.

Arthritis is another chronic condition that robs us of the quality of our lives. There are many forms of arthritis, the most common being "osteo", or osteo-inflammatory arthritis. This form of arthritis is so common that many physicians expect and assume that everyone over the age of 50 has it. In fact I recently went for a physical exam and in the process of filling out the copious paperwork involved in seeing a doctor these days; I answered the question as to whether I suffered from arthritis with an honest no. Upon seeing this response on the form the doctor questioned me, asking if perhaps I had made a mistake. I asked him why and he said, "everyone over 50 has a 'little' arthritis"!

Arthritis is rampant in virtually every industrialized nation on earth. When I was in Europe on lecture tour a few months ago, I was amazed and dismayed to find that arthritis is a major concern for almost every member of the population over the age of 50. In cold, damp climates, arthritis complaints are worse, since this type of weather makes the condition much more uncomfortable.

Presently it is estimated that there are over 100 million people in industrialized countries suffering from arthritis. This figure could rise to more than 150 million sufferers in the next twenty years.

If you are beginning to see a common thread running through these chronic disease conditions, you are very observant. That commonality is the fact that virtually all these diseases are on the epidemic rise, because medical science has no cure or effective method of management.

There are several chronic conditions that are classically related to old age. Conditions such as osteoporosis, primarily, although certainly not exclusively, in females and chronic prostate inflammation in older males

91

are classic examples. You might be amazed to learn that these conditions have practically nothing to do with old age. In fact, both osteoporosis and prostate problems are occurring in younger and younger people all the time.

Osteoporosis affects an estimated 20 million people in the United States alone. Worldwide, the numbers exceed 40 million. This problem accounts for about 2 million fractures in people over 45. In the next ten years, osteoporosis is expected to increase by more than 400 percent!

Prostate inflammation, or benign prostatic hypertrophy (BPH), is another condition that is being diagnosed in increasing numbers. Statistics in 1997 indicated that there were some 33 million men, in seven major industrialized countries, suffering from moderate to severe BPH. Projections, based on populace age and lifestyle, indicate that by the year 2007, just around the corner now, that the figure will exceed 43 million!

All of these dismal statistics make turning middle age nothing less than frightening!

If conventional medicine had the solutions to these problems, they would certainly be selling those latest wonder drugs or surgical procedures to us. The truth is that they don't exist. Medical science has virtually no idea how to stop the explosive epidemic of virtually every one of these conditions.

If you are 40 years old or older, your chances of developing one or multiple chronic diseases is much greater than not. It is vital that you understand that medicine, in the midst of all its genuine past achievements in the areas of trauma, emergency and acute disease response, cannot prevent, manage, or reverse any chronic degenerative disease. If you want to greatly reduce your risk of contracting these conditions, or if you have any of them already and would like to improve your condition, you must resign yourself to look elsewhere. That is the purpose of this book. Once again, it's all about options.

What is the answer? If drugs and surgery don't solve the problem, what will? The answer lies deep within the biochemistry of this most amazing human body of ours.

This body we call home is, in fact, the most complicated chemical laboratory ever invented by anyone. With all our medical insight and accomplishments, we have only begun to understand its infinite complexity. One thing that we do know for a fact however, is that any machine, be it an automobile, a home appliance or the human body, needs raw materials with which to operate as well as a good maintenance program to keep it operating in peek condition. In the case of the body, those raw materials are a group of chemicals we have come to call nutrients. Not merely the simple vitamins and a few minerals, oh no, science has revealed that presently, we need about 120 nutrients and nutrient compounds in order for the body to perform optimally in our present environment.

Further, science has identified numerous nutraceutical compounds and combinations, which can provide the body with sufficient raw material to actually rebuild living tissue and rebalance chemistry to the point where chronic disease may be improved or, in many cases, reversed altogether.

In the case of the arthritis sufferer previously mentioned, the use of a complete nutrition program, along with what we call targeted nutrition specifically for arthritis, can rebalance the chemistry of the body. Substances such as glucosamine sulfate and chondroiton sulfate not only improve the condition, but may even reverse it.

The choice is ours. Many people will only follow the advice of their medical doctors. The statistics just provided prove that this "advice" has not been effective. The explosive increase in the diagnosis of chronic degenerative disease should encourage people to explore alternatives. Conventional medicine has simply not served our needs in the areas of prevention and/or reversal of these diseases.

Through our work with hundreds and hundreds of people here at our Institute, we see first hand, how effective these alternative concepts really are. For us, they are no longer theories on the pages of dusty clinical journals. Every day we see people who are improving the quality of, and extending the quantity of, their lives. You, too, can achieve similar results.

In the chapters ahead we will examine some of the most prevalent chronic illnesses facing societies worldwide. I will show you how you may, with minimal lifestyle revision, take charge of your health through preventive measures. If you already suffer from one or more chronic diseases, I will show you how you can greatly improve the situation, and in many instances, completely reverse the disease. Once again, and I cannot stress this enough - "Others have accomplished this, and so can you!"

Part II: Fixing The Problem

Chapter 5

Heart Disease: The Number One Cause of Death... Still

Heart disease and stroke take more people from their life prematurely than any other cause. These killers strike a new victim every two seconds!

During the last 15 years, we have followed the low fat diet. In fact, almost everything labeled 'healthy' is also low fat or non-fat. Yet, despite this fanaticism, heart disease has not diminished. To make matters worse, one of the leading factors in heart disease, obesity, has risen in greater numbers than at any other time in history!

While awareness as to the importance of such factors as diet, stress management and exercise have helped people deal with this killer, these factors have never been fully understood.

One of the areas of greatest confusion must be diet. Atherosclerosis, the cause of most heart disease is caused by diet. But we have not been correctly informed as to which dietary factors are to blame.

Other than by-pass surgery, are there solutions to heart disease? Yes! As with most chronic disease conditions, its cause is an altered biochemistry. When the biochemistry is corrected, the disease process is interrupted and the body is in the best possible position to help itself.

At the heart of this change in biochemistry must be diet. The dietary recommendations of The American Heart Association have failed miserably in curbing the epidemic of heart disease, yet its protocol, with its dismal history, is still preached from every medical alter in the world. Watch your cholesterol. Reduce the intake of animal fats. Eat margarine. Eat less protein and eat more starch.

It might surprise you to know that cholesterol, that evil terrible substance, or so we are told, supposedly gets into your arteries and kills you, has NEVER caused one case of heart disease or death! Further, there has never been even one clinical study to show that cholesterol has ever been at fault. Yet we are still being brainwashed about this natural essential fatty substance.

In order to gain control of this runaway horse called heart disease, we must look towards its cause. You may be both surprised and disgusted to find out that the real cause of heart disease was first identified in 1974. Yet despite this discovery over 25 years ago, NOTHING has changed in the conventional medical programs ostensibly designed to prevent or manage this condition.

Through the application of medicine's reactive methods to this chronic disease, the bypass operation was developed. While this procedure can save lives in an emergency, it does NOTHING to stop the progression of the illness, leaving most bypass patients facing the same procedure again in 5 to 7 years.

It's time we examine the REAL causes of heart disease and how you can intervene, at almost any stage, and begin reversing the process which got you to that point in the first place. As with all chronic disease, heart disease is best prevented rather than treated. But take heart, (pun intended) even if you have been diagnosed with heart disease, there is a tremendous amount you can do to help your body heal.

Coronary Thrombosis - The Twentieth Century Killer

As we look to a new millennium and the twentieth century passes into the history books, it will have to be written that it was the century of the heart attack. Prior to the twentieth century, coronary thrombosis or the 'heart attack' was virtually unknown. With a bit of luck, the new century ahead will bring a greater awareness of the real causes of this problem and subsequently it's return to obscurity.

Death rate from coronary thrombosis (an occlusion of one or more of the main arteries, usually surrounding the heart) in 1890 was roughly 0 - no recorded cases. Even as late as 1914, the four most common forms of heart disease were rheumatic, hypertensive, enlargement, and syphilitic - no mention of heart attack. In the 1930's, the four most common forms were hypertensive, coronary, rheumatic and syphilitic. Suddenly coronary heart disease makes its appearance.

By the early 1970's, deaths from coronary thrombosis rose to almost 340 per 100,000 people, killing more people than all other forms of disease put together.

Current statistics reflect an interesting phenomenon. By 1996, deaths from heart disease dropped to 135 per 100,000, giving rise to the medical industry's claim that they are beating this condition. A closer look at the statistic, however, reveals a much different picture. Death rates have dropped dramatically due to the bypass operation, which can intervene and prevent death. But we must forever keep in mind that the actual number of heart disease cases has risen! This means that the bypass operation, while forestalling the inevitable, does nothing to prevent the problem from occurring!

This is reflected in the 1994 statistics showing that there we 22.3 million cases of heart disease reported that year, keeping heart disease the number one cause of death (733,834 deaths in 1996.)

The biggest argument against these statistics is that during the 19th century, people did not live as long. This is, however, not the case. If you factor out infant mortality and juvenile deaths from infections, the average life expectancy today is only 8 years longer than it was in 1900!

Another argument is that doctors were not trained to recognize the disease. Yet the heart attack is usually not subtle in its symptoms. What physician could overlook severe chest pain and pressure, a dull pain which travels down the neck and into the left arm, cold sweats, nausea, a fall in blood pressure, rapid weak pulse and so on? Yet, even as late as the 1930's, it took a specialist to identify coronary thrombosis because of its rarity. Today, most members of the general public would recognize its symptoms for what they are.

To summarize, heart attacks have been the leading cause of death for only the last thirty years, killing over 700,000 people annually, compared with the few who died of the same cause in 1900.

What is The Real Cause of the Epidemic?

If cholesterol is the cause of heart disease as we have been told, the last 15 years of the low fat, low cholesterol diets should have made a marked improvement in the statistics. It has not. Diet does play a significant role in the formation of atherosclerotic plaque, but not in the way we have been taught. More on this a little later.

What then is the real cause of this dreaded disease?

Present research shows that deposits form on artery walls. Eventually, these arteries are occluded completely caused by a proliferation of muscle cells within the artery wall.

This research, first conducted between 1970 and 1974 by Dr. Earl P. Benditt and his associates at the University of Washington School of Medicine, clearly shows that the cells in the artery wall proliferate because of a mutation in their DNA. This altering of the structure of DNA is caused by a variety of factors such as cigarette smoke chemicals, low-level radiation, epoxides of fatty substances, chlorine, and most importantly, free radicals from certain foods.

These data were confirmed again in 1975 through studies conducted by Dr. Robert Heptinstall of the Johns Hopkins School of Medicine.

It is this mutation of cells, which causes them to explosively multiply, eventually creating a lesion that ruptures into the inner wall of the artery.

There are many natural substances, most of them nutrients, which can help to reduce this cellular damage by protecting the artery cell DNA from oxidative and radioactive damage.

It is important to understand that no one single factor can lead to heart disease or a heart attack. But when two or more of these factors are present at the same time, disaster is a distinct possibility.

For example, autopsies performed on mummies from both Egypt and China show that many of these people had plaque build-up in their arteries, however none of them showed signs of ever having a heart attack.

The 20th century lifestyle was characterized by lack of exercise, improper diet, poor food quality, excess stress, and environmental poisons from chemicals and radiation. These factors created an atmosphere conducive to an epidemic of coronary thrombosis.

To put this further into perspective, we quote from an article which appeared in Family Circle magazine in 1971. Dr. Paul Dudley White, an early cardiologist, stated, "First of all, I want to emphasize that heart disease truly is an epidemic today, a fact that many people seem to refuse to accept... Your generation has become so used to the specter of heart attacks, you don't even conceive of life free from this danger. But remember, when I was an intern at Massachusetts General Hospital in 1911, there was no Department of Cardiology."

When Dr. White first set up his cardiology laboratory in 1920, coronary thrombosis was still so uncommon that most medical students did not know of the disease.

What About Cholesterol?

Today, professionals in the medical industry, and especially the American Heart Association, cling to the concept that cholesterol causes heart disease. Their philosophy continues to dictate that, in order to reduce heart disease, less cholesterol must be consumed.

The problem with this theory is that firstly, it does not stand up to evidence uncovered over the last twenty-five years, and secondly no clinical study has ever proven that cholesterol causes heart disease! In fact there are numerous studies, some of them very famous, that prove just the opposite, namely that dietary cholesterol has nothing to do with this disease process. Even the famous Framingham study proved that the cholesterol concept is a myth. In fact, each of the following studies, a few among many, have shown that low-cholesterol diets do not reduce heart disease:

St. Mary's Hospital Trial, ... 1965.
The London Research
Committee Trial 1965
The Norwegian Trial 1966
The London Medical Research
Council Trial 1968
The National Diet Heart Study 1968
The Finnish Mental Hospital Trial
1968
The Los Angeles Veteran's Trial
1969
The Framingham Study 1970
The Ireland-Boston Heart Study
1970
The Edinburgh-Stockholm Study
1975
The UCLA Study 1975
The Honolulu-Japanese Study 1975

In addition to this list, the Coronary Drug Project in 1974 was the first of many studies showing that drugs employed to reduced blood cholesterol were of no value in preventing heart disease.

It is now known that arterial deposits are not caused by cholesterol. By the time cholesterol begins sticking to your artery walls, 90 percent of the damage has already been done. It is now well established that how much cholesterol you eat or don't eat only minimally affects cholesterol levels in the blood.

Cholesterol is a natural substance; it is formed in the body and performs a variety of life-sustaining functions. Cholesterol is responsible for liver function, nerve insulation, brain function (your brain has the greatest concentration of cholesterol in the body), and many other vital tasks.

In a healthy body, the less cholesterol that comes from diet the more the body makes and vice versa. If you have elevated cholesterol, especially if accompanied by an improper ratio of High-Density Lipoprotein (HDL) to Low-Density Lipoprotein (LDL), it is due to a liver problem. A good cholesterol range is somewhere between 165 to 220, provided that the HDL reading is higher than the LDL reading.

If your cholesterol is high, or the ratios out of line, you need to support your liver. Nutrients of significant value are choline, inositol, methionine, essential fatty acids, and glandular extracts (especially adrenal and liver). Also, be sure and check for thyroid function as this can alter blood cholesterol levels as well.

The concept that dietary fat intake does not raise cholesterol levels nor does it cause heart disease is further evidenced by studies of many populations, which have little or no heart disease in spite of the fact that they follow a diet very high in saturated fats and cholesterol. Some of these groups and studies include:

The Maasai of Tanzania
The Samburu and Punjabis of Northern Kenya
Swiss of the Loetschental Valley
Benedictine Monks
The Northern Indians
Primitive Eskimos
The Atiu and Mitiaro natives of Polynesia
Jews living in Yemen
Sweden (where heart disease is less than one-third that of the United States and their fat consumption is almost three times as high!)

Almost all of the cultures and tribes previously listed are sustained by diets high in fat, high in protein and naturally low in carbohydrates.

Fat only becomes a significant factor in the presence of sugar or highly refined carbohydrates. Even then, fat does not cause heart disease, but it can cause you to become overweight when consumed with high amounts of sugar. Obesity is a genuine factor in the development of heart disease and therefore a diet high in both fat and sugar is very unhealthy.

Low Cholesterol Diets
Fail to Reduce Heart Disease

In their desperate attempt to blame cholesterol for the cause of heart disease, the medical industry has been on a fanatic cholesterol-fighting war for decades. To this day, heart disease has not been lowered through any of these efforts. Why do we stick to a concept that we know is scientifically unsound?

To find this answer we must look toward whom might have the most to gain from the perpetuation of such propaganda. The food industry has made a multi-billion dollar industry out of the sale of polyunsaturated fats. Their popularity grew rapidly out of the 'cholesterol scare' and is, to this day, being maintained in order to keep the sales of vegetable oils high. Yet, as we will soon see, vegetable oils actually contribute more to the pathology of coronary thrombosis than any other single dietary factor. Despite these findings, vegetable oils are being promoted by the American Heart Association and they advise us to use them 'for our good health'.

What about margarine and hydrogenated vegetable oils? What liquid vegetable oils do to destroy your arteries, these solidified, synthetically combined fats do ten times faster since all fats must be processed by the liver. When artificially assembled fats are ingested, the liver cannot recognize them and they are subsequently poorly metabolized.

If everything you have been told about fats is wrong, what should you eat? How about taking a lesson from our grandparents and great grandparents? What did they eat? Remember, before the 1900's, heart disease was virtually unknown, yet their diet was higher in fat than ours. They ate lard, butter, and other natural fats. Vegetable oils were not available commercially and margarine had not yet been invented.

It is interesting to note that if you chart the rise in heart disease, it increases at the same rate as the consumption of vegetable oils increased. Should that not be telling us something?

What about eggs? The long-suffering egg has been the staple of human diets around the world for thousands of years. The late Adelle Davis, pioneer nutritionist, often said that the egg was the most perfect food for man. Since cholesterol doesn't cause heart disease, neither does the cholesterol in eggs. Additionally, eggs contain a substance called lecithin, which naturally metabolizes the fats in eggs including the cholesterol.

We will now explore the real cause of heart disease and show you how you can prevent and even reverse the ravages of atherosclerosis, thereby reducing your risk of coronary thrombosis by at least 80 percent.

If Cholesterol is O.K., What's the Problem?

Since science has proven that cholesterol doesn't cause heart disease, what does? Remember the studies conducted in the 1970's at leading medical centers that we mentioned earlier? Let's take a closer look at what they found out:

- Atherosclerosis occurs only in arteries - never in veins
- Atherosclerosis occurs primarily near the junction of two arterial branches and only select arteries are usually involved.
- Cholesterol is the last substance to stick to the artery wall. By the time cholesterol arrives, 90 percent of the damage leading to the disease process has already occurred.

Let's analyze these findings in order to illustrate the real cause, and subsequently, the method for reversing this problem.

The idea that cholesterol doesn't cause heart disease is further supported by the fact that even though the same amount of cholesterol circulates in both the veins and arteries, atherosclerosis never occurs in the veins but only in the arteries. The reason this happens is the answer to the cause of the condition.

When we look at a 'cross section' of a vein, we find that it contains two layers, an inner and outer layer. An inspection of an artery, however, shows us that it has three layers, the inner and outer layer as with veins, but also a middle layer of muscle tissue.

This muscle layer is responsible for ensuring that blood leaving the heart reaches the furthest extremities while maintaining proper blood pressure. Also, under stress, this muscle wall constricts, increasing the pressure of blood and oxygen flowing to all parts of the body. But it is this same muscle wall that allows atherosclerotic plaque to begin to build.

Of all the various types of tissues found in the human body, one of the most susceptible to what we call free radical DNA damage is the muscle cell.

The deoxyribonucleic acid (DNA) of each and every cell in your body carries your genetic code. When the molecular structure of DNA cells is attacked by chemical 'free radicals', they can change, mutate, and multiply out of control.

There are numerous free radicals formed in the body under various conditions, but the specific free radical action that appears to attack arterial muscle tissue comes primarily from the oxidation of polyunsaturated vegetable oils. This would explain the reason why heart disease has risen at roughly the same percentage rate as the consumption of these oils. Furthermore, the heating of vegetable oils can triple the formation of 'free radicals'.

Once the free radical is circulating in the blood stream, it attaches itself to the inside of the artery wall and begins to literally drill a hole into the inner layer of the artery. Once it reaches the middle muscle layer, it attaches itself and begins to alter the structure of the cell. Changes occur in the outer lipoprotein layer of the cells first and, over time, slowly change the structure and genetic code of the entire cell. When this cell eventually dies, as all cells do, it will replace itself not as it was, but as the mutated, altered variety it has become.

One of the characteristics of these mutated muscle cells is that, similar to cancer cells, they multiply at a much more accelerated rate than the healthy cells around them. This creates a thickening of the middle muscle wall of the artery. Over time, this thickening ruptures the inner wall of the artery, creating a bulge.

This concentration of cells causes an increase in the production of cholesterol at that site. The final step in the disease process is what has been called calcification of the artery. Calcium circulating in the blood stream is attracted to the fibrous plaque formed at these damaged arterial sites. The calcium is held to the plaque by an electrical-charge. The addition of this alkaline, rocky calcium further hardens the artery.

This plaque building process continues as the calcium attracts additional material from the bloodstream, including cholesterol, triglycerides, and carotene, all naturally present in healthy people. Again, this attraction is created by a positive / negative electrical process. The calcium is very positive in this divalent form and it draws, like a magnet, various blood lipids. If this process continues unabated, the plaque will grow in size and become thicker and thicker, eventually closing off the blood flow.

It is important to understand that even if the cholesterol levels in the blood stream are normal or low, it will still be attracted to the calcium now lining the arteries in strategic places. This is why we say that cholesterol does not cause this disease and lowering cholesterol will not prevent or stop it!

Let's review the most common causes of free radical formation in the body. You can then begin to avoid them as if your life depended upon it, because it does.

Consumption of Unsaturated Oils.

These oils promote free radical formation, especially if they have been heated. Instead use saturated fats in moderation. For cooking, use only olive oil. This wonderful oil may be used cold, or heated in cooking, with complete safety. Throw all other vegetable oils away!

Cigarette Smoking.

Most cigarette manufacturers add numerous chemicals to the tobacco they use. Tars ingested and smoke inhaled from these chemical laden cigarettes are the problem, not the nicotine. If you smoke cigarettes, quite now, or switch to a chemical free brand (i.e. Nat Sherman or American Spirit).

Ingestion of Toxic Chemicals.

Tens of thousands of toxic substances routinely found in the air, food, water, and our business and home environments are the biggest causes of free radical damage. For example, chlorine, as found in many household and industrial cleaners and our water supplies, produces some of the most dangerous free radicals known.

Radiation Exposure.

Over exposure to the sun, x-rays, microwave ovens, high frequency electronic equipment, etc.

Chronic Health Conditions.

Long term and chronic disease such as arthritis, heart disease and cancer. Even conditions such as constipation, which releases methyl cholanthrene into the blood stream, are a source of free radical formation.

With few exceptions, and with little modification of lifestyle, these factors can be addressed, reduced, or completely avoided. Smoking cigarettes and using vegetable oils other than olive oil are the two greatest factors, something all of us can correct if we truly value our health.

Well-documented information concerning the dangers of cigarette smoking is widely available, so we will not delve into it here. But, because the idea of avoiding vegetable oils is so new and contrary to virtually everything we have ever been taught, let's take a closer look at the clinical evidence and find out what these dangerous oils really do in the body.

As early as 1974, the real dangers of polyunsaturated oils (corn, safflower, peanut, sesame, and others) began to be realized. Studies at that time involved animals and the feeding of various groups of swine. Swine were used because their cardiovascular system is similar to that of humans.

The results of the studies were shocking. Researchers found that, overwhelmingly, the pigs fed a diet of margarine and other hydrogenated fats had the greatest degree of hardening of the arteries. The next greatest group was the one fed a high sugar diet. Conversely, the group fed butter as the main fat had almost no arterial damage at all and the group fed a diet high in eggs had virtually clear arteries altogether!

The tests further showed that it was not just polyunsaturated oils and hydrogenated fats, like margarine, that were to blame, but egg substitutes as well. These products became very popular for a time during the height of the "cholesterol scare". Fortunately, their popularity is declining. Studies done on various animals fed egg substitutes showed severe upset in their blood lipid profiles and these animals all died very prematurely.

Further evidence against the use of polyunsaturated oils comes from studies done on aging and wrinkling of the facial skin. The group of test subjects who consumed high amounts of polyunsaturated oils showed marked clinical signs of premature aging, while looking physically older as well.

Yet another study involved patients who adhered to the American Heart Association's published diet, which suggests a 15 percent intake of polyunsaturated oils. The results showed that they developed a significant increase in uric acid in the blood. Elevated uric acid levels are a risk factor in heart disease and indicate the destruction of cellular nucleoprotein.

The Sugar Connection

While attention has been fixated upon the cholesterol myth regarding heart disease pathology, we have totally overlooked an increasing dietary factor, which contributes to more heart disease than cholesterol ever will.

The over consumption of sugar and sugar-forming foods in the diet may be linked to virtually every chronic degenerative disease process. Outside of the obvious connection between sugar consumption and such diseases and conditions as hypoglycemia, diabetes and obesity, sugar has been linked to arthritis, osteoporosis, and most definitely, to heart disease.

Triglycerides, the largest fat molecules in the blood stream, are formed exclusively from excessive carbohydrates. While these fats are normally stored in the fat cells of our bodies, they can circulate in the blood stream and reach dangerously high levels.

Work done by John Yudkin and others have clearly linked the consumption of sugar with an increase in ischemic heart disease as far back as 1957, yet our focus remains on cholesterol. According to the findings of Yudkin, excess sugar consumption is just as great a risk factor in the progress of coronary heart disease as is the practice of cigarette smoking.

The following graphs illustrate the direct relationship between dietary factors such as an increase in vegetable oil consumption and sugars along with a decrease in egg consumption. All of these problems were caused by the complete misunderstanding of the cause of heart disease. By making these dietary changes we have actually contributed to a dramatic increase in the incidence of this condition.

Sugar and Atherosclerosis:

As this graph clearly illustrates, annual increase in sugar consumption corresponded to a similar increase in the number of deaths from cardiovascular disease.

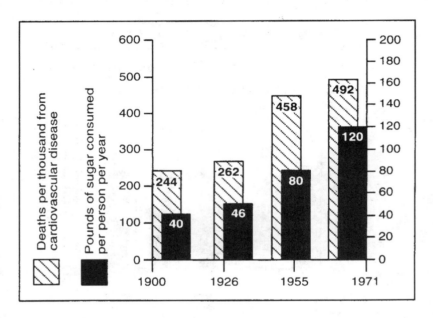

Vegetable Oils vs. Lard and Butter:

These two graphs compare the trend of replacing natural saturated fats, such as, butter and lard, with polyunsaturated vegetable oils. You can see once again that as vegetable oil consumption increased, deaths from heart disease rose almost at the same rate.

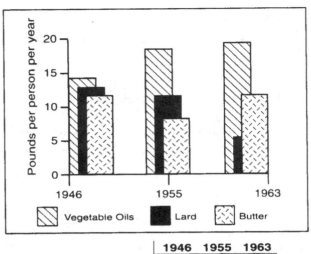

	1946	1955	1963
Total Animal Fat	22.3	19.1	13.3
Total Vegetable Oil	14.4	17.7	19.0

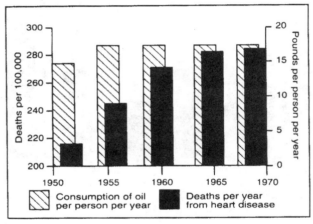

Correlation Between Egg Consumption and Deaths from Heart Disease:

One of the saddest outcomes of the cholesterol scare was the drop in the consumption of eggs. Eggs are the most perfect food for humans. Clinical studies have shown that a diet high in eggs and other quality protein foods can lower cholesterol levels in the blood faster than all the leading drugs combined. You can see by the graph below that as egg consumption decreased, coronary heart disease increased at a corresponding and proportionally inverse rate.

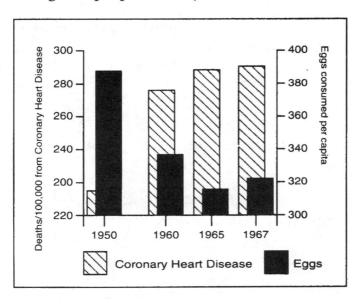

Now that we have made our case concerning what does not cause heart disease, let's take a look at what does.

There are eight major risk factors, which directly lead to atherosclerosis:

Heredity - If heart disease runs in your family you have a much greater chance of developing this condition yourself.

Calorie Imbalance - Consuming the wrong type of fats and oils as well as the over consumption of sugar and sugar forming foods.

High Blood Pressure - This condition damages the arteries and inner workings of the heart muscle, making them more susceptible to free radical damage and increased site cholesterol formation.

Smoking - Cigarette smoking and the chemicals put into most cigarettes make the tars a prime source of free radical formation. Nicotine is not the problem in spite of what we have been told.

Antioxidant Deficiency - These nutrients protect the cells of the body from free radical damage as well as preventing the formation of the oxidative free radical in the first place.

Vitamin E Deficiency - In the absence of adequate vitamin E, plaque formation within the arteries leads to coronary thrombosis.

Lack of Exercise - A sedentary lifestyle further deteriorates an already damaged cardiovascular system.

Stress - I have often said that stress is the cardinal or major cause of all disease and disorder within the body. We find it as a factor in almost every condition, and here it is again! Stress can wreak havoc with the cardiovascular system through over stimulation of the adrenal glands. This leads to excess adrenaline in the bloodstream, which constricts arteries and accelerates free radical proliferation.

By incorporating simple routines into our lives, many of these risk factors may be eliminated or greatly reduced. Of greatest benefit is taking supplements containing the Full Spectrum of nutrients. An emphasis should be placed on antioxidants and specialized nutrient combinations designed to help reverse the plaque forming process (A list of which follows). A little exercise and reducing or managing stress will further improve your odds of beating atherolsclerosis.

What About Cholesterol-Lowering Drugs?

Drugs that have been designed to lower blood levels of specific lipids such as cholesterol and triglycerides do not have any effect on preventing heart disease, nor have they ever demonstrated a benefit in preventing a recurrent heart attack. This we are told by the United States Department of Health, Education and Welfare through a report from the National Heart, Lung, and Blood Institute's Coronary Drug Project.

Drugs that block the absorption of cholesterol from foods can be very dangerous since they would prevent the absorption of fat-soluble vitamins, essential fatty acids and other fat-like nutrients.

It is important to remember that the body needs fats for proper metabolism and life function. The fanatic elimination of fats from the diet, combined with drugs that further prevent fat absorption, will lead to a variety of health conditions as time progresses.

Heart Disease Prevention & Management Program

Probably one of the most important nutrients in the prevention of heart disease, from its many causes, is vitamin E. For over 50 years, Drs. Wilfrid and Evan Shute have been achieving great results in the prevention of cardiac disease and the treatment of cardiac patients. Their program revolves around the use of vitamin E. After over 50,000 or more patients, they believe that vitamin E is essential in any cardiac program.

Vitamin E provides multi-functional benefits. Tocopherols, the active compounds found in vitamin E, provide several important benefits to the cardiovascular system.

Tocopherol, an anti-clotting agent, prevents blood clots throughout the entire cardiovascular tree. It helps dissolve existing blood clots and increases the blood's supply of oxygen. Tocopherol improves the efficiency of the heart, thereby reducing the demand for available oxygen. It also prevents scarring of the heart muscle after a heart attack and it accelerates the healing process. In addition, Tocopherol is a vasodilator and strengthens capillary permeability.

Vitamin E has also been shown to be beneficial in the treatment of angina. In a clinical study reported in the New England Journal of Medicine, patients given 400 IU of Tocopherol, four times per day, were able to reduce their need for nitroglycerin significantly.

Other Anti-Oxidant Nutrients

Since the prevention of free radical formation by oxidation is essential to our goal, the anti-oxidant nutrients must be a part of our program.

In addition to vitamin E, other nutrients can also offer this much-needed protection.

Vitamin C, an antioxidant, provides protection against free radical substances by keeping them in solution, thereby allowing the kidneys to better eliminate poisons. Vitamin C stimulates the production of the enzyme lipoprotein lipase (LPL), which acts as a cleansing agent against the artery wall. Lastly, vitamin C is essential in our over-all program, as it is a co-factor with several other ingredients in the protocol.

The B-Complex nutrients, Vitamins B1, B2, Niacin, Pantothenic Acid, B6, and PABA, are collectively synergistic and provide antioxidant benefits in their own right. They all work hard to prevent the formation of free radicals within the body.

The mineral selenium is one of the most powerful antioxidants known. It is estimated that it provides from 200 to 500 times more antioxidant benefits than even vitamin E. both vitamin E and selenium prevent free radical damage to tissues.

The Amazing Amino Acids

Recent research into the science of applying isolated amino acids to specific disease conditions continues to prove both beneficial and rewarding. Heart disease and the processes by which it develops are no different.

One of the most well known amino acids relating to the cardiovascular system is L-Carnitine. This amino acid helps the body to utilize fats at virtually every level. L-Carnitine has been used, clinically, in both the prevention and treatment of heart disease and in other cardiac related conditions. L-Carnitine is essential in the management of congestive heart failure because it strengthens the stroke or beat of the heart and it naturally lowers or regulates blood fats as well. One note of caution: Carnitine can be purchased in two forms L and dl. DO NOT USE THE dl FORM! Because the dl form of Carnitine is less than one/tenth the cost, most companies elect to use this form. The bottom line is that only the L form has any effect upon your heart.

Another amino acid, much less known than L-Carnitine, is called Cysteine Hydrochloride. This wonderful amino acid protects against damages caused by radiation of all types by actually terminating the free radicals through ionizing the radiation. Further, Cysteine hydrochloride is a powerful chelating agent, attaching itself to a variety of minerals and carrying them out of the body via the urine.

Other Essential Co-Factor Nutrients

In addition to the amino acids and antioxidants, there are several other nutrients and nutrient co-factors which have been shown to be of benefit in both the prevention and treatment of heart disease.

Vitamin A must be both considered and included in any program for heart disease and cardiovascular health. This vitamin protects the mucosal linings, your body's first line of defense against invading microbes. It also increases the size of the thymus gland, the center of your immune system, allowing for greater antibody production. Lastly, vitamin A works with selenium, and together they are much more powerful than either one alone.

Choline and inositol are two B-Complex factors and together with another amino acid, methionine, they form a group of nutrients call lipotropics. Lipotropics are responsible for metabolizing fats in the liver. If you have elevated cholesterol to an excess, it is a liver problem not necessarily a dietary imbalance. The lipotropic group will improve liver function and lower blood lipid levels naturally without the side effects of many of the cholesterol lowering drugs. Further, methionine is needed by the body for its powerful detoxification properties.

Another very effective free radical inhibitor is the mineral zinc. Vitamin A cannot function in the body without zinc so they must be present simultaneously in order to be effective.

The late J.I. Rodale, a pioneer in the modern nutrition revolution and a heart patient himself, often said that the greatest heart tonic in the world was Hawthorne Berry. He was so impressed with the ability of Hawthorne Berry to improve cardiovascular health that he wrote an entire book on the herb.

Gingko Biloba and *Dimethyl Glycine* are two compounds which have the ability to increase the oxygen content of body tissues. The oxygenating benefits of a good exercise program are worthless if the cells of the body cannot absorb the oxygen from the blood stream. Gingko Biloba and Dimethyl Glycine dramatically increase the cell's ability to assimilate oxygen.

Co-Enzyme Q10 is another nutrient that we believe is vital to cardiovascular health. CoQ10 actually reduces angina and improves cardiac function. Heart patients taking CoQ10 consistently have better exercise tolerance than those who do not.

For those who already have heart disease, increasing available oxygen to the cells of the body is critical. Along with some of the nutrients we already mentioned, germanium, a rare trace mineral, increases the oxygen of each cell, thereby decreasing oxygen deficit symptoms such as angina.

Chondroitin sulphate, a nutrient known for its benefit to the connective tissues of the body and therefore widely used in the management of arthritis-like problems, is also beneficial to the heart. Chondroitin sulphate has natural anti-coagulant and anti-thrombogenic properties, which prevents blood fat clumping, while being a natural anti-clotting agent.

Other Nutrient Factors To Consider

In addition to adding nutrients for their cardiac benefits, we must consider one of the most important factors in the progression of atherosclerosis, namely calcium buildup on the artery walls. One of the most effective ways of assisting the body in the removal of this unwanted form of calcium is to increase the acidity of the body and to, temporarily, reduce the available calcium. Under this condition, the body is able to take the calcium off the artery wall and put it back into solution in the blood stream. Once the calcium has been 'chelated' off the inner artery wall, the cholesterol and other blood lipids can no longer adhere to the site. Since copper and manganese are necessary for the absorption of calcium they too must be included.

Because the immune system of the body is important in the management of abnormal cell formation, and since the explosive multiplication of cells is at the root of the atherosclerosis problem, supporting the immune system is important. Two ways in which we can further stimulate the immune function naturally is through the use of extracts of spleen and thymus nucleoprotein.

Lastly we must not forget the role that fatty acids, especially the omega-3 group, play in maintaining good blood chemistry. Also, fatty acids from marine lipids act to prevent blood fats from sticking together to form clots.

It may easily be seen that while the science of nutrition can offer many things to help prevent and manage modern society's most deadly killer, the program can be a bit overwhelming. Because of the many factors that both directly and indirectly affect cardiovascular health and well-being, the list of nutrients and nutrient co-factors is rather complex.

If you were to go out and try to purchase all of the nutrients we have discussed it would be challenging, time consuming, and costly. In addition, ratios are extremely important in any program wherein we hope to create a 'chelating' environment. Too much or too little of certain nutrients can dramatically reduce the effectiveness of this program. For this reason we have assembled a Master Protocol which reflects what we believe to be the ideal diet and nutrient combination in the management and promotion of cardiovascular health.

Dietary Protocol for Cardiovascular Support

The following steps should be taken to modify your dietary habits as soon as possible.

1. Eliminate ALL polyunsaturated vegetable oils from your diet. This includes restaurant foods cooked in these refined oils.

2. Eliminate the use of all 'plastic' fats such as margarine, hydrogenated oils and other synthetic products, which are rapidly becoming popular.

3. Limit the calories from fat to no more than 25 or 30 percent unless you are very active.

4. Use olive oil for both cold and hot food applications/preparations.

5. Eat fruits and vegetables as close to their raw, natural state as possible.

6. Ensure that you get at least 60 grams of high quality protein every day.

7. Avoid the over-consumption of processed protein foods such as cold meats, cheeses and other foods containing nitrates.

8. Reduce the amount of refined carbohydrates and sugars in the diet.

Lastly, while not dietary in nature, begin a regular exercise program according to your fitness level and physical condition. If you have not exercised for some time, consult a professional for advice regarding what type of exercise would be appropriate for your situation.

Nutrient Protocol for Cardiovascular Support

Vitamin A (beta carotene) 15,000 IU
Vitamin D (Fish Liver Oil) ...... 240 IU
Vitamin E (d-Alpha Tocopherol) . 360 IU
Vitamin C (Calcium Ascorbate) 2,000 mg
Vitamin B1 .... 100 mg
Vitamin B2 .... 30 mg
Vitamin B6 .... 90 mg
Niacin .... 60 mg
Pantothenic Acid .... 100 mg
Vitamin B12 .... 150 mcg
Folic Acid .... 240 mcg
Biotin .... 60 mcg
Choline .... 450 mg
Inositol .... 60 mg
Para Amino Benzoic Acid..... 90 mg
Calcium .... 240 mg
Magnesium .... 300 mg
Iodine .... 135 mcg
Iron .... 4.5 mg
Copper .... 150 mcg
Zinc .... 15 mg
Potassium .... 240 mg
Manganese .... 6 mg
Chromium........................ 120 mcg
Selenium .... 120 mcg

Cysteine HCL	450 mg
dl-Methionine	120 mg
Gingko Biloba	30 mg
L-Carnitine	50 mg
Bilberry	25 mg
Hawthorne Berry	15 mg
Dimethyl Glycine	50 mg
Thymus Nucleoprotein	50 mg
EPA/DHA (Essential Fatty Acids)	50 mg
Co-Enzyme Q-10	2 mg
Chondroitin Sulfate	50 mg

The exact combination, outlined in the preceding formulation, has been tested and used with excellent results since 1979. While it represents what we have found to be an optimal preventive dosage, those suffering from more acute cardiovascular conditions can achieve accelerated benefits if they increase the dosage by 50% during the first 90 days of use.

Conclusion

As with all chronic degenerative diseases, heart disease can be prevented. Once it has developed, the condition still may be greatly improved. But we must take action. Conventional medicine has been approaching these conditions in a reactive manner. They fail to see the cause of the problem, and therefore do not understand the implications involved in the prevention, management, or reversal of this deadly disease.

Every degenerative disease, without exception, is the result of an imbalance of the body's internal biochemistry. Often years, or even decades, pass before symptoms exhibit themselves and we become aware of the problem. Through providing the raw materials needed by the body for health, and through eliminating the artificial and excessive factors provided by a modern junk food diet, we can reverse the tide towards degenerative disease. We can then focus on a course of action which will enable us to maintain or regain optimal health.

We will now turn our attention to another chronic disease, which has become epidemic word wide, diabetes. If you suffer from diabetes and are also concerned about your heart health, there is a definite link between the two. Those with diabetes have a much greater chance of developing many forms of cardiovascular disease. For optimal wellness, it is necessary to address both problems, if they exist.

Chapter 6
Diabetes: The Fastest Growing Epidemic Worldwide

If someone were to ask you what the most epidemic disease of the so-called 'civilized' world was, what would be your answer? You might say cancer. Cancer is certainly the most feared of modern-day diseases. You might choose heart disease. This condition still kills more people around the world than any other single cause. Yet, neither of these conditions is the most epidemic. When we refer to an epidemic, we mean a disease or condition which is on the rapid rise and is spreading with unusual speed.

Adult onset diabetes or Type II non-insulin dependent diabetes is the epidemic of the twentieth century. It is rising in numbers faster than all other chronic degenerative diseases combined and promises to be an even greater problem in this new century ahead.

Diabetes is so common that almost everyone knows someone who has the disease. According to the National Institutes of Health, there are about 12 million diagnosed diabetics in America and it is estimated that there are at least that many more undiagnosed cases. According to 1997 statistics from the Centers for Disease Control and Prevention's diabetes division, 798,000 new cases are diagnosed every year. That amounts to one new case being diagnosed every 30 seconds! To make matters worse, each year tens of thousands of diabetic Americans lose their eyesight, compromise their circulation, suffer irreversible heart damage, and/or require the amputation of a lower limb. Each year, many of these people die prematurely due to diabetes.

Of all these cases of diabetes, ninety percent of them are the adult-onset, Type II variety. Only ten percent are the genetically induced Type I juvenile-onset version.

The saddest part about these statistics is the fact that adult-onset, Type II diabetes, is completely controllable and very often reversible WITHOUT the need for dangerous drugs, or worse yet, the misuse of insulin.

Type II diabetes is, almost exclusively, caused by dietary abuse. It steals a long and healthy life from millions and millions of people. We will examine the cause, progression, and reversal methods of this needless, chronic disease.

Even more common in occurrence is hypoglycemia, or low blood sugar. It is frequently the precursor to adult-onset Type II diabetes. If left unchecked, hypoglycemia can devastate the lives of its victims, while providing them with better than a nine to one chance of progressing to diabetes later in life. This condition, like diabetes, is completely dietary induced and can be controlled. Let's find out how.

Hypoglycemia: The Undiagnosed Disorder

For many decades, hypoglycemia was both shunned and denied by the mainstream medical profession. Millions of people went to their physicians with a long list of debilitating symptoms, only to be told that their symptoms were psychological in nature. These patients were also advised to seek psychiatric help if their symptoms persisted. This 'mis-diagnosis' only led these people to further and further desperation. Many of them even resorted to such drastic measures as suicide. This, in turn, further fueled the argument that these people were suffering from a mental disorder.

Today, we know that hypoglycemia or low blood sugar is both real and very common. It is a chronic condition of the twentieth century. As is the case with many chronic illnesses, hypoglycemia was virtually unknown at the turn of the last century. This means that these conditions have escalated to epidemic proportions in less than 5 generations! Recent findings portray how severe the problem is. In October 1997, federal officials stated that the number of people in the USA diagnosed with diabetes had increased sixfold. The numbers had jumped from 1.6 million in 1958 to 10 million in 1997. The reason, in part, was due to Americans being too fat.

Whenever we see such an incredible rise in a non-contagious disease condition, we cannot help but look towards our environment and lifestyle for answers. We know that one of the greatest and most direct factors influencing human biochemistry is food consumption.

At the turn of the last century, the average person consumed 10 to 15 pounds of sugar per year. Today, we all consume at least our own body weight in sugars every single year! Further, the refining of whole wheat into white flour has produced a substance that is, chemically, one small step away from sugar. This means that eating foods made from white flour contributes to the overall consumption of sugars. The internal biochemistry of the body must regularly contend with this fact.

After months or years of this continual onslaught against normal chemistry, the body loses the ability to regulate sugars. This produces rapid fluctuations in the glucose levels in the bloodstream.

Low blood glucose levels are an indication of hypoglycemia and high blood glucose levels are an indication of diabetes. Two seemingly opposite problems, but with the same basic cause, namely excess sugar and sugar-forming foods in the diet.

While there can be several causes for clinical hypoglycemia, such as excess alcohol consumption, stress, or the use of certain prescription drugs, ninety-nine percent is the result of dietary abuse.

The symptoms of hypoglycemia are many and can come and go with great regularity. This often makes the disorder difficult to diagnose. The only scientific way to determine clinical hypoglycemia is through the six- hour glucose tolerance test (anything less than six-hours is non-conclusive).

The number and frequency of certain symptoms is also a valid determining factor for the presence of hypoglycemia. Let's look at these many symptoms, keeping in mind that you may experience more than one of these symptoms at the same time. They may come and go, only to return again. If you experience any significant number of these symptoms on a some-what regular basis, you can be fairly certain that you have hypoglycemia, and if left unchecked, will likely progress to diabetes.

Anxiety
Breathing (shallow and rapid)
Chill (cold and clammy)
Emotional Outbursts
Fatigue or Tiredness
Headache
Hot Flashes
Insomnia
Irritability
Mental Confusion
Nausea
Nervousness
Nightmares

Obesity (overweight by more
than 25 pounds)
Physical Coordination (reduced)
Pulse Rate (elevated)
Restlessness
Sleep Disturbances (insomnia, night
sweats, sudden awakening)
Tinnitus (ringing in the ears)
Tingling Sensation (in the fingers,
toes, or tongue)
Vision problems (blurred or double)
Weakness

If you experience eight or more of these symptoms on a regular basis, and other possible causes have been ruled out, you can consider yourself a hypoglycemic.

There are two types of hypoglycemia. The most common form occurs along with excess bodyweight. The second, more obscure form, produces normal or likely an underweight condition. The cause of both is the same, namely excess insulin in the bloodstream, but the manner in which we manage the conditions differs slightly (see the management protocols for both Type I and Type II hypoglycemia later in this chapter).

Medically, the cause of hypoglycemia, adult-onset diabetes and most obesity, is called hyperinsulinemia, or excess insulin.

In the hypoglycemic patient, the pancreas produces excess insulin. This drives the blood sugar level down below an optimal level. This dip in blood sugar levels, over prolonged periods of time, produces the many side effects and symptoms previously listed.

Typically, when we feel weak and flushed from loss of blood sugar, our first reaction is to eat some more sugar. When we do this, the blood glucose once again rises rapidly, stimulating another insulin response, which in turn lowers blood sugar below normal again. This produces the yo-yo effect of "highs and lows" so common with hypoglycemic individuals.

There are three phases of what we call carbohydrate intolerance. Each level is progressively worse than the one before it and the side effects also become more severe. Let's take a closer look.

1. **Carbohydrate Intolerance:** This condition produces a craving for starches and sugary foods. Frequently, the subsequent consumption of starches contributes to obesity through excess insulin converting most carbohydrates to triglycerides and storing them as body fat. These individuals have a better than 10 to one chance of progressing to phase two, hypoglycemia.

2. **Hypoglycemia:** As "carbohydrate intolerant" individuals continue to consume excess sugars and starches, periods of low

blood sugar levels become more and more frequent. The symptoms previously listed begin to appear. The hypoglycemic individual has an eight to one chance of progressing to phase three, diabetes.

3. **Diabetes:** This dreaded chronic degenerative disease is the final outcome for those traveling along this pathway.

The powerful hormone behind this process is called insulin and an understanding of both what it is and what triggers its excess production is essential.

What is Insulin?

In order to more clearly understand carbohydrate intolerance, hypoglycemia, and diabetes, it is essential to understand their cause. Each is caused by an excess of the hormone "insulin". Produced by the pancreas, insulin circulates in the blood.

Insulin is the glucose-regulating hormone. In healthy individuals, it is produced on an as-needed basis according to the levels of glucose present in the blood.

Many people are of the erroneous thought that insulin burns up excess glucose. It does not! Insulin serves to transport excess glucose to the body's various storage sites.

The first and normal site for glucose storage is in the liver and muscles. Insulin converts the blood glucose into a substance called glycogen, which is 'stored sugar'. This is then transported to the liver and muscles. This is unfortunate for those following the 'sugar-filled' Standard American Diet (SAD), because the body's ability to store glycogen is very limited.

Once all of the body's storage sites for glycogen are full, insulin further converts blood glucose into another substance called triglycerides and these are then carried by insulin to the fat cells of the body. This is why most hypoglycemics, and virtually all Type II diabetics, are overweight.

In order to control hypoglycemia, Type II diabetes, and most obesity, we must control the amount of insulin present in the bloodstream. Currently, there are no drugs that are able to reduce or limit the production of insulin. It can only be accomplished by avoiding the foods which cause an 'insulin response', the production of insulin by the body.

All sugar and sugar forming foods (carbohydrates) eventually break down into glucose. The key is the speed with which this breakdown occurs. The faster the conversion, the more insulin is secreted into the bloodstream, setting the stage for the insulin disorders of obesity, hypoglycemia and diabetes.

Our body needs a certain amount of glucose, but far less than the average junk food diet provides. Through this constant excess, insulin is not only over produced but the receptor sites for that insulin become de-sensitized, requiring more and more insulin to do the job. (See the next section on diabetes)

Unfortunately, this cycle of insulin response and production can develop into a terrible downward spiral. As more and more insulin is produced from excess sugars in the diet, more and more of it is converted to triglycerides and stored in the fat cells. As the fat cells increase, the body becomes increasingly overweight. As the body weight rises, insulin becomes less and less effective, requiring the body to produce higher and higher amounts, which in turn cause a greater and greater weight gain, which starts the cycle all over again.

The Importance of Weight Control

After the first few weeks of infancy have passed, we have all the fat cells we will. You cannot make anymore. The fat cell, however, has the ability to continue to increase in size depending upon how much stored sugar, or triglyceride, it must hold. As the fat cells become larger and larger, their responsiveness to insulin decreases, causing the need for ever higher amounts of insulin in order to remove excess sugars from the bloodstream. Since it is the excess insulin that causes obesity, hypoglycemia, and diabetes, controlling and normalizing body weight is essential in the regulation of the insulin/glucose cycle.

For those persons who are overweight and also have either hypoglycemia or diabetes, a reduction in bodyweight frequently reduces symptoms. In some individuals, a reduction in body weight eliminates the symptoms completely without any other protocol.

These individuals respond extremely well to a controlled carbohydrate diet, which counts and limits the amount of sugar-forming foods eaten each day. With a reduction in available carbohydrates, insulin production is greatly reduced. With the normalizing of insulin levels, excess bodyweight is slowly removed. Through reducing the bodyweight and the insulin production, hypoglycemia and diabetes are easily controlled with the help of a few assisting co-factors (see protocols latter in this chapter).

There are many effective exercise programs, which will simultaneously help accelerate fat loss and help the body to use insulin more effectively.

When we exercise, several physiological benefits occur. Muscles need energy to perform. When we exercise, we increase the need for fuel for the muscles. That fuel is glucose; therefore, exercise increases the uptake of glucose by the muscle cells. This in turn naturally reduces blood glucose levels. This means that the body needs less insulin to regulate blood sugar, reducing the peaks and valleys so common in all these blood sugar disorders.

Diabetes:
The Final Insult of Excess Insulin

As discussed previously, very few people are born with diabetes. Those that are, are called juvenile-onset, or Type I diabetics, and they constitute only about ten percent of the total number of diabetes cases worldwide.

The remaining cases of diabetes, which has reached epidemic proportions, are the result of continual dietary abuse over years or even decades of time. Almost all adult-onset diabetics were first hypoglycemic. But since that condition went undiagnosed and untreated, they progressed ever onward to the final phase of insulin-induced disorders, namely, diabetes.

Clinically, diabetes is *hyper*glycemia, or excess blood sugar. In the adult-onset Type II diabetic, hyperglycemia is almost always caused by a defect in the insulin receptor sites, not by lack of insulin.

Years and years of continual dietary abuse created a situation in which there was excess sugar in the body. Insulin was then forced to convert that sugar into triglycerides and store those molecules within the fat cell. In order to accomplish this, insulin must attach itself to "insulin receptor sites" on specific cells of the body. Through years or decades of continual dietary abuse involving excess sugar consumption, these receptor sites become de-sensitized. More and more insulin is then required to remove the excess sugar.

This is why most all Type II diabetics have normal or even higher than normal levels of insulin in their bloodstream. Treating these individuals with drugs that increase insulin production, or treating them with insulin itself (by injection), only serves to make the disease ultimately worse.

Type II diabetics need to reduce the amounts of sugar and sugar-forming foods in their diets. This will take the demand off of the insulin receptor sites, which constantly have to convert and store this excess sugar. This will reduce the presence of insulin in the blood stream, thereby reducing the symptoms of diabetes and the other related insulin disorders.

Excess sugar, or glucose, in the blood is one of the body's true emergencies and it will attempt to lower that blood sugar by almost any means. Individuals with constant high blood sugars levels have a much greater chance of developing a variety of other chronic degenerative diseases and do so much earlier in their lives. Osteoporosis, poor skin condition, inflammation of the joints (arthritis), poor circulation, amputations, and heart disease are just some of the side effects that occur much more frequently when the body's balance of blood sugar and insulin goes astray.

It is important to remember that Type II diabetes develops slowly over the years. This is one of the reasons why this disease is so insidious. Often, by the time the disease has been diagnosed, the patient has already suffered considerable damage to nerves, blood vessels, the heart, the eyes and even the brain.

I have often called Type II diabetes the non-contagious leprosy of the 20th century. Diabetes eats away at multiple organ and tissue systems. Slowly and steadily, inch by inch, destroying the quality of life for the sufferer.

The symptoms of diabetes are often very subtle in nature and can begin so slightly that we hardly even notice their presence.

Common Initial Warning Signs of Type II Diabetes:

Excessive thirst
Frequent urination
Wounds which heal slowly
Fatigue and excessive tiredness,
    especially after eating
A breath which smells like 'acid'
An increase in infections
Abnormal weight loss
    without an obvious cause
Loss of libido (sexual desire)

While there are certainly other signs of this disease, if you have even one of these on a regular basis, you should have your blood sugar levels tested. You can do this quite accurately by obtaining any one of a variety of glucose test strips, which are available without a prescription, at any pharmacy. If the test strips show any deviation from normal, you should have a blood test to determine a more accurate blood sugar level.

Factors that Worsen Diabetes

In addition to the obvious dietary factor of excess sugars, which we have been discussing, there are other situations, both environmentally and chemically, which can make diabetes worse.

I have often said that stress is the cardinal cause of

all illness and certainly it plays a direct role in the process of diabetes. During periods of stress, it is not uncommon for a diabetic to observe sudden rises in blood sugar. This phenomenon can occur even if the stress was brief but severe. Life changing events, such as the loss of a job, spouse or relative, can produce such stress as to cause the onset of diabetes in someone who has not yet even been diagnosed with the illness.

For this reason, any program that wishes to address the complete needs of the diabetic should include nutritional support for the nervous system as well as support for glucose metabolism.

Other common circumstances which can adversely affect insulin and subsequently insulin-induced disorders include anesthesia, anti-inflammatory drug abuse, and infections in the body. Under each of these circumstances, a person prone to insulin-induced diseases should pay particular attention to their blood sugar levels and have them checked more frequently than at other times.

Summary of Insulin-Induced Disorders

It can now clearly be seen that excess insulin in the body causes numerous health challenges at varying levels. Let's summarize the levels of what we call carbohydrate intolerance, or hyperinsulinemia, in their progressive order of severity.

Carbohydrate Intolerance. As the first level of insulin resistance, carbohydrate intolerance produces excess body weight. In fact, this is the primary cause of at least seventy-five percent of all obesity! At this stage, the individuals affected may experience some fluctuation in blood sugar but likely those symptoms will be few and far between. Fatigue, cravings for sugars and poor appetite are the likely symptoms of this phase.

Hypoglycemia. Low blood sugar levels, caused by the body's inability to regulate insulin production, is the second phase of carbohydrate intolerance. These individuals begin to experience some or many of the symptoms listed earlier in our discussion of hypoglycemia.

There are two types of chemistry involved in low blood sugar. First there is the hypoglycemic with obesity. This is the most common form and, fortunately, the easiest to   control.

The second form of hypoglycemia produces an underweight condition. These individuals must follow a modified program which we will outline shortly.

Diabetes. The final insult to the human chemistry in the process of insulin excess is diabetes. There are also two forms of this condition as well. Firstly, there is juvenile-onset, or Type I diabetes. This is genetically driven and virtually all these individuals will be insulin-dependent for their entire lives. This is the most difficult form of diabetes to manage, but fortunately, it accounts for only about ten percent of all diabetes cases. Even with the delicate manner in which it must be handled, Type I diabetics can still benefit immeasurably from the following program.

The second form of diabetes is, of course, adult-onset, or Type II diabetes. It is this form, which occurs usually after the age of 30, that makes up the epidemic numbers of diabetes cases we are seeing every year. These individuals do not suffer from a lack of insulin but rather have too much insulin, producing a host of side effects. It is the type II diabetic for which this program has had the greatest life-saving effect. This condition is one hundred percent dietary induced and therefore, can be reversed through proper diet and dietary supplement programs such as the program we will be outlining a little later.

No matter what stage of this disease process you may find yourself in, you can greatly improve or even reverse your condition if you make the following program a part of your life.

What Do You Do Now?

Let's assume you have an insulin-induced disorder such as obesity, hypoglycemia, or Type II diabetes. Where do you go from here? With a few small modifications, the management of all these conditions is basically the same. We will do so with a combination of dietary restrictions and specific dietary supplementation. The following section will explain the full protocol of diet and supplementation necessary for the control or reversal of your hypoglycemia or diabetes. The protocol will work only if you follow it exactly.

Any variation from this basic program will produce less than optimal results. We will note accordingly any specific factors applying to certain conditions. Otherwise, all participants having any of the insulin-induced disorders we have discussed will benefit from the same program.

Protocol for Managing and Reversing Hypoglycemia & Diabetes

Dietary Factors:

As with most chronic degenerative diseases, diet plays a significant role in the development and subsequent reversal or management of hypoglycemia and diabetes.

If we are ever to master these conditions, it will be essential to regulate the amount of sugar and sugar-forming foods in the diet. This is best accomplished by not counting calories but rather by counting carbohydrates. Since all carbohydrates eventually turn into blood glucose, the amount and type of carbohydrates consumed plays a direct effect upon the levels of blood sugar and subsequently the amount of insulin secreted into the bloodstream.

There are several excellent books which cover carbohydrate restricted diets in detail. If you are also overweight, you may wish to choose one that also places emphasis upon weight management as well.

A good guideline for determining the amount of sugars and refined carbohydrates often hidden in common foods may be found in the book called *Calories and Carbohydrates* by Barbara Kraus. This book is published by Signet Paperback Books, and the current twelfth revised edition is available in most bookstores for $5.99 US.

I strongly recommend that anyone wishing to gain control over the amount of sugars and sugar-forming foods in their diet obtain this handy book. It even lists favorite fast food restaurant items, giving the calorie and carbohydrate count for each.

In your case, you will want to pay attention only to the carbohydrate count of each food, because, for practical purposes, you will not be concerned with calories.

It is essential that you begin the program by reducing your total daily carbohydrate intake to less than 40 grams. (Note: an exception for underweight Type II hypoglycemic appears below)

As your available carbohydrates begin to fall, if you are a hypoglycemic, you will experience cravings for sweets, which can sometimes be almost overwhelming. I know that this will be a difficult time but you must persevere. It will only last a few days, and once the cycle of sugar has been broken, the intense cravings will subside. Lingering cravings for sugars will be controlled by specific dietary supplements, which we will discuss later in the program.

If you are a diabetic, your blood sugar levels will very likely fall steadily as you continue to restrict your carbohydrate intake. For this reason, if you are taking medications, and especially if you are taking insulin, you will need to monitor your blood glucose levels regularly. In the beginning, testing 4 to 6 times per day is not excessive.

As your blood sugar falls, if you are taking medications, you doctor will want to slowly and correctly begin to reduce the amount of medication you are taking since you will not be needing it in the quantities you were before.

If you add an exercise program to the dietary program, you will achieve results much faster, but you will also need to test your blood sugar more often since it will likely fall even faster.

As your blood sugar normalizes over the next few weeks, you can gradually increase the number of carbohydrates in the diet. Eventually you will get to the point where, if you are a hypoglycemic, your symptoms will begin to return. If you are a diabetic, your blood sugar will once again begin to rise. This is called the carbohydrate threshold. It is usually different for each person, so you will have to establish what that number of carbohydrate grams would be for you, each day.

Once you know your threshold for carbohydrate intake, you must simply confine your daily consumption of carbohydrates to an amount approximately 20 percent below that figure. This will enable you to keep your symptoms and/or blood sugar levels in check.

Special Note for Underweight Hypoglycemics: If you have hypoglycemia and are of normal weight, or especially if you are underweight, you cannot totally restrict your carbohydrate intake. To do so would produce even greater weight loss and subsequent fatigue.

You need to count carbohydrates, but you will have to keep the level above one which will produce further weight loss. To make this calculation, determine your 'carbohydrate threshold' by using the preceding method. Once you begin reducing your total carbohydrate intake, at some point you will start loosing weight. Then, increase your carbohydrate consumption to 10 percent above the level which produces the weight loss.

In order to keep your weight up, but still produce a minimal insulin response, you must learn how to choose carbohydrate foods wisely. The faster carbohydrates break down into simple sugars, the quicker and greater the insulin response. For this reason, you must choose complex carbohydrate foods, which take several hours to slowly break down into simple sugars. Examples would be whole grains (such as black wild rice), breads that are truly whole grain, legumes, and certain vegetables.

Foods you need to avoid are those containing sugar, honey, molasses, corn syrup or any other forms of simple sugars. Additionally, you must avoid highly refined starches such as anything made with refined white flour, refined grains and pastas as well as over-cooked root vegetables such as potatoes. All of these foods will convert to glucose too rapidly causing an insulin response, throwing you into a state of low blood sugar.

As I said earlier, there are sugars hidden in virtually everything that you eat. You may not think that the foods you eat contain any sugar or sugar-forming ingredients, but think again. The following are examples of commonly consumed foods and their sugar content.

Food	Sugar content in Teaspoonfuls
Soda Pop (12 oz)	3-12
All Cakes & Cookies (4 oz serving)	5-10
Candies (1 piece)	1-5
Canned Fruits (1 cup)	2-4
Ice Cream (3 oz)	3-5
Malted Milk Shake	10-16
Jams & Jellies (1 oz)	1-6

You can see how it adds up. Sugars are hidden in other foods as well, including breakfast cereals, breads, rolls, and anything made from refined white flour.

Speaking of breakfast cereals, the leading cereals are between eight and fifty-two percent pure sugar! No wonder our children are hyperactive!

(For further information on attention deficits and hyperactivity in children refer to The Institute's publication entitled *Drug Free Answers to Correcting Learning Disabilities*)

I will be the first to tell you that it is difficult to

abstain from the very foods you not only crave, but are actually addicted to; carbohydrate sensitivity is a genuine addiction. Instead of leaving you to your own frustrations, I will tell you about several specific nutrients and nutrient co-factors which will both help you win your battle with sugar addiction and make your body function more effectively as you pursue your program of glucose and insulin management. These nutrients are outlined in the following section along with specific protocols for their use.

Do I Have To Do It All Alone?
Dietary Supplementation for Hypoglycemia & Diabetes.

For the person afflicted with insulin-related disorders, one nutrient, a mineral, offers unparalleled promise and is a pivotal element of support. That mineral is chromium. Yet, chromium alone is far less effective than when properly combined with other nutrient cofactors which provide a Full Spectrum approach to the problem. Together, they contribute a synergistic and infinitely greater assurance of an appropriate solution.

As with any chronic degenerative disease, those suffering from hypoglycemia or diabetes need more of certain nutrients, not less. However, we cannot provide mega-doses of isolated nutrients without first ensuring that all of the nutrients, needed by the body on a daily basis, are being provided in the right ratios.

To simply and effectively ensure that these needs are met, we use a liquid multiple vitamin, mineral, amino acid, phytonutrient formula. It provides all of the 100+ nutrients needed daily for optimal health. The formula provides a synergistic combination of nutrients, in their correct natural ratios, insuring that they are bio-available. This means they can be easily digested, absorbed, and assimilated by the body.

Components of an Ideal Full Spectrum Nutrition Formula

8 - 12 Essential Amino Acids
3 Fatty Acids
16 Vitamins
75 + major, trace and micro trace minerals
Phytonutrients from fruits and vegetables

Once this base line nutrition has been met, we can proceed with the aggressive supplementing of specific nutrients and nutrient groups. This will assist the body in re-balancing the relationship between blood sugar and insulin. Such a protocol will not only provide the specific nutrients necessary for proper glucose regulation, but will go far in reducing the cravings for sugars and sugar-forming foods so common in individuals with these disorders.

Nutrient Support for Glucose/Insulin Regulation

In addition to chromium, the mineral vanadium and the amino acid, aspartic acid, have been shown to be very helpful in assisting the body in the regulation of glucose and insulin. Following are the ratios of these nutrients which we have used with tremendous success at The Institute. This formula, along with Full Spectrum Nutrition, has helped tens of thousands of people live a normal life, free from hypoglycemia and diabetes. Together with the proper diet as outlined earlier, it can ensure that you will not have to progress to further stages of these diseases. Further, you will not have to suffer the numerous and debilitating side effects which arise from excess insulin in the blood.

Components of a Comprehensive Glucose/Insulin Regalating Formula

Aspartic Acid	500 mg
Chromium	100 mcg
Vanadium	500 mcg
Bilberry Extract	20 mg
Bitter Melon	200 mg

This represents the potency of our 'formula of choice' in a 'per capsule' dose. We then use six capsules per day (two with each meal) for two to four weeks. This is followed, by using one capsule three times per day indefinitely.

Glandular Support

As with all chronic diseases, hypoglycemia and diabetes can affect many organs and organ systems either directly or indirectly. For this reason, we recommend the short-term use of a multi-glandular formulation, which provides the DNA, or genetic code of specific organ tissues. When taken, these substances serve to strengthen not only the specific organs in question, such as the liver and pancreas, but ensure that the various organ systems are working in proper harmony or synergy with each other.

There are two specific formulas generally available, one for men and one for women. The formulas we are currently using at our Institute are as follows...

Female Formula

Pantothenic Acid	150 mg
Adrenal	75 mg
Brain	75 mg
Heart	75 mg
Kidney	75 mg
Liver	75 mg
Pancreas	75 mg
Pituitary	75 mg
Spleen	75 mg
Thymus	75 mg
Ovarian	75 mg
Para-Amino Benzoic Acid	75 mg

RNA	75 mg
Glycine	75 mg
Choline	75 mg

Male Formula

Adrenal	75 mg
Brain	75 mg
Heart	75 mg
Kidney	75 mg
Liver	75 mg
Pancreas	75 mg
Pituitary	75 mg
Spleen	75 mg
Thymus	75 mg
Prostate	75 mg
Testes	75 mg
Para-Amino Benzoic Acid	75 mg
RNA	5 mg
Glycine	75 mg
Zinc	25 mg

The preceding multi-glandular formulation potencies represent a maintenance type dosage. First time users may wish to double the dosages for the first four weeks and then have their situation re-evaluated. If deemed necessary, continue using a maintenance dosage for an additional four to eight weeks.

Managing Stress

As illustrated earlier, stress, especially un-manageable stress, can wreck havoc with the glandular systems of the body. Since both hypoglycemia and diabetes are endocrine disorders, stress has a rapid and intense negative impact on these conditions. If we are to gain control over these problems, managing stress is very important.

During periods of stress, the body can consume very high amounts of certain nutrients. When these nutrient levels are depleted, the nerves become irritated and additional stress becomes impossible to manage.

For this reason, we always use a combination of nutrients in higher amounts when working with hypoglycemics and diabetics. These nutrients, in the following combinations and ratios, have proven time and time again to stabilize the body's many chemical functions through calming and nourishing the central nervous system.

Stress Management Formula

Vitamin C	1000 mg
Vitamin B1	50 mg
Vitamin B2	50 mg
Vitamin B6	50 mg
Vitamin B12	500 mcg
Pantothenic Acid	1200 mg
Calcium	400 mg
Magnesium	100 mg
Adrenal Substance	200 mg
Valerian Root Extract	200 mg
Kavakava	100 mg

The preceding protocol has been thoroughly tested. I have used it with great results for over 15 years. While it is relatively simple, it is important that you follow it exactly as presented.

If you have hypoglycemia, or most especially, adult-onset Type II diabetes, don't be told by Doctors, loved ones, or anyone else that your condition is hopeless.

Most physicians do not understand how to treat either of these conditions. Because of their misunderstanding of the biochemical processes involved in these disorders, they often treat them in exactly the opposite way in which they should be managed.

Believe it or not, there are medical doctors who believe that the best way to treat hypoglycemia is by giving the patient a little sugar every two hours! This is a sure-fire way for them to guarantee themselves a patient for life!

These same doctors treat diabetes much the same way by force-feeding refined carbohydrates to diabetics in order to keep their blood sugar levels up. Why have they never thought of lowering the consumption of sugar-forming foods in these people's diets so that they would not need all those drugs or insulin? Conventional medicine is often not founded on logic!

A Case In Point – Tom M.

Tom, who was referred to us by a third party, first contacted our Institute in April of 1998. When he called, the voice on the other end of the telephone was a desperate one. Tom had been diagnosed with Type II diabetes about two years ago. While taking down his information, we discovered that he was taking 14 different oral medications daily! Further, his body weight was nearing 300 pounds. Tom was desperate. His doctor told him that his blood sugar was still too high and that if it did not come down in 30 days, he was going to put him on insulin by injection. Tom had done enough reading to know that was not a good recommendation for a Type II diabetic and he was really scared.

The first thing we did was evaluate his diet. He told us that the diet he was following came from his doctor's office. He said he followed it very strictly. This was our first clue into Tom's dilemma. We asked if he had a copy of his diet handy and sure enough, he faxed it to our office that afternoon. Upon reviewing his diet, one endorsed by the American Diabetes Association, we found that it was 68 percent sugar-forming foods! On this diet, Tom was guaranteed to remain a diabetic the rest of his short and miserable life!

After reviewing his case, I called Tom and suggested some lifestyle changes, the very ones outlined in this chapter. We put him on a diet that was low in carbohydrates and high in protein and fresh vegetables. We started him on a maintenance program of Full Spectrum nutrition plus targeted nutritional support for his specific needs. We cautioned him to monitor his blood sugar level at least three times daily because we expected it to begin to fall.

To make a long story short, within three months, Tom was medication free. He went from 14 pills to no pills in ninety days! Other exciting changes were occurring for Tom as well. He lost almost 75 pounds. As his bodyweight lessened due to the decrease in the amount of insulin circulating in the bloodstream, his insulin receptor sites began to function better. Today, Tom remains disease free, as declared by his physician. Sadly, Tom doesn't see that doctor any longer. Upon hearing how Tom achieved his remarkable metamorphosis from disease, his doctor told him never to come back. When Tom questioned why his doctor did not share his excitement over his return from disease, the doctor coldly said, "You did not follow my diet and take my advice."

The reason we say that this is 'sad' is because if

Tom's doctor had learned from his patient's case, think how many other patients he might have influenced in a positive way.

For those suffering with conditions such as these, I am telling you that there is hope, plenty of hope. But you must TAKE ACTION and DO IT! If you follow the guidelines we have provided, you will succeed.

Program Summary

Dietary Restriction. It is imperative that you follow a dietary program that reduces the amount of total sugar-forming foods in the diet.

Exercise. A regular exercise program, designed for your age and level of fitness, will accelerate your victory over virtually any phase of hyperinsulinemia.

Dietary Supplements.

<u>Full Spectrum Nutrition</u> – Provide your body with the 100+ nutrients it needs every day. (See Chapter 15).

<u>Glucose Metabolizing Nutrients</u> – Use Chromium, Vanadium, Aspartic Acid, and Bilberry Extract in *mega-dose* amounts.

<u>Glandular System Support</u> - The DNA from specific glands and organ tissues serves to boost endocrine system function, thereby giving you a jump start to your overall program.

Stress Reducing Nutrients - Since stress plays such a direct role in the pathology of carbohydrate intolerance, the addition of stress reducing nutrients is of vital importance. The body's reserves of nutrients such as vitamin C, Vitamins B1, B2, B6, B12, and pantothenic acid are rapidly depleted during times of physical and emotional stress. Carbohydrate intolerance produces both forms of stress and they exert a negative effect on the entire endocrine system through the action of the adrenal glands.

While this program seems simple enough, it is powerful in the results it can deliver.

It is important to remember that carbohydrate intolerance, at any level, is a progressive, degenerative process. The longer you ignore your problems, the worse they will become. They will progress from one stage of hyperinsulinemia to another. Each step is more debilitating to the body and more difficult to reverse.

For this reason, time is of the essence. You must make a conscious decision *now* to change your lifestyle, or resign yourself to a life filled with disease.

*C*hapter 7

Arthritis: Destroyer of Life's Quality

There are various foundations and associations involved in the research and treatment of arthritis and many forms of joint and connective tissue disorders labeled as arthritis. Collectively, these organizations have never admitted or acknowledged the fact that nutrition and diet have an impact on these conditions. They continue to subscribe to an obsolete, 30-year-old doctrine, which dictates only the use of aspirin or other over-the-counter medications for relieving the pain of this chronic and debilitating disease.

This is unfortunate, because the United States is about the only country that still clings to that philosophy with stubborn blindness. Most other countries not only acknowledge the diet/nutrient connection in the prevention and treatment of arthritis, but routinely advise those suffering from these conditions to use nutrients on a daily basis.

There is overwhelming evidence to show that arthritis is a complex breakdown of internal biochemistry. As will be demonstrated in this chapter, arthritis can be dramatically improved or even reversed without the use of drugs and/or invasive surgery.

First of all, we must understand that every form of arthritis evokes some type of inflammatory response. An initial approach should be one which assists the body in reducing that inflammation. This, in turn, would automatically reduce the pain.

Secondly, as with all chronic disease processes, it is important to look at the cause of the chemical changes within the arthritis sufferer, not merely the chemical changes themselves. This reveals to us that, at minimum, the most common forms of arthritis have their roots in an imbalance of the body's acid/alkaline balance, as well as a gross deficiency of several essential nutrients, including calcium.

Lastly, if a program for arthritis is to be truly successful, it must include factors for those who already suffer from moderate to advanced forms of the disease. These issues include relief from pain as well as factors that can help the body rebuild damaged cartilage and connective tissue, which has been lost through perhaps years of the disease process.

The program we propose in this chapter is designed to meet all three objectives. Whether you have just been diagnosed with some form of arthritis or whether you have suffered for some time, this program can help you! While naturally, the longer you have had the problem, the greater the chances of permanent damage, I have never seen an arthritis patient who wasn't significantly improved through the use of this program and I have been practicing nutrition for over 27 years.

So take heart. Just because arthritis is practically expected after age 45 you can both reduce your odds of getting it and go far towards reversing it if you have the condition already. In 1994, it was estimated that over 43 million people in the United States and Europe have arthritis. A new case is diagnosed every 60 seconds. You don't have to become, or remain, a victim of this epidemic. The choice is yours, but you must act if you expect results.

What is Arthritis?

It seems like a simple enough question to answer. Everyone knows what arthritis is, don't they? The answer, surprisingly, is NO! Medically, there are no known specific causes of arthritis!

Arthritis is not even a specific disease, but rather the generic name for a group of conditions, likely having individual or multiple different causes. The word 'arthritis', comes from the Greek word which means 'joint'. We have come to interpret the word as meaning inflammation of the joints.

Some researchers and health care practitioners would like us to believe that these conditions are caused by latent virus and bacteria in the body, past infections, rotten teeth and many other remotely connected factors. While these conditions may be linked to a few isolated cases of arthritic-like conditions, they cannot account for the multi-millions of cases diagnosed every year.

Dr. Francis Pottenger clearly established the relationship between a diet of highly cooked foods and arthritis in animals. This work was done many decades ago and yet the establishment continues to cling to the concept that diet does not affect this disease. Animals fed diets of raw foods showed no evidence of arthritis. Their counterparts, having been fed a diet of cooked and processed foods, developed a variety of arthritic symptoms at an early age. One of the worst of all the offending foods for the arthritic patient is processed, pasteurized dairy products such as milk, ice cream and processed cheeses. Every arthritic patient I've ever counseled had been on a diet of over-cooked and over-processed foods for decades.

We have been able to link such a diet to the proliferation of numerous chronic degenerative diseases. Arthritis is no exception. We will be discussing diet in greater detail later on.

While no one really knows what causes arthritis, we do know that we can interrupt the disease process and stop the disease from progressing.

There are several types of arthritis. The most common is called osteo-arthritis. It concerns the breakdown of the cartilage tissue that cushions and lubricates the joints. Over time, this material is lost from a variety of assaults, which may include infections to the joint itself, excessive wear & tear (athletics), and numerous nutritional deficiencies.

Another form of arthritis is called rheumatoid arthritis. This is not a degenerative disease in the clinical sense, but rather an autoimmune disorder. It is a condition wherein the body's immune system launches an attack upon the cartilage and connective tissue proteins. Eventually, this abnormality will destroy every joint in the body.

While the cause of osteo-arthritis and rheumatoid arthritis vary greatly from each other, the end result is the same. Both produce a loss of cartilage and connective tissue through repeated inflammation and irritation of the joint and surrounding physiology.

As the synovial membrane of the joint tissue becomes repeatedly inflamed, the blood supply increases. White blood cells proliferate at these sites, indicating the presence of some form of infection. This increase in cellular activity causes the surrounding tissue and joint to swell. The swelling pushes the bone joints further apart, creating a larger and larger space. As the space between them increases, the risk of further infection and subsequent inflammation occurs.

It is now believed that the acute inflammation and pain experienced by most arthritics is due to damage caused by the proliferation of free radicals. In thinking about this process as we have described, please keep in mind that many free radicals can be eliminated or neutralized through the use of a variety of antioxidant nutrients.

PROSTAGLANDINS AND INFLAMMATION

For those of you who are chemically minded, we will briefly discuss the role prostaglandins play in this particular disease process.

Prostaglandins are a group of chemicals which are primarily derived from polyunsaturated fats (vegetable oils) in the diet. They may be divided into two basic groups. The prostaglandin-1 family members are desirable and carry out a variety of beneficial functions within our biochemistry. For example, prostaglandin E-1 is necessary for the normal function of the T-cells of the immune system. These E-1 prostaglandins also prevent the second group of prostaglandins, called E-2 prostaglandins, from causing inflammation within the joints of the body.

Aspirin, an over-the-counter non-steroidal anti-inflammatory, works temporarily in reducing inflammation because it greatly slows down the formation of the prostaglandin E-2 grouping which cause inflammation in the first place.

Now that we have a little better idea of what we are dealing with, let's take a look at how modern medicine manages this condition.

Conventional Treatment for Arthritis

If we follow the standard medical model of diagnosis, drugs and ultimately surgery, we pretty well understand conventional medicine's approach to this condition. It varies little.

Arthritis is usually first diagnosed as a result of patient complaints of pain, stiffness, and loss of motion in specific joints of the body. The physician then customarily recommends taking an over-the-counter pain- killer. Almost all painkillers belong to a family of drugs known as non-steroidal anti-inflammatory drugs. (NSAIDs) The only popular exception to that group would be acetaminophen (Tylenol ® Datril ® and Liquiprin ®) Acetaminophen is not often recommended for arthritis because it contains no anti-inflammatory properties but consumers, unaware of this, take it thinking that it is safer than other over-the-counter pain killers. Unfortunately, it is not.

While NSAIDs are wonderful for occasional aches, pains, or headaches, their constant use renders them increasingly less effective and can produce a variety of potentially serious side effects. The use of NSAIDs is completely out of control. Last year, $2.5 billion worth of these analgesics and anti-inflammatories were sold in the United States alone!

It is estimated that there are at least 100 different NSAIDs either available or in development at any given time. Some of the more popular NSAIDs include: Indocin®, Advil®, Motrin®, Aleve®, Nuprin®, Excedrin®, Midol® and Orudis®.

By taking continual high doses of NSAIDs, we interfere with vital bodily functions at a chemical level. Some of the symptoms of NSAID abuse include:

Allergic reactions
Anxiety
Cramps
Diarrhea
Drowsiness
Edema
Headache
Hypertension (high blood pressure)
Indigestion
Kidney problems
Nausea
Nervousness
Sensitivity to sunlight
Ulcers and stomach bleeding
Wounds which heal slowly

Another common side effect of NSAIDs is their ability to inhibit the synthesis of proteoglycans. These molecules are responsible for carrying water to the cartilage tissue to keep it soft and pliable. This means that the very drugs we most commonly take to relieve the discomfort of arthritic symptoms are actually contributing to the disease process!

Further, the black picture of NSAID misuse doesn't stop here. Many of the deaths that occur each year can be directly linked to excessive NSAID use. Common conditions, which can result in death, involve the kidneys, stomach, and liver, all organs damaged by NSAID abuse.

As the disease of arthritis progresses and the pain

and inflammation worsens, medical doctors resort to using more and more powerful NSAIDs, available by prescription only. Their side effects are the same as we have already discussed with one exception - there are more of them.

When the NSAIDs fail to relieve the patient's discomfort, the doctor moves to the next group of drugs, the corticosteroids. Drugs such as cortisone and prednisone, are the most commonly used. They work, but not without a potentially terrible price. They depress the immune system to the point of failure. They thin the bones, cause hypertension, diabetes, osteoporosis, and even mental disturbances! For this reason, legitimate physicians will only use them for very short term or in the case of life-threatening conditions.

The final method of treatment for arthritis in the 'physician's bag' is, as always, surgery. Joint replacement has become such big business that many hospitals rely upon this type of surgery to stay in business. The problems with surgery are numerous. The pain, the recovery time, the side effects and the cost must all be considered. Worse yet, just because you have one joint replaced doesn't mean you are out of the hot water. Arthritis is a systemic disease and will, eventually affect all the joints of your body. How many do you want to have replaced?

While the picture of the treatment and prognosis of arthritis painted is not pretty, the good news is that there is an alternative. Through proper nutrition and subsequent detoxification of the body, even more advanced cases of many types of arthritis may be successfully improved or reversed.

Nutritional Support for Managing & Reversing Arthritis

Several specific nutrients have repeatedly proven to be of exceptional importance in the prevention, management, and even the reversal of arthritic conditions. Before beginning a discussion of these nutrients, it is important to emphasize the fact that the body works on the principles of synergy and balance. It requires well over 100 nutrients daily to accomplish the task of not only keeping you alive, but healthy as well. To 'mega-dose' on individual or 'isolated' nutrients, without the simultaneous intake of a Full Spectrum supplement, is unwise. It can lead to drastic biochemical imbalances within the body. (See Chapter 15).

Simply stated, for optimal results in any nutritional support program, use a Full Spectrum dietary supplement as a foundation on a daily basis. Then add the specific nutrients which have demonstrated their effectiveness in improving the condition at hand. Following is a listing of select individual nutrients which have helped many arthritis sufferers dramatically improve the quality of their lives. Each is accompanied by an explanation as to why that nutrient is of profound value. Later in the chapter, you will also find recommended protocols indicating suggested potencies.

Essential Fatty Acids (EFA): It was heart disease that first drew our attention to the importance of Gamma-linolenic acid (GLA) and eicosapentaenoic acid (EPA) in the prevention and management of chronic disease. Since that time, these essential fatty acids have continued to demonstrate their relevancy in reference to numerous chronic conditions. In 1985, an article appeared in the publication Clinical Research reporting that these essential fatty acids significantly improved rheumatoid arthritis in many patients. Further, they are absolutely essential in the management of common or osteoarthritis.

Remember our discussion of prostaglandin's earlier? Well the good varieties are made through the conversion of GLA in the body. In order for this to occur, you must have adequate GLA available. The best sources of essential fatty acids include fish oils, borage oil, flax oil and evening primrose oil. It is important to note that all of these oils, especially the vegetable sources, are highly subject to rancidity when they come in contact with the oxygen in the air. Rancid oils produce tremendous amounts of free radicals, the very substances we are trying to curtail due to their active role in the arthritis process. For this reason, you should be very cautious about the source of the fatty acids you choose. Once exposed to air, they do more harm than good. If you must buy the oils in bottles, they MUST be refrigerated. Much better still would be to purchase the fatty acids which have been extracted from the various oils and then placed in airtight gel capsules. One further step against free radical formation would be to look for capsules that are opaque in nature. Avoid the clear, see-through capsules. They allow light to penetrate, causing some breakdown of the delicate fatty acids within.

Calcium and Magnesium: Arthritis is caused, in part, by a long term, sub-clinical calcium deficiency. Therefore, taking extra calcium is a logical adjunct to a full spectrum nutritional approach. Calcium requires several co-factor minerals in order to be properly absorbed. Mal-absorption of calcium, due to lack of proper acidity or imbalances in nutrient intake, is the cardinal cause of such problems as kidney and gall stones, bone spurs, and of course, arthritis. The best calcium supplements are comprised of the chelated calcium-cittrate and malate and contain supporting mineral co-factors such as magnesium, boron, copper, manganese, and zinc.

Copper: In addition to being an essential co-factor in the absorption and retention of calcium, copper has long been associated with the relief of stiff and aching conditions. The practice of wearing copper bracelets for relief of arthritis pain is an old remedy, but the science behind it is sound. Organic source copper, that which comes from plant sources, is much more absorbable by the body at the cellular level and is therefore the preferred source.

Vitamin B-6: This is the universal 'transport vitamin'. Virtually every nutrient combined with enough vitamin B-6 is transported readily to the cellular level. Additionally, vitamin B-6 plays a direct role in reducing pain from inflammation as well as preventing the nighttime cramps frequently suffered by arthritis patients. The complete research relating to vitamin B-6 and arthritis may be found in an old book by Dr. John M. Ellis, MD entitled The Doctor Who Looked At Hands. This book is, unfortunately, out of print but may still be available in libraries and used bookstores.

Pantothenic Acid: Another B-complex vitamin, pantothenic acid, has proven to be highly effective in relieving the symptoms of both osteo and rheumatoid arthritis. Many researchers around the world believe that arthritis is caused directly by a deficiency of this essential B vitamin. The body is easily depleted of Pantothenic acid by excess stress and the consumption of over-processed foods.

Quercetin: A very powerful specific anti-oxidant, Quercetin inhibits the lipoxygenase pathway of arachidonic acid metabolism which is responsible for some of the most powerful inflammatory chemicals in the body, while at the same time producing anti-inflammatory prostaglandins. Quercetin further inhibits the release of histamine, which can exacerbate inflammatory conditions such as arthritis.

Glucosamine Sulfate: In order for cartilage to maintain its integrity, and not break down because of excessive use, it needs adequate amounts of water. Proteoglycans, structures that bind the collagen within the cartilage, are also the structures that attract the water and keep the joint and surrounding tissues lubricated with moisture. Glucosamine sulfate is a major building block of proteoglycans. Glucosamine is, therefore, necessary for making the proteins that bind water in the cartilage matrix. Glucosamine sulfate not only initiates the production of the key elements of joint and cartilage integrity, but also protects the existing cartilage. Glucosamine can actually help the body repair and replace lost cartilage thereby reversing the disease process!

Chondroitin Sulfate: Many of you may be familiar with an age old 'Grandma's Remedy' of eating gelatin if you suffered from stiff joints. It worked because gelatin contains a substance called Chondroitin sulfate. While Glucosamine sulfate forms the proteoglycans that fit within the collagen of the cartilage, Chondroitin sulfate provides a magnetic attraction for water. Chondroitin's long chain of repeating sugars attracts fluid to the proteoglycan molecules. This accomplishes two things. The fluid acts as the cushion or shock absorber, protecting the cartilage tissue from further assault and breakdown and since joint cartilage has no blood supply, the fluid transports nutrients into the cartilage, keeping them healthy. Without such constant nutrient immersion, the cartilage becomes mal-nourished and dries out. This results in a thinner, more fragile, cartilage structure. Because gelatin is an incomplete protein, it is very hard to digest for many people. Further, the amount of Chondroitin sulfate in gelatin is minimal, requiring the need for consuming very large amounts. For this reason we recommend using concentrated Chondroitin sulfate. The best source is from sea cucumber since this is not only the most concentrated source but is also 'hypo' allergenic as well.

dl Phenylalanine: This amino acid has the ability to subdue the pain response thereby providing a natural pain relief without all the side effects of NSAIDs or corticosteroids. Since it is a naturally occurring amino acid, the side effects of taking it, even in larger quantities, is minimal.

*Note: You should not take Phenylalanine if you have high blood pressure.

Vitamin C: Since the process of arthritis involves free radical formation and subsequent tissue damage therefrom, antioxidants play a powerful role in the prevention process. Vitamin C is an antioxidant which delivers protective benefits because of its antioxidant properties. It also acts as a natural diuretic and helps the body to more quickly rid itself of toxins that can build up rapidly in the arthritic patient.

Selenium: Another powerful antioxidant, selenium must be found in most well rounded Full Spectrum nutritional programs. If your Daily Foundation nutrition program does not provide this essential antioxidant mineral, you will need to add it to your program as well.

By combining these specific nutrients with a Full Spectrum foundation, you provide your body with all of its daily nutritional requirements. Remember, at the end of this book, we will provide you with a list of nutrients and the exact potencies and ratios used to successfully achieve positive results.

Methyl-sulfonyl-methane: While this nutrient is still relatively new and many of the promoters selling it are making often rather wild claims for its efficacy, MSM is effective in the management of many health challenges. For the purpose of our disscussion here, MSM is an important adjunct to an overall arthritis support program due to the fact that it relieves both pain and inflammation. Further, MSM has shown benefits for athletes in relieving stress-induced conncetive tissue injuries. Clinical studies have repeatedly shown that mega-doses of MSM are more effective in relieving pain than the leading NSAID's, with none of the common side effects of those drugs. It seems that MSM accomplishes this feat by helping the cells of the body eleimnate toxins through an acceleration of fluids through cell membranes. This in turn, increases cellular detoxification, eleminating waste matter. Since all forms of arthritis are linked directly to excess toxicity within the body, the connection is both sound and important.

Cetyl-myristoleate: A member of the fatty acid group of nutrients, CMO is only beginning to receive the proper attention and recognition that it deserves. Like many natural substances derived from foods, fatty acids perform hundreds of functions within the internal biochemistry of the body, which are absolutely essential to life. CMO, a member of this powerfrul group of nutrients, also performs many essential functions, one of which is the specific rebuilding of cartilage, tendons and ligaments, which have deteriorated through abuse and free radical damage. In a pioneer clinical study, a group of matched subjects were divided into three groups, the first group was given CMO alone, and the second group received CMO plus Full Spectrum Nutrition (See Chapter 15), and the last group, the control group received the placebo.

At the end of the study the results were as follows: The placebo group had an 8 percent improvement. Those taking CMO alone reported a 58.l percent improvement in that grouping. In the last group, an amazing 84.2 percent of those taking both the CMO *and* the Full Spectrum Nutrition supplement reported at least a 75 percent improvement in their arthritis symptoms! Not only does this prove that CMO must be part of a total approach to arthritis management, but that the concept of totality that I am stressing, namely using ALL the known nutrients in the right ratios to each other, is essential for maximizing the results.

Other Factors Affecting Arthritis

Whenever we address a chronic degenerative disease of any kind, we must not rule out the possibility of allergic reactions, which can contribute significantly to almost any disease process. Such is the case with arthritis.

There is a group of foods which have been directly linked to the formation and aggravation of arthritis in many people. These foods all belong to a specific group called the nightshades. In fact, many members of the nightshade family are so poisonous that they can produce rapid and unpleasant death. Those that do not immediately make you sick are routinely consumed as foods and include: white potatoes (including foods containing potato starch), tomatoes, peppers and eggplants. All these foods contain a chemical called solanine, which causes delayed inflammation in some people. If you are having trouble managing your arthritis after following this program, you may wish to consciously eliminate the nightshades from your diet on a permanent basis.

Other allergies to a wide variety of foods may also play a part the genesis of arthritis. Therefore, if allergies to foods of any kind are suspected, it is a good idea to have an allergy test and to subsequently avoid all offending foods.

The cleansing fast discussed in Chapter 13 will

help to rid the body of many of these offending compounds. If you continue to avoid the offending foods, your system should remain fairly clean of histamine. It is also important to realize that anyone suffering from arthritis for any length of time will have an overload of toxins in their system. The specific byproducts of the process that causes arthritis in the first place also produces toxic byproducts, which must be safely removed in order for management or recovery to be achieved. This is another reason why we recommend the Liver, Kidney, Colon, Bowel and Bladder cleanse outlined in detail in Chapter 13.

Oxygen: The Universal Cleanser

For many arthritis sufferers, relief from pain is the first thing on their minds. Pain from arthritis goes deep into the body and can be severe. In our search for alternatives to drug therapy in the management of arthritis, we discovered an all natural substance that not only accelerates healing and detoxification of the joint tissues but actually relieves the pain and stiffness connected with all forms of arthritis.

For over 100 years, we have known about the beneficial effects of super oxygenating the body. In fact, medicine has used super oxygenation in a variety of forms for the treatment of numerous disease conditions. Hyperbaric oxygen is often used in accelerating the healing of wounds or burns. Intravenous oxygen is routinely used by alternative hospitals around the world as part of an overall program of health building rejuvenation, allowing the body to better heal itself from the ravages of virtually all chronic diseases.

While these two forms of oxygenation are effective, they are not readily accessible or affordable to the average person. Because of the work of several pioneers in the field, the use of oxygen for conditions such as arthritis became somewhat well known. Arthritic people would mix food grade 35% hydrogen peroxide (the only safe form to take internally) with water and drink it. Hydrogen peroxide, in that concentration, has a particularly nauseating taste that is almost impossible to cover up. However, if it is mixed with anything but distilled water, the pathogens and enzymes naturally present in juice and food will cause the oxygen to disassociate. This renders the mixture virtually worthless for oxygenation purposes.

Some time ago, we developed a method whereby the hydrogen peroxide could be buffered, or protected, from disassociation when mixed. Subsequently, there are now products available which contain buffered 35% hydrogen peroxide along with aloe vera and sterilized natural fruit flavors. This makes a very palatable drink and may be consumed several times per day. This is especially helpful during the initial stages of the treatment program when the pain and stiffness from arthritis is most severe. One word of reminder concerning any hydrogen peroxide or oxygen product. They must be consumed on an empty stomach in order to prevent the premature release of the oxygen. (For further information on the use of oxygen therapy for chronic and degenerative diseases we refer you to The Institute's publication entitled **Effective Oxygen Therapy for Chronic Conditions.**)

The Role of Exercise in Recovery from Arthritis

When you are stiff and hurting from the pain of arthritis, the very last thing you wish to think about is exercise. In fact, some forms of exercise could actually make your arthritis worse by further damaging compromised cartilage tissue. Yet without exercise, your stiff joints will continue to bind up, even reducing their range of movement and mobility.

The answer is in the proper form of exercise. For those with moderate arthritis, low impact aerobics on a very cushioned surface are beneficial. Those with more advanced arthritic conditions should avoid even low impact exercise. Weight resistance exercises, together with stretching exercises, are the best possible combination for the arthritis sufferer. If you are unfamiliar with exercise and exercise equipment, we suggest that you consult with a physical therapist or exercise physiologist for a program that's right for you. Many of the better gyms and health clubs have personnel who are trained in these areas of specialty. They can get you started on the correct program that will increase your flexibility while ensuring that your delicate joint tissues are not further compromised.

Light Therapy: A Hidden Secret Revealed

Over 50 years ago, Dr. John Ott and others conducted studies that indicated the sun's many hidden healing properties. These properties were shown to be beneficial in treating a variety of chronic and immune related disorders. These finding have been reconfirmed in recent years.

With all the negative publicity surrounding the sun and the link between its radiation and some forms of skin cancer, you see people avoiding the sun like some evil plague. Yet, the key to everything in life is, and always will be, moderation. The sun is the great energy turbine that fuels our entire solar system. All life on our planet is directly dependent upon the sun. Plant chemistry ceases without sunlight, and without plants, all life as we know it would end.

How, then, can something so beneficial be so dangerous? There are several reasons. We know that the incidence of skin cancers have been steadily on the rise over the past few decades. We also know that certain layers of insulation in our upper atmosphere have either been altered, or in some areas, destroyed. The ozone layer of the upper atmosphere serves as a filter and thereby screens out many of the harmful rays striking the earth from cosmic space. As the ozone breaks down, increasing amounts of these potentially dangerous energies make their way to the Earth's surface.

With moderation as the key, you can still enjoy the health giving benefits of sunlight without going to the extremes that place your body at risk.

Your skin produces a substance called melanin which protects your body from the sun. It is also the substance that makes some peoples' skin darker than others and causes lighter skinned people to tan. If you nurture the production of melanin through gradual exposures to the sun, you can build up a protective layer within the skin.

What, you ask, has this to do with arthritis? Research has shown that many chronic diseases, such as arthritis and allergies, are tremendously improved by routine and regulated exposures to the sunlight. Sunlight is known to be a powerful immune stimulant, but excess exposure has an adverse affect on the immune response, hence the need for moderation. (For further information on the management of allergies through natural means we refer you to our Institute publication entitled **Naturally Controlling Allergies.**)

In applying sunlight therapy, specifically to arthritis, the following program has been very helpful. While participating in this program, NEVER LOOK DIRECTLY AT THE SUN!

To begin the program, expose your eyes to unfiltered sunlight for 15 to 30 minutes each day. For those who are not accustomed to being out in the sun, begin with five minutes at a time, gradually working up to the full amount of time.

Once you are accustomed to this, close your eyes in a relaxed and non-squinting manner and face directly into the sun. Your eyelids will protect your delicate eye tissue, yet the energy will still penetrate through.

While you are following this program, it is also beneficial to expose your skin to the sun as well. Your body produces vitamin D when sunlight makes contact with the exposed skin.

Many of our patients reported that they received significant relief from their arthritic stiffness and pain simply through use of this program alone.

A Special Note for Those Suffering from Gout or Rheumatoid Arthritis

Persons suffering from gout, a genetic disorder which prevents the proper excretion of uric acid from the body, can benefit from the basic arthritis program outlined in this book as well as the following suggestions.

Add vitamin C to your daily diet until bowel tolerance is reached. To do this, begin with 1000 mg and increase each day by an additional 500-mg until you develop diarrhea. Then reduce your intake to just below that level. Furthermore, eating cherries or drinking cherry juice is very beneficial for the gout patient. This, along with avoiding purine-forming foods such as red meats, organ meats, sweet breads, shellfish and beer, can help the gout sufferer live a relatively normal life.

In addition to our basic arthritis protocol, those suffering from rheumatoid arthritis need to add one extra supplement to their program and that is chicken cartilage. Fortunately, chicken cartilage is now readily available in capsule form, which saves attacking every chicken in sight! Since potencies for chicken cartilage vary from one manufacturer to another, follow the dosage as outlined on the individual label. Be sure that the product you take is from chicken cartilage, NOT shark cartilage. They are NOT THE SAME! Shark cartilage should ONLY be used in the management of cancer since it prevents the replication of healthy cells.

In our many years of working with thousands of cases of arthritis, we can assure you that the program outlined in this book is very effective. The fact that the various nutrients are both potent and synergetic makes this program work extremely well. Following is the exact protocol we have used at The Institute of Nutritional Science with great success. We suggest that you adopt our program if you wish to have optimal results.

Protocol for the Prevention and Management of Arthritis

Diet: It is important to begin a diet consisting of raw foods. Eat at least one serving of raw cabbage every day as well. Reduce or eliminate the consumption of over processed foods and lifeless foods. Eliminate the consumption of nightshades (discussed earlier in this chapter) and if further problems persist, check for food allergies by having an allergy blood test. If it reveals any severe food allergies, be sure to eliminate those foods from your diet as well.

Detoxification and Cleansing: We cannot stress the importance of properly cleansing the 'organs of elimination' in your plan to treat your arthritic condition. A Full Spectrum cleansing/detoxification program must address all the organs involved including the liver, kidneys colon and bowel. The following formulation is what we have used successfully on hundreds and hundreds of patients.

Psyllium Husk (fiber)	as needed
Cascara Extract	2 mg
Rhubarb Root	10 mg
Buckthorn Berry	10 mg
Elderberry	15 mg
Licorice Root Extract	50 mg
Garlic Bulb...........................	75 mg
Quassia Bark	50 mg
Black Cohosh Root	25 mg
Red Sage Root.....................	50 mg
Goldenseal Root...................	10 mg
L-Glutamic Acid HCl	25 mg

The above formula should be contained in a single capsule and you should take the specific number of capsules as outlined in the 'fasting' section of this book. (See Chapter 13).

After completing the fast or cleanse, it is important to replenish the healthy, good bacteria in the intestinal system. This is best accomplished through the use of a full spectrum acidophilus product, which provides all the various bacterial strains naturally occurring in the gut.

Specific Nutrient Program: The following dietary supplement program represents both the potency and the ratio of nutrients used with the greatest success at our Institute.

Full Spectrum Nutrition (preferably in liquid form)
Provides the 120 nutrients which make up the foundation for daily intake.

Essential Fatty Acids (best taken in airtight opaque capsules)

Then add the following specific nutrients:

Vitamin B6	100 mg
Pantothenic Acid	500 mg
Copper (chelate)	1 mg
Calcium (chelate)	100 mg
Magnesium (chelate)	50 mg
Zinc	6 mg
Evening Primrose Oil	100 mg
Quercetin	100 mg
Glucosamine Sulfate	500 mg
Chondroitin Sulfate	500 mg
Cetyl-Myristoleate CMO	300 mg

Methyl Sulfonyl Methane MSM	....	200 mg
Bosuellic Acid	....	200 mg
Nettle Leaf Extract	....	400 mg

If pain and stiffness is considerable, add liquid oxygen at the rate of one ounce three times per day on an empty stomach (30 minutes before or three hours after a meal).

If you do not get adequate calcium from your diet, or if you are a female over the age of 45, you need at least 1200 mg of supplemental calcium daily. It should be taken simultaneously with the mineral co-factors boron, copper, magnesium, zinc, and manganese.

In severe cases, this formula may be doubled for the first 30 to 60 days. It is wise to work up slowly, however, since all arthritics are toxic and may otherwise experience symptoms of rapid detoxification which could include headache, nausea, diarrhea and fatigue. Should these symptoms occur, simply reduce the dietary intake dosage of these nutrients and begin more slowly. Gradually increase the dosage until the optimal levels stated above have been reached.

Well that's the program. Nothing has been left out and there are no secrets. While some of what we have told you may be familiar, likely, other parts of the program will seem foreign. Nonetheless, it works. We have literally hundreds of case histories of people whom have benefited immensely from this exact program. You must follow it faithfully and regularly. Arthritis is a chronic condition, meaning that you have it for life. This means that you will have to begin to take a more active role in maintaining and/or regaining your health. If you had known this information years ago, perhaps you would not be in the position you find yourself today. Only you can make the difference by beginning and continuing this program.

Chapter 8
The Aging Female

The human body is much like a very sophisticated machine. For illustrative purposes, we will compare it to an automobile. When new, a car can perform flawlessly for 50,000 or 100,000 miles before requiring a major tune-up. As long as you change its oil, lubricate the chassis joints, and rotate the tires, most new cars will require very little in the way of repairs. However, as the miles accumulate on the 'machine', an increasing amount of maintenance is required to keep it operating properly. In many respects, the human body is much the same.

When our bodies were young, we felt invincible, and in some respects were. We could devour copious amounts of junk food. We could also combine and comfortably consume foods which did not 'agree with each other'. It all went down, and stayed down, with little or no discomfort. If we were to do that today, most of us would find ourselves running for some form of 'designer' anti-acid.

Remember when you could work two or more jobs and still have the stamina and energy to go out and party till the wee hours on Friday and Saturday nights? Most of us can't do that anymore; just the thought of such a thing makes us tired!

Why is this so? As the body ages, it does not operate as efficiently and effectively as when it was younger. The extent of maintenance problems a given body will have is, like the automobile, directly related to the manner in which it was cared for throughout its earlier life. If you follow the manufacturers maintenance recommendations for auto maintenance, as your car gets older, you will have minimal repair problems. However, the owner who neglected maintenance procedures on an identical model would have significantly more repair problems. The same applies to our bodies, which is why some 'senior citizens' are in much better shape later in life than others are. Yes, genetics have an influence on health and longevity, but forty or fifty years of stress, dietary abuse, lack of exercise and proper rest take their toll. Like the automobile that wasn't properly maintained, if your body is a 'high miler', it too, needs extra care.

Further, as we age, there are some specific changes that will also begin to occur in addition to the expected results of normal aging. In the female, menopause is the largest chemical and physiological change to be expected. Other problems include emotional disturbances and osteoporosis, which may or may not be linked to menopause. We will take a close look at these concerns and, by explaining how the maturing female body works, show you how to minimize the adverse side effects of these natural changes. What you learn will not only help you through the 'change of life', but will enable you to live your life to the fullest during the years ahead.

Menopause

Menopause and 'the change of life' are terms used to describe the transition in a woman's life; a transition from a period of reproductive function to one of expanding horizons. The last half of a woman's life should never be perceived as 'the end' or as a loss of 'womanhood', but as an opportunity for her to modify her role in life.

Usually by the time menopause has set in, a woman has raised children and is now ready to experience the many joys and opportunities that the future holds. The time that follows can be joyous years filled with travel, leisure, grandchildren, and time to enjoy all the best life has to offer. Sadly many women face this period with considerable worry and even fear. They have heard the horror stories of the complications both during and after passing through menopause.

Unfortunately, many of these fears are often justified, since innumerable women do indeed suffer from both the physiological and psychological phenomena, which can make this period less than pleasant for some and down right miserable for others.

If this were an inevitable part of aging, and nothing could be done about it, we would somehow bear up under the load and endure. But thankfully, unlike many issues over which we have little or no control, that is not the case here. If we are properly informed and advised, we will discover that there is much we can do to make the transition a smooth and pleasant one.

While many menopausal women exhibit symptoms typically associated with menopause, many others pass through this phase of life virtually unaffected. Therefore, we must deduce that these unpleasant manifestations are not inevitable.

Taking this viewpoint, this chapter will serve to explain the process of menopause and to offer safe and highly effective solutions to those who need them.

If you suffer from the ravages of menopause, take heart, there is a great deal of hope. You are now in one of the greatest times of your life. The opportunities that life affords you, now that many of your family obligations have been fulfilled, are only as limited as your imagination and your goals.

In order to fulfill those goals, you must have the energy, stamina, and good health to really enjoy the journey.

What happens during Menopause?

There are still many things we don't fully understand about the process of menopause. What we do know however, is enough for most women to gain complete control of their physiological chemistry and hence live a normal fulfilling life.

The average age in which the menopause process begins to occur is usually somewhere between forty and fifty years of age, the most common period being from 45 to 48. Interestingly, research has shown that there is some connection between the onset of puberty and the onset of menopause. If you began to menstruate early, you will have a greater chance of entering the menopause later in life than those who went through puberty at a later age. Further, there appears to be a connection between late menopause and women who have had multiple children.

At some point, as the body nears the end of its reproductive period, the ovaries are supposed to gradually become inactive. This process should be slow and virtually undetectable in the healthy woman, provided her diet is adequate and she is using Full Spectrum dietary supplementation on a regular basis. Even women whose ovaries cease producing hormones rapidly can still be relatively symptom free, providing their health has been maintained.

There are literally thousands of women who go through this process with little or no ill effects. Sadly, there are an equal number of women who do not. For them, this period of glandular change produces distressing or overwhelming side effects.

The most frequent symptom experienced during and post menopause is called the 'hot flash'. This vaso-motor event can occur many times during the day and night and most often involves the face, neck, and upper chest area. The skin becomes bright red and very hot, often producing profuse perspiration and a feeling of suffocation. If the attack is severe, the woman can experience feelings of anxiety and panic, having to 'get up and move around', or 'go out for a breath of fresh air'.

As these hot flashes proceed, they not only become more intense, but the periods of sweating also become more profuse, often requiring a complete change of clothing. Women suffering from these uncomfortable episodes are forever trying to open windows and doors to get some air, while others are cool or uncomfortably cold.

Some of the other symptoms frequently associated with the menopause include dizziness, headache, difficulty in breathing, shortness of breath, and heart palpitations. In more severe cases, mental depression, mood swings, insomnia, and erratic behavior begin to develop. This combination of both physiological and psychological side effects can act as a 'double whammy', taking their toll not only on the unfortunate female, but her entire family and circle of friends. Sadly, many women go untreated for these devastating side effects either because their doctors do not fully understand the severity of the problem, or they genuinely do not understand how to address the condition.

Of all the possible problems associated with the menopause, the psychological or mental side effects can be the most devastating. The depression, agitation, insecurities, anxiety, and inability to concentrate frequently result in the women entering a destructive downward spiral of loss of self-esteem. In turn, this leads to her feeling that she is 'no longer a woman', or that she has lost her appeal to the opposite sex.

Many women become fixated upon the idea that they have lost their beauty and that it is just a matter of time before they will age, their skin will wrinkle, they will lose their sex drive, and they will become a saggy, flabby bag of flesh.

This does not have to be the case however. With a proper diet, a regular exercise program, emphasizing strength training, and a daily Full Spectrum dietary supplement program, any woman can maintain her attractiveness and her physical attributes. There is no reason why a woman who makes the decision to properly take care of herself cannot enjoy an active sex life to a very advanced age. Frequently, healthy women remain sexually active longer than most men do.

Of the numerous myths associated with a woman's 'change of life', many may stem from the fact that estrogen is the predominate hormone giving women their feminine attributes. When estrogen is no longer being produced by the ovaries, the assumption is that her femininity is over.

The human body is the most complicated and yet amazing chemical laboratory ever invented. It constantly performs checks and balances to ensure that the internal functioning remains effective. This case of estrogen balance and replacement is no different.

The female body has an excellent backup system called the adrenal glands. They are supposed to take over, producing a hormone similar to estrogen, when the ovaries cease their work. This hormone provides enough chemical support to carry out all of the functions that estrogen would normally perform, except for those which prepare the body for conception.

When women have difficulties and unpleasant physiological and psychological symptoms during and after menopause, the blame can be directly attributed to a failure of the adrenal glands to function properly while serving as a 'back-up' system.

What Else Does Estrogen Do?

In order to achieve a better understand of the importance of both estrogen and 'estrogen-like' hormones, a brief discussion of their roles, excluding fertility, follows.

The word estrogen is an all-inclusive term for a group of hormones produced by the ovaries. These hormones govern sexual development during, and immediately after, puberty. They determine sexual characteristic, such as body form and mammary development. During adulthood, they are responsible for maintaining fertility and the proper functioning of the sex glands, including uterine changes during menstruation.

These powerful hormones carry out many other,

often unnoticed, functions within the women's bio-chemistry as well.

In addition to the more obvious functions of the estrogen hormone family, they serve to delineate other physiological aspects of the body. These include skin tone, body form, skeletal structure, fluid balance and the integrity of mucous membranes. Many of the most powerful functions of the estrogen group involve their inter-reactions with other hormones and glands in the body. They frequently serve as balancing factors by either increasing or decreasing the amount of other hormones being produced. It is in this area that much of the trouble begins for women after menopause. When the ovaries cease producing estrogens, these other hormones, some of them very powerful, are left unchecked and can act in considerable excess.

Now lets take a look at what causes this problem to occur and how we can, safely and effectively, inter-vene to help restore biochemical balance within the body.

The Cause of the Problem

As indicated before, the adrenal glands, two very important glands situated just above the kidneys, play a major role in the transformation from metabolic regulation by ovarian estrogens to metabolic regulation by 'estrogen-like' hormones. It is the adrenal glands that are responsible for taking over the job of producing these hormones to carry out all of your important bio-chemical activities, except the menstrual cycle.

The problem with this pretty picture is that many women suffer from moderate to severe adrenal hypo-activity. This is because the adrenals have many responsibilities within the body chemistry, and they often become overworked and undernourished.

One of the biggest jobs of the adrenal glands is to engage the 'fight or flight' state during periods of danger or perceived danger. We say perceived danger because most of the time when the adrenals are stimulated to secrete these powerful 'fight or flight' hormones, it is a false alarm and no real immediate danger is actually present.

This over-stimulation of the adrenal glands, by perceived dangers, causes these glands to become exhausted. Repeated stimuli from our environment leads to further and further exhaustion, and subsequent greater inability for the adrenal glands to produce the vital 'estrogen-like' hormones needed after menopause. (For further information on this stress-induced fight or flight syndrome, get our Institute's publication entitled, **Stress Can Kill You!**)

If you suffer from moderate to severe symptoms of menopause, your adrenal glands are not functioning properly. This generally is due to the fact that they are continually being over-stimulated by external stresses, which you are not able to mentally or emotionally cope with. Consider the following examples and how often these or other, similar, events occur during your day.

Behavior problems with children
Worrying over money problems
Negative stimuli from TV, radio, or newspaper articles
Marital differences
Time management
Not enough time in the day
Retirement
Fear of the threat of old age and disease
Behavior of others which you find offensive
Job security or job change
Illness of a family member
Death of a family member or friend
Worry over appearance
Fear of the future
And... Peer pressure, to name just a few.

The constant stress produced by these circumstances keeps the adrenal glands stimulated. Because of this, they are almost continually in a state of fatigue. During these perceived threatening situations, the adrenal glands prepare the body to either fight for survival or run for its life. Yet, virtually all of these situations are emotional or psychological stresses, requiring no 'fight or flight' response.

When we do not physically act upon these stimuli, the powerful hormones produced by the adrenal glands circulate in the bloodstream and are never consumed. These hormones can cause severe damage to several systems within the body, the most susceptible being the nervous system. Constant over-stimulation of the nervous system, by these adrenal hormones, causes them to over-react; in time, they lose their ability to properly assess the degree of seriousness of a situation. Once this stage is reached, such symptoms and anxiety, depression and nervousness can occur. Perhaps you can now begin to see how the adrenal glands are at the heart of virtually all the annoying symptoms of menopause.

These 'false alarms', which trigger a constant adrenal response, keep the body in a state of emotional tension leading to many of the psychological side effects of menopause. There are, however, some physical chemical situations that can further exhaust the adrenal glands.

The Curse of the SAD Diet

Over the past few decades, the American diet has deteriorated into one of mostly sugar, the wrong type of fats, and little protein. This eating pattern has come to be known as the Standard American Diet (SAD). Abbreviated SAD, this eating regimen is truly worthy of its acronym. Evidence of the detrimental effects of this diet may be seen in the rapid, almost epidemic, increase of chronic degenerative diseases in our society. The correlation between the diets and the disease is indeed a strong one. Further, as this SAD diet has spread to other countries, Europe in particular, the quality of overall health has begun to decline there as well. Thus far, only the poorer, so-called 'third world' countries have escaped the wrath of our terrible eating habits, mostly because their populace cannot afford it. I hope for their sake, they never can, for when they do, they too, will suffer the detrimental effects of an increase in chronic degenerative disease. Now, you ask, what does this have to do with menopause? Plenty, I assure you.

The Standard American Diet consists mostly of highly refined carbohydrates and sugars, all of which raise the blood glucose levels in the body, causing insulin to be secreted from the pancreas. This process, in and of itself, does not adversely affect the adrenal glands, but what follows does.

The mechanisms involved in regulating blood sugar include the pancreas and the insulin receptor sites upon which insulin acts. Over time, they become exhausted, causing fluctuations in blood sugar levels. As the irregularities worsen, the individual develops what is known as hypoglycemia, or clinical low blood sugar.

Every time the body's blood sugar dips below normal, the adrenal glands are called upon to produce a hormone, which will convert sugar stored in the body (glycogen) back into active glucose, which is useable for energy. This constant demand upon the adrenals further overworks them, reducing their ability to meet estrogen hormone needs.

At the time when the ovaries cease to produce estrogens and the adrenal glands must take over, the stresses and the diet of many women prevent these all-important glands from doing their much-needed job.

When the adrenals are so overworked that they can produce only a fraction of the estrogen-like hormones needed, symptoms of menopause are the result. What are the symptoms of over-exhausted adrenals?

Dry mouth
Circulatory system stimulation - hot flashes and/or chills
Elevated blood pressure
Lowered blood pressure
Hypoglycemia - low blood sugar
Excessive perspiration
Nervousness and shakiness
Anxiety
Mood Swings
Depression

If you take a close look at these typical symptoms of adrenal exhaustion, you will see that they are virtually the same as those of menopause!

Most of these symptoms are the result of an over-active sympathetic nervous system. Estrogen, and later on in life, the estrogen-like hormones from the adrenal glands, are responsible for modulating the sympathetic nervous system. If these are deficient or missing, the problem can accelerate out of control. One example of this sympathetic nervous system response is to force the blood, normally pooled in the interior of the body, to the surface, causing the common hot flashes.

There is virtually no way to control the symptoms of menopause without addressing the needs of the adrenal glands. If you are under an excessive amount of stress or if you are a high strung type of personality, it will be impossible for you to manage your menopausal symptoms and regulate your body without first addressing these issues.

Fortunately, there are many nutrients and foods, which when taken properly, can help to nourish the adrenal glands and the sympathetic nervous system, thereby helping to bring the body back into a normal chemical balance. In the following section, we will discuss some of the ways you can help rebalance your body and begin to live the kind of life you want and deserve.

Helping the Body to Transform Gracefully

Since the adrenals are at the heart of the menopause problem, and stress is at the heart of the adrenal problem, we must begin with a discussion of stress management if we wish to achieve optimal results.

Learning to relax is something we all talk about but very few actually practice. Our society, for some strange and perverse reason, almost worships stress. We honor and reward those who can seem to withstand high doses of stress and survive. If we really understood the detrimental effects of stress upon the body, we would reward and recognize those who have learned to manage the stress in their lives rather than those who have not.

All stress is cyclic in nature. Once stress is produced, it alters the body chemistry, causing more physical stress, which in turn causes more emotional stress. Menopause is no different. It is stress which further weakens the adrenals. If this condition is left untreated, the cycle repeats itself ad infinitum.

Hopefully, you can see the picture. In order to break this cycle, we must approach the problem from two separate angles. First of all, we must manage emotional stress through relaxation techniques and time management. Secondly, physical stress must be managed by adding to our diet specific nutrients, which have been shown to calm the sympathetic nervous system and nourish the adrenal glands.

Managing Emotional Stress

If we sit down a few minutes and take stock of our lifestyle, we can all find ways in which, through a little forward planning, we could reduce the amount of daily stress in our lives.

So often, people try and cram 90 minutes into every hour of the day. Then they cannot understand why they are constantly under pressure and always behind schedule by the end of everyday. Time management is a very important skill to develop.

Another enormous source of internal emotional stress comes from the formation of, and stubborn attachment to, opinions. These opinions are usually about things we see or hear, and our reactions to them. In most cases the opinions we form serve little purpose except to excite our emotional nerve centers, putting more and more stress on our adrenal glands. If you sit back a moment and analyze just how the many opinions you form, and desperately cling to, affect life, you will have to admit that they do not really serve much purpose. Opinions have never changed anything for the better, only positive actions have. Incidentally, positive activity rarely produces stress because it sets up a free flow of human energy, which can actually energize and rejuvenate the body.

Another major area of stress in our lives comes from a lack of proper forward planning. For example, many of us worry excessively about money problems. Most money problems come from over-extending ourselves and not planning properly for the potential financial ups and downs of life. We often get in over our heads and, subsequently, have to endure tremendous pressure in trying to meet all of our obligations. By having a forward plan for your life, much as a business man would have a business plan for success, you can often save yourself untold amounts of stress by looking forward.

All of this comes down to discipline. Looking forward, managing time, and controlling reactions over opinions, most of which are worthless in the grand scheme of things, can go a long way in reducing the overall total stress load upon the body. Once this has begun, the adrenals can once again get on with the real job of producing hormones and regulating your complex chemical hormonal laboratory.

Diet and Nutrition to the Rescue

Any nutritional program that seeks to address and improve the symptoms of menopause must place strong emphasis upon the nutrients involved in stress. Since the adrenal glands are the stress glands, these nutrients can be effectively used to provide adrenal support.

When we think of the stress nutrients, the B-complex must come to mind first. While all of the B-complex nutrients are not directly involved in the stress cycle, those that are directly involved will be consumed in great volume during periods of high stress.

Pantothenic acid, a B-complex nutrient, is the chief stress-relieving nutrient. In the absence of Pantothenic acid, the adrenal glands begin to shrivel up and become filled with dead, inactive cells. Under this condition, the adrenals cannot produce cortisone or the estrogen-like hormones.

So important is Pantothenic acid that even a slight deficiency reduces adrenal function. The more stress you find yourself under, the greater the consumption of Pantothenic acid will take place. It is not uncommon, under periods of severe stress, for the body to consume in excess of 2000-mg of Pantothenic acid per 24-hour period!

The twin stress relief nutrient to Pantothenic acid is vitamin B-12. This essential nutrient is also consumed in much higher amounts during stress. By taking extra vitamin B-12, it not only replaces this loss, but also feeds the nervous system and helps to prevent the sympathetic nervous response so common in uncontrolled menopause.

While adrenal hormones are produced without the aid of vitamin C, the need for this antioxidant nutrient rises during the menopause. When the adrenal glands are over-worked, they are subject to internal hemorrhage. Vitamin C prevents this breakdown of the integrity of the cardiovascular system. One obvious sign of a vitamin C deficiency is the breaking of the small capillaries in the legs and on the face.

We must also consider vitamin B-6 in any approach to menopause. Vitamin B-6 is the universal carrier nutrient, helping all other nutrients in its presence to be better absorbed where specifically needed.

Herbology, the science of plants for health and healing, has made some powerful contributions to the management of menopause. There are many herbs and herbal extracts, which have been used for hundreds of years and remain today, some of the best sources for re-balancing the body chemistry of the menopausal woman.

Black Cohosh is the first herb that deserves our attention. Used widely by native Americans, and indigenous peoples of Central America, Black Cohosh has long been a favorite in the relief of menstrual cramps and symptoms of menopause. Studies show that the use of Black Cohosh, as part of a total program, can increase the estrogenic effect of other herbs.

The next herb of mention is Dong Quai. In Asia, Dong Quai is regarded as the 'female' tonic of choice. Clinical studies conducted on this herb support the efficacy of Dong Quai in reducing and eliminating hot flashes, so often occurring during the menopausal years.

Licorice Root is an ancient herb used for its positive effect upon the adrenal glands. Since the adrenals are at the heart of the solution, Licorice Root should always be included in the management program.

One of the most annoying complaints from women of menopausal years is the drying out of vaginal tract. This uncomfortable condition frequently leads to a decreased libido and all the self-esteem issues connected with that problem. Red Raspberry, the leaves of which are important, have been used by the ancients to encourage easy labor. Why is this important during menopause? It is because Raspberry exercises a relaxing, lubricating effect on the longitudinal muscles of the uterus, helping the body to reduce the symptoms of vaginal irritations.

Mexican Wild Yam is probably the best known herb for managing menopause. Creams made from this herb have been shown to increase progesterone, an important hormone group, in post-menopausal women. Many excellent preparations are available.

Although not a vitamin, lecithin is another important nutrient. This fatty substance, along with fatty acids such as Omega 3 and Omega 6, is essential. It provides the sterols, which are the raw materials, or building blocks needed by the adrenals when making hormones.

Many who suffer from menopause have trouble sleeping at night. This lack of satisfying rest further contributes to the central nervous system irritation and subsequent symptomology. If sleeping is a problem, it can be addressed in several ways through the use of specific herbs.

Firstly, natural calming herbs such as Kava Kava, are highly recommended if you find yourself high strung and anxious. Secondly, if you take Valerian Root an hour or so before bed, along with some calcium, you will fall asleep more easily.

Finally, I recommend the herbs Damiana, Suma, and Schizandra for their long-standing female properties, which include vaginal support and increased libido.

Another factor often greatly affecting the menopause is a lack of protein. All hormones in the body are constituents of protein and a lack of this body building substance can result in overall hormone deficiencies. Everyone needs a minimum of 60 grams of high quality protein every day; you will require more if you are active.

Enter the Phytoestrogens

Absolutely essential to hormone regulation during menopause is another group of nutrients called phytoestrogens. These substances, which come from plants, are capable of producing mild estrogenic effects. These effects can be greatly enhanced by using a phytoestrogen product composed from a variety of sources. By providing these estrogen effects, symptoms of menopause can be greatly reduced.

Dietary phytoestrogens and other phytoestrogen-containing herbs, some of which we have already discussed, offer other significant advantages as well.

What About Estrogen Therapy?

I am sure most women have heard about the potential health problems associated with the use of either synthetic or even natural estrogen replacement. The significant health risks associated with this therapy include an increase in cancer, gallbladder disease and the thrombo-embolic diseases, such as strokes and heart attacks. If your physician determines your need for hormone replacement therapy, seek another opinion. If you discover that you must have this treatment, always insist upon receiving both estrogen and progesterone. This will greatly reduce the risks involved with this type of treatment.

The good news is that the plant derived phytoestrogens we discussed do not carry any of these increased health risks. Therefore, they should be used as the first treatment of choice. Remember, as with nutrients and supplements, phytoestrogens work best when in proper combinations rather than separately or individually. Currently, we are successfully using phytoestrogens from flavones, flavonols, flavanones, isoflavones, saponins, and ligans.

Studies affirming the direct connection between estrogen therapy and increases in disease continue to surface in scientific literature. Today, there is a better, and very effective, option for most women. The protocol outlined at the end of this book has proven to be very effective in the safe management of menopausal symptoms for thousands of women.

A Word About Hysterectomy

The hysterectomy can bring about all the same symptoms of menopause with additional problems and increased nutritional needs. There are several different types of hysterectomy procedures. Those having a 'full' or complete hysterectomy enter what could be called 'instant menopause' because the ovaries have been removed. This means that your body has not had the chance to gradually adjust to the hormone and glandular changes.

In this situation, we can further help support the body by increasing the potencies of some of the nutrients and compounds previously discussed. We can also add other nutrients to help mitigate some of the short-term side effects of the surgery. Itemized later in this chapter is an excellent protocol, listing ingredients and potencies recommended for an initial program.

After a complete hysterectomy, two of the big problems are fluid retention and electrolyte imbalance. Potassium can be very helpful in this situation since it will help accelerate the sodium/potassium pump and rid the body of excess fluid and built-up toxins. By using a supplement that provides not only potassium but calcium and magnesium as well, all the major electrolytes are addressed and any deficiencies can be eliminated.

Multi-glandular therapy is frequently of benefit since many glands and organs are affected during 'instant menopause'. Desiccated, or dehydrated, nucleoproteins, from a broad spectrum of glands and organs, can provide the much-needed boost these ladies need.

Women who undergo a total hysterectomy, and hence enter 'instant menopause', can be very sensitive to glucose metabolism. When blood sugar levels rise and fall erratically, the typical result is frequent mood swings, anxiety and loss of energy. This being the case, special attention should be given to the amount of sugar and sugar-forming foods in the diet. A diet consisting of high amounts of these foods should be eliminated. If these dietary changes do not solve the blood sugar level problems, supplementing with aspartic acid, bilberry extract, and the minerals chromium and vanadium, should prove to be extremely helpful.

Osteoporosis
Another serious menopause related condition is

osteoporosis. This condition is caused by the lack of calcium in the diet and/or the body's inability to properly digest, absorb, and assimilate calcium. This results in the loss of bone density.

Several myths are associated with osteoporosis. Firstly, we are always told it is a woman's disease. It is not. Men also get osteoporosis; it is just more common in women. Secondly, we are told it is a hormone problem. That is not exactly accurate. However, severe hormone imbalances can accelerate osteoporosis and should be addressed by the methods outlined in this book. If you do not have severe imbalances and related symptoms, you do not need hormone replacement therapy, or anything else, to prevent osteoporosis. This disease usually begins at a much younger age and by the time you are middle age, the stage for this debilitating disease is already in place.

There are two major causes leading to the development of osteoporosis. First and foremost it is a calcium deficiency. Calcium is the most difficult mineral for the body to absorb and hence many people, especially women, can be more or less constantly in a deficient state. The most common form of calcium sold as a dietary supplement, is calcium carbonate and may be found in products labeled egg shell, dolomite, and coral calcium. This form of calcium is very inexpensive and therefore very popular. The problem with this form of calcium is that it is also very alkaline, making it nearly impossible to absorb.

In order for calcium to be absorbed into the body

tissues and thereby returned to the bone, it must be acidic. Having a pH of 6.0 or lower is ideal. Calcium carbonate has a pH around 11, making it very alkaline. The only way the body can absorb and utilize this calcium is by acidifying it down to a much lower level. Natural hydrochloric acid, produced in a healthy stomach, serves this purpose nicely. The problem is that most people, after the age of 40, no longer produce adequate amounts of hydrochloric acid. This is due to the over consumption of dead, lifeless foods that have been over-cooked, canned, frozen, or otherwise adulterated from their natural state.

This dietary abuse, for years or decades, leaves the body deficient in hydrochloric acid and enzymes. If you suffer from indigestion, heartburn, gas, bloating or belching after meals, you can rest assured that you are not absorbing calcium either.

The second major cause of osteoporosis is the lack of natural stomach acids. If you take calcium carbonate, for example, and you have a hydrochloric acid deficiency, your absorption of this form of calcium will be only about 10 percent. This means that if you are taking a 1000-mg tablet of calcium, you are actually getting only about 100-mg of useable calcium. That is nowhere near enough to prevent osteoporosis.

Therefore, in addressing osteoporosis from a nutritional standpoint, we first use a form of calcium that has been pre-acidified. The combination of calcium we use successfully at The Institute is a 50/50 blend of calcium citrate and calcium malate. This is the only combination proven in double blind, placebo-controlled studies, to both prevent further bone loss and to increase bone density in post-menopausal women!

To this combination, we add the six co-factor nutrients necessary to carry the calcium back to the bone and increase absorption. They include Vitamin D, Magnesium, Boron, Manganese, Copper and Zinc. Since these nutrients must be present at the same time as the calcium, we have combined them into one single capsule to ensure absorption.

If we suspect a pH imbalance in the body, we know it would be impossible to achieve adequate calcium uptake. For those individuals, we conduct a pH test to determine acid and alkaline ratios. If the individual is indeed too alkaline, we use a preparation consisting of betaine hydrochloride (natural hydrochloric acid), and a variety of precursor substances used by the body to build enzymes.

Lastly, we use a synthetic version of a plant compound called ipriflavone. This nutrient has demonstrated an enormous role in preventing and treating osteoporosis, especially in women. Ipriflavone prevents bone breakdown, while enhancing the bone-building process. Over 150 studies have examined the effects of ipriflavone and most all were very positive. In one study, 79 post-menopausal women were given either ipriflavone or a placebo. After the one year period, the results showed that ipriflavone was just as effective as estrogen!

The great thing about ipriflavone is that it doesn't

have any estrogen effects, so it will not contribute to the side effects often seen with that therapy.

The Menopause Protocol

In summarizing the many factors which can positively improve symptoms of the menopause, we offer the following protocol. We start with the basic, or foundation program, and offer suggestions on how to proceed if adequate control is not achieved.

Step 1: The Foundation.

Before beginning any dietary supplement program aimed at mega-dose amounts of specific nutrients, the foundation of the internal biochemistry must be addressed. We do this through a concept developed at The Institute. It is called Full Spectrum Nutrition and it addresses the complete daily nutritional needs of the human body.

Every day of your life you need at least 120 nutrients in order to maintain bio-chemical activities within your body. These nutrients include amino acids, fatty acids, vitamins, major minerals, trace minerals, phytonutrient chemicals from plants and extra-strength, heavy hitting antioxidants to protect the body from free radical damage caused by toxins in the environment. Regardless of lifestyle or physical condition, everyone over 12 years of age needs this combination of daily baseline nutrients.

Once this has been attained, we then add the following nutrients for specific menopausal support.

Vitamin B6 .... 25 - 50 mg
Vitamin B12 .... 100 mcg
Pantothenic Acid .... 250-1000 mg
Lecithin .... as needed
Ipriflavones .... 300-600 mg
Red Raspberry .... 25 mg
Black Cohosh Root .... 20 mg
Damiana Leaf .... 30 mg
Don Quai Root (4.1) .... 100 mg
Licorice Root .... 25 mg
Mexican Yam Root .... 200 mg
Suma Root .... 25 mg
Schizandra Berries .... 25 mg
White Peony Root .... 100 mg
Hesperidin .... 100 mg

Phytoestrogen Compounds including:

Flavons - bioflavinoids
Saponins - Sarsaparilla, Muira Puama and Wild Yam
Phytosterols
Isoflavons
Ligans

If you or your loved ones are suffering needlessly from menopausal or post-menopausal symptoms, this formula may solve the problem.

Step 2: Adjunct Nutrients for Specific Support.

If considerable stress, mood swings, and/or anxiety is involved, we add another high potency stress formula, providing more B-complex with a continued emphasis upon Vitamin B12 and Pantothenic Acid.

If there are blood sugar problems, we add a combination of chromium, vanadium, bilberry extract, and aspartic acid. This helps to regulate blood sugar and reduce cravings for concentrated sugar foods.

The 'golden years' are supposed to be the best years of life. They should be filled with time to expand your horizons, take on projects, and fulfill interests that had to be postponed earlier in life due to other commitments.

In order for you to be able to really 'live' these years to the fullest, they cannot be filled with the annoying and often debilitating symptoms and side effects of the menopause.

By following the guidelines set forth in this chapter, every woman can look forward to enjoying the post-menopausal years and reap the rewards, which they deserve for a lifetime of hard work.

In closing this chapter, I must remind you that the protocols given in this chapter are only as good as how faithfully you follow them. Since they are based upon natural nutrients and nutrient co-factors, they will not, suddenly and instantly, transform your body chemistry overnight. Conversely, they will not put your body and your health at risk as do many other forms of drug therapy.

You can truly have the quality of life and experience the joy you have waited for. Take responsibility for your health by caring for the only real house you will ever have - the body in which you live.

Chapter 9
The Aging Male

L ike the women we discussed last chapter, men too, become 'high milers'. If they haven't taken care of themselves down through their years, they can expect a similar amount of problems in later life. These problems will require a much more ridged care and maintenance program in order to achieve any reasonable quality of life in the later years.

Over and above these obvious problems of poor maintenance, which will be addressed for everyone in Part III of this book, the male body also goes through some natural biological changes. As with the female, these can be prevented, minimized, or even reversed through proper application of nutrition principles.

Some of the problems men routinely face later in life include a diminished libido or sex drive, prostate problems, which include benign prostatic hypertrophy (BPH) - an inflammation of the prostate gland, prostate infection, and of course, prostate cancer. Well guys, take heart; there are solutions for these problems.

Impotence: Rekindling the Fire in the Furnace

I have long had the reputation of openly addressing issues which many people have felt embarrassed or uncomfortable discussing. Such areas include male impotence and prostate problems. Yet despite this taboo subject, these problems affect many millions of men every year.

The age of the magic pill seems to be upon us. What a great time for an aging man to be alive! The new 'sex pill', soon to be sold under many different names, is the greatest - or is it?

With every wonder drug there is often a dark side. The sex drugs are no exception. Sadly, many people who are taking these drugs often should not be doing so. Further, many of the side effects can go from merely annoying to fatal in the presence of other medications. Is there a safer way? Oh yes!

As a man ages there are several factors that can adversely affect both his sex drive as well as his physiology. For example, about 85% of Erectile Dysfunction is caused by organic or physical circumstances while 15% are caused by psychological problems such as depression, performance anxiety, and stress.

Factors Leading to Impotence

Drugs:
Alcohol
Antihistamines (allergy medicine)

Antihypertensives (blood pressure medicine)
Antidepressants
Antipsychotics
Tobacco
Tranquilizers

Endocrine Disorders:

Diabetes
Hypothyroidism
Decreased male sex hormone production
Elevated prolactin
Elevated estrogen

Other Disorders:

Cardiovascular Disease (atherosclerosis)
Depression
Hypertension

These obvious, and not so obvious, factors should be ruled out and/or eliminated before further steps are considered. Once these have been addressed, there are several nutrients, mostly herbs, which can assist in both increasing sex drive as well as improving physiological performance.

Building a Safe and Effective 'Sexual Potency' Formula

Nutrients, specifically herbs, are not only generally safe but in most cases, very effective as well. Following is a list of ingredients you should consider if you are suffering from impotence and lack of sexual drive.

Vitamin E: You should ensure that you are taking at least 400 IU daily.

Vitamin B3 (Niacin): This nutrient will cause dilation of the capillaries, helping to increase blood flow to the penis.

Zinc: Long associated with sexual prowess, zinc is the main constituent of all male hormones. The seminal fluid contains the highest amount of concentrated zinc in the male body.

PABA (Para-aminobenzoic acid): This B-complex nutrient also increases specific hormone production.

In addition to these specific nutrients, the following herbs should be considered in a balanced ratio. (See Chapter 17 on specific protocols under impotence for details.)

Helpful Herbs

Fo Ti Root
Gotu Kola Nuts
Aveena Sativa Leaves
Damiana Leaves
Ginseng Root
Rubi Fructus Leaves
Muira Puama Extract
Tribulus Terrestris

If erectile dysfunction is caused by circulatory problems consider the following...

Dimethylglycine - a potent oxygenater
Octacosanol
Gamma Oryzanol
Ginkgo Biloba

There is one other herb, which we have left out of the above list because it is a double edge sword. I have used it very successfully with many of our clients, but it first must be determined that you do not suffer from uncontrolled, silent hypertension as the herb yohimbe can raise blood pressure in some individuals. If hypertension is not a problem, by all means add yohimbe to your program. The active ingredient in yohimbe bark, called yohimbine, is available generally, only by prescription. For most men however, you will obtain adequate response from the concentrated herb, without the need for the prescription variety.

The use of these herbs and nutrients is exceedingly safer than the pharmaceutical choices. These alternatives should be considered BEFORE resorting to more invasive treatments.

Another thing to remember is that natural products don't work quite as fast as drugs. You can't expect to take a natural product and be ready, willing, and able in an hour. If you have an ongoing problem, consider taking these nutrients and herbs on a daily basis, right along with the rest of your health building program.

The Prostate

Every man dreads the pain, annoyance, and embarrassment caused by the problems that surface when the prostate gland no longer functions properly. We are all too aware of those annoying problems such as painful burning upon urination, or having to get up three or four times a night, disturbing what otherwise might have been a restful sleep. Then there is the constant feeling that we can never ever quite empty our bladder, no matter how many trips we make to the bathroom. These are classic signs of a condition called benign prostatic hyperplasia, or simply put, a swelling of the prostate gland. There are many reasons why this condition occurs and it strikes about 60 percent of all men over 50 years of age.

Left unchecked, prostate problems and related symptoms continue to increase. Other annoying conditions can develop, such as being unable to sit through a movie or business meeting without excusing yourself to make a trip to the bathroom.

One of the most devastating symptoms, which often develops as prostate problems continue, is painful sexual intercourse. If this persists or if you are taking certain medications, you can loose your desire to have sex altogether. This impotence leads to a whole host of other problems, both physical and emotional. Should you elect to turn to surgery for your prostate problems, this could end your sex life completely and forever. The prostate is an integral part of every man's sexuality, but when prostate problems arise, it can rapidly become a burden.

If left unchecked, inflammation of the prostate can lead to prostatitis, a potentially painful and serious infection. This infection can spread to the bladder and even the kidneys.

Another area that strikes terror by the mere mention of the word is prostate cancer. You need to recognize the early warning signs of this potentially fatal form of cancer as well as your options for both preventing and controlling this condition in your life.

The good news is that there are safe, natural and effective ways of handling this and other classic prostate problems without the need for ineffective and often harmful drugs and painful, risky surgical procedures. If you have a prostate condition, read this section carefully BEFORE you elect a more invasive procedure. If you have already begun pharmaceutical treatment and it has proven less than effective or the side effects of the medication are less than desirable, consider the protocols outlined in the pages ahead. They have been well researched and clinically tested on thousands of men with excellent results.

This chapter will help you to identify the early warning signs of prostate trouble and offer a step by step program of natural methods of managing and even reversing prostate disease. The point of this chapter is to encourage you to seek and insist upon natural prevention and control rather than the standard method of management and treatment that has failed so many men before you.

You will also learn why conventional medicine mocks prevention. You see, the entire financial stability of allopathic medicine in many countries lies in treatment - sadly often avoidable treatment - rather than prevention.

Facts about Your Prostate and what can go wrong

Your prostate consists of both gland and muscle tissues, covered with a fibrous outer coating. Its glandular function is primarily to produce semen, the lubricating and transport fluid which carries your sperm from the testicles out through the urethra. The muscular action of the prostate provides power for the seminal fluid, increasing the force of the ejaculation. Another part of its muscular action includes assisting the bladder in the flow of urine.

Anatomically, the prostate gland is located right under your bladder. It surrounds a portion of the urethra, a tube which carries both urine and semen through the penis.

As we age our prostate naturally grows. This is due to the muscular tissue, since all muscles grow with age and use. Prior to puberty your prostate is quite small, about the size of a small marble. After puberty it goes through a rather rapid growth spurt. During young and middle adulthood the prostate is roughly the size of a golf ball. Under healthy conditions, it should remain about this size for many, many years. Then after about age 50, it begins to grow again. How much it grows and if it becomes inflamed depends upon a variety of factors.

As the aging process takes place, several problems relative to the prostate gland can occur. It is essential that you understand and be able to identify these problems in their early stages. For it is at this time when preventive methods have their greatest effect.

Some prostate conditions which can develop include congested prostate, inflamed prostate (prostatitis), an abnormal enlargement of the prostate (benign prostatic hyperplasia), and, of course, prostate cancer.

Congested Prostate

A congested prostate is a condition that can occur if your normal sexual rhythm is altered. Extremes in sexual habit, either too much or too little, can cause this often painful condition to lead to other, more serious prostate problems.

Prostate congestion occurs if there is excessive sexual stimulation, such as foreplay, without the eventual ejaculation. As the seminal fluid increases without release, the prostate can become swollen, causing pain, which can spread to the testicles. This same condition can also occur if you reach orgasm too early, thus not allowing for the full voiding of the seminal fluid.

This problem can also develop if you go for long periods of time without sexual release.

The key to both the prevention and relief of this condition is to expel the accumulated fluid and then try and develop a regular rhythm for sexual activity.

A congestion of the prostate is often the first problem men experience. In fact it can happen almost any time after puberty.

Recommended Protocol for Prostate Congestion

1. Full Spectrum Nutrition covering all 100 plus nutrients in both balance and potency.

2. Since a congested prostate is caused by extremes, establish a fairly regular schedule of sexual activity. If you have a problem

you can either ejaculate it away or in the case of excess, give it a rest!

3. Avoid the conditions under which prostate congestion can occur

Abstinence from ejaculation for prolonged periods
Long periods of foreplay without ejaculation
Early ejaculation without sufficient foreplay
Impotence
Coitus Interruptus
Prolonged Intercourse (heroic sex)

4. If all else fails, you may need to ask your doctor for a prostatic massage to empty the seminal fluid.

Prostate Inflammation.

This condition, identified by an often acute swelling of the prostate, can easily develop into what we call prostatitis, an infection of the prostate gland.

Prostatitis can be caused by either invading bacteria or virus but almost always it's from bacteria found in the intestinal tract. This is why it is important to maintain proper balance of the friendly bacteria in the intestinal tract through eating foods which are high in natural bacteria such as cheese and yogurt or better still, taking a dietary supplement of multi-source bacteria. Other possible causes for prostatitis could be tuberculosis, yeast infections from the female vaginal tract and other opportunistic infections.

Acute prostatitis may be identified by a rapid onset of symptoms, which quickly increase in severity. (Following this discussion is a list of warning signs.)

Chronic prostatitis is the same condition but usually in lessor intensity while reoccurring on a varying basis.

The problem, as with most infections, is once you have had the first one, subsequent infections are easier to get. If you have already had one attack of prostatitis, you have roughly a 30 percent chance of getting another. If you have had two or more attacks, you have better than a 60 to 70 percent chance of another down the road. It is for this reason that we should look at aggressively preventing this condition from occurring.

Prostatitis is often incredibly painful, causing a heavy feeling in the lower bladder and bowel area, with a frantic urge to urinate. When you urinate it can cause a deep burning pain through the penis, which may spread to the lower back, the scrotum, and even the rectum. Left unchecked, the infection can rapidly spread to the bladder and kidneys.

Warning Signs of Prostatitis

1. Hot Pain in Your Groin
2. An Almost Uncontrollable Urge to Urinate
3. Painful Urination
4. Fever and/or Nausea
5. Lower Back Pain
6. Pus or Blood in Urine

The standard treatment for this condition is an aggressive course of antibiotic. Because of the severity of both the infection and the symptoms, antibiotic therapy for an acute attack may be necessary. There are measures you can take to reduce your risk of prostatitis and prevent a reoccurrence.

Protocol for Chronic Prostatitis

1. During an attack drink copious amounts of water to flush out the infection. One glass every hour.

2. Use natural antibiotics and immune stimulants such as Echinacea, Goldenseal, garlic, concentrated collostrum from organically raised cattle, and mushroom extracts.

3. Full Spectrum Nutrition which includes

all 100 nutrients your body needs on a daily basis.

4. Extra amounts of prostate friendly nutrients such as vitamins A, C, E, Beta-carotene and the mineral zinc. (See nutrient protocols for combinations and potencies in Chapter 17.)

5. Cranberry juice should be consumed regularly since it causes bacteria to be flushed from the bladder wall. Cranberry juice also helps prevent infections of the bladder, kidney and prostate and should be a regular part of your daily program if you have reoccurring problems in these areas.

6. A light massage of the groin area will help to increase circulation to the prostate area, lower inflammation and increase urination.

Prostate Enlargement

This condition is the most common prostate problem, making it the number one reason why men over 50 visit their doctor. Medically the condition is called either benign prostatic hyperplasia (BPH) or benign prostate hypertrophy. The use of the term benign in the name means that it is a condition which is not cancerous. But that's the only good news about it.

BPH can be very distressing and painful. In some rare instances it can lead to a life-threatening situation.

The symptoms of prostate enlargement or BPH, are inconvenient, painful and often debilitating.

Warning Signs of Benign Prostatic Hyperplasia

1. A weak stream of urine - even though the urgency is there.
2. Dribbling after the initial urine stream subsides.
3. Frequent nocturnal urination. (getting up two, three, or more times per night)
4. Feeling of fullness in the bladder
5. Total inability to urinate due to blockage of the urethra.
6. Inability to empty the bladder.
7. Stopping and starting during urination
8. Painful orgasm
9. Impotence or diminished libido
10. Fatigue

Left unchecked, these symptoms can worsen to the point of misery and result in frequent infections due to the inability to completely empty the bladder of waste matter.

As we mentioned earlier, BPH is one of the most common complaints of men from middle age forward.

In the United States alone, 2 million men visit their doctors every year for this condition. These visits result in hundreds of thousands of prescriptions to be written for medications that not only have a fair amount of side effects, but have been shown to be only about 30 percent effective in the long-term management of the problem. Further, these doctor visits result in over 400,000 prostate surgeries annually. It is estimated that conventional medical treatments of BPH exceeds $2 billion annually.

A Simple Test For Early BPH

Respond to each statement with either a yes or no answer. We will only be concerned with the yes responses.

1. Urination has become more difficult than it used to be.
2. Many times I have to 'push' to start the flow of urine.
3. I awake two or more times each night to urinate.
4. When urinating, the stream stops and starts again several times.
5. I have a feeling that after urination, my bladder is not fully empty.
6. It is harder to wait, when I have to relieve myself, than it used to be.
7. My urinary stream is weaker and less forceful than before.

If you answered yes to just one question on this test, you should pay close attention to signs of additional complications. If you answered yes to two or more statements you likely have early BPH. This is not a cause for concern. Most all these are early warning signs and you are still in an excellent position of managing and even reversing this problem through the use of completely natural methods.

The Role of Hormones.

When your prostate naturally begins to grow again around the age of 45 or 50, hormones are essentially responsible for this problem. Testosterone, the male sex hormone, reaches its peak between the ages of 16 and 20. After age 20, it slowly begins to decline while the production of other hormones such as prolactin, estradiol and follicle related hormones increase.

Once we reach middle age, production of an enzyme, which has been labeled 5-alpha-reductase, increases, oftentimes dramatically. This enzyme converts testosterone into another hormone called dehydrotestosterone, a relative. During our younger years, this hormone is essential. It is responsible for our sex drive and sexual development. Later in life however, an excess of this hormone produces a variety of negative manifestations including excessive body hair, a loss of hair on the head, adult onset acne and excessive growth of the prostate gland.

Studies continue to show that those men with higher amounts of dihydrotestosterone during middle age will have a much greater chance of developing all of the above symptomology, including prostate enlargement.

Medicine to the Rescue but... Is Life Really Better Through Chemistry???

As soon as the apparent cause of BPH had been identified, the drug companies wasted little time in coming up with a chemical which could be sold to the many millions of men suffering with this problem. It seemed simple, just find a drug that inhibits the formation of 5-alpha-reductase, and everybody will be happy - and rich!

In 1992 Merck & Company released a chemical drug called finasteride. It is sold to you as Proscar ®. Early clinical trials with the drug seemed to be promising. Proscar ® caused considerable decreases in BPH symptoms. What was not celebrated or even talked about in the interviews and press releases were the terrible side effects of Proscar ®. Merck never mentioned the tremendously high incidence of impotence and decreased libido as well as numerous ejaculatory disorders in men taking the drug.

To further the sales of their new 'wonder' drug, Merck issued statements to the effect that their new 'pill' could reverse male pattern baldness. Now at last vanity had entered into the picture and every guy from age 35 forward was willing to stand in line for the stuff.

Today Proscar ® is being taken by over 650,000 men in 25 countries at a cost of about $80.00 per month. This means that these desperate men are increasing the revenues of Merck's bank accounts by more than a half billion dollars every year.

Taking a closer look at the side effects and warnings for Proscar ® is discomforting at best. It warns that women who are pregnant with a male child could seriously risk the child's health by even touching tablets of Proscar ®. These women are also advised, for the same reason, against having intercourse without a condom if the man is taking Proscar ®.

The other commonly used drug for BPH is called terzosin hydrochloride and is made and sold by Abbott Labs under the trade name Hytrin ®. This medication was originally used for hypertension. Side effects for this drug are also very annoying. They include erectile dysfunction, fatigue, dizziness, heart palpitations, sinus congestion, and in some cases, severe low blood pressure.

To make matters worse, neither of these drugs do one single thing to help your body reverse BPH. They may help alleviate some of the annoying symptoms, but the cause of the disease remains and the progression continues unabated.

What About the Knife?

When drugs fail to curtail either the symptoms or progression of BPH, the physician turns to his or her next line of defense, which is surgery.

Between 1984 and 1990 prostate surgery boomed. Today, urologists generate over $5 billion dollars annually by performing over 400,000 prostate operations. It is estimated that there are over 13,000 urologists in the United States that derive 50 percent of their business from the prostate operation alone!

Fortunately there are a number of safe and highly effective supplements available, which in clinical studies and practical applications, have been proven to be far more effective than drug therapy and far safer than surgical intervention.

The Natural Way to Prevent & Reverse BPH

The toughest part of this whole concept for me to understand is the waste of money, time and compromised health for tens of thousands of men when a safe, natural method of prostate management exists. This program has been clinically and empirically tested over and over again. The results continually show that not only is the natural program safer, but it is at least 50 percent more effective than drug therapy!

You can probably see by now why the big drug companies don't want you to have this information. Yet choice is of utmost importance, especially when you are making choices about your health. These choices, right or wrong, can affect the quality and even the quantity of your life ahead. You have the right to be informed.

In the protocol for BPH, we find benefit from vitamins, minerals, and especially selected herbs. Let's talk about some of the major players in the natural fight against BPH. Then we'll give you the complete protocol.

Enter the Herbs

Herbology is mankind's oldest form of medicine. In our desperate search for answers to many devastating diseases, we are once again returning to nature, seeking plant derived chemicals for the management of sickness. I often wonder what the state of human health might be today if we had not strayed so far away from nature and a natural way of life.

The first herb that must be considered in any prostate program is known as Serenoa repens. You may be familiar with it as saw palmetto.

We actually use the berry produced by this plant for the magical effects it has upon prostate health. If you remember our discussion of the role hormones play in the evolving process of BPH, then you know that testosterone alone is not a bad thing, but when it is converted to dihydrotestosterone we have a problem. Concentrations of extracts from the Serenoa repens berry actually block the conversion of testosterone into dihydrotestosterone! The herb is not only all-natural but it is safe and inexpensive as well. The pharmaceutical industry produces chemicals to try and block the production of the enzyme 5-alpha-reductase, causing terrible side effects; nature has given us a natural method of accomplishing the exact same thing with absolutely no side effects whatsoever!

How long has this plant been used for health? Longer than the drug companies have even been in existence! American Indians routinely used the berries from the saw palmetto plant to help with genitourinary tract problems.

Saw palmetto has been used by herbalists, both ancient and modern, for its natural aphrodisiac properties.

In recent years, at least 16 scientific double-blind, placebo controlled clinical studies have been conducted on the extract of this ancient plant. Every single study has shown that it improves urination, urine flow, reduces pain, and reduces prostate size.

Despite this overwhelming body of clinical evidence, the Food and Drug Administration concluded that the results were insignificant. Why did they take this position? To answer that, at least in part, we must consider the position taken by drug industry leaders regarding safe, inexpensive, natural substances. Not surprisingly, with billions to loose, the drug companies conducted their own studies with the obvious conclusion that the natural plant extracts were nowhere near as effective as their pharmaceuticals.

Serenoa repens has been in use in many countries of Europe for at least 15 years. Yet despite this lengthy track record of results and satisfaction, drug companies still suppress this information in the United States. According to clinical studies conducted by Merck themselves, less than 50 percent of the men taking the drug Proscar ® evaluated it as effective. By the same token, similar evaluation studies conducted with Serenoa repens indicated that 90 percent of the men taking it were completely satisfied with the results!

Nature comes to the prostate rescue once again in the form of another plant called Pygeum africanum. A native of Africa, it too has been used for decades in many places around the world to successfully treat and reverse BPH.

One clinical study involving Pygeum africanum showed that 80 percent of the participants reported significant improvement in their symptoms after just 30 days into the study.

In the United States many physicians have been reluctant to become overly excited about these herbs because the drug companies are spending so much time and money to ensure that they think otherwise.

On the one hand, progress is being made because many nutritional companies are now formulating products containing one or both of these excellent herbs. Unfortunately, in our haste to bring these products to market, many companies have overlooked some of the other important co-factors which not only help the herbs to work better but also contribute healing and preventive properties of their own.

The amino acids Glycine, Leanne, and Glutamic acid have shown to help relieve prostate symptoms such as getting up at night, frequency and urgency of urination, and impaired urine flow. In one clinical study, men using these three amino acids alone, with no other treatment, observed that they had an 80 percent reduction in night time awakenings and over 70 percent of them reported a reduction in the urgency to urinate.

These amino acids have never been shown to help reverse or cure BPH. That's why you need to take them with the herbs we have already discussed. Their importance and contribution, however, lies in the rapid alleviation of annoying symptoms which is why we recommend them.

Although we earlier introduced you to several specific nutrients paramount to the treatment of BPH, they are worth reviewing. The vitamins B-6, C, and E are crucial for several reasons. Vitamins C and E are powerful antioxidants, important in the prevention and mitigation of most chronic disease conditions. Vitamin B-6, the universal catalyst or carrier, helps all other nutrients to work better. Additionally, Vitamin B-6 has a direct effect upon prolactin levels, reducing them safely and naturally. A reduction of prolactin prevents the conversion of testosterone to dihydrotestosterone.

Lastly, we have a single mineral, but a very important mineral. Zinc has long been associated with male sexual health. This is because zinc is an integral part of hormone structures and a major constituent of seminal fluid and is involved in the production of sperm. When boys hit puberty, their hormone levels rise, oftentimes rapidly. This causes a depletion of zinc in the body, which can lead to a depressed immune system and such annoying side effects as acne.

As we age, a zinc deficiency can lead to impotence

and prostate enlargement because the prostate tissue requires zinc to maintain its health and integrity. Further, adequate zinc also prevents the formation of dihydrotestosterone, making it a multi-purpose mineral for total prostate health.

If you have begun to notice some of the symptoms of BPH (see the self-test appearing earlier in this chapter), you should begin the following protocol at once. If you currently have BPH, you may use the same protocol but in higher potencies, at least for the first few months.

Protocol for the Prevention, Management, and Reversal of Benign Prostatic Hyperplasia:

Following are our recommendations for the management of BPH. Please see the protocol section in the back of this book for additional information regarding formulation and product suggestions.

1. Serenoa repens extract should be taken daily in doses of about 150 mg for prevention, and 200 mg to 300 mg for treatment of BPH.

2. Full Spectrum Nutrition providing 100+ nutrients in a balanced formulation which considers potency and ratio.

3. Essential Fatty Acids, especially the Omega

3 and Omega 6 groupings, are very important to good prostate health. Take three capsules of these oils daily.

4. Zinc is the single most important mineral for the prostate. I recommend zinc gluconate. A good dose would be about 30 mg per day.
5. Amino acids, Glycine, Alanine, and Glutamic acid should be taken daily in dosages of 200 mg each. If you already have BPH, you might want to double that amount for the first four to six weeks.
6. Pygeum africanum should be taken at the rate of 100 mg per day. If you already have moderate to severe BPH, consider 200 mg per day for the first four to six weeks.

7. Vitamin B-6, over and above the amount found in your Full Spectrum supplement, should be taken daily. We have found that an extra 50-mg, works very well.

8. Vitamins A, E, and C should also be taken in extra amounts because of their antioxidant properties.

9. Pumpkin Seed and Stinging Nettle Leaf should also be included at 150 mg or much of each.

Note: While this program has been clinically tested at the Institute and has been used with great success for many years, if you have BPH, you should be working in conjunction with your health care provider to establish a program that is right for you.

Prostate Cancer: The Big Fear

In the United States alone prostate cancer kills 45,000 men every year, with about 250,000 new cases of the disease being diagnosed annually.

There are some basic facts you should know about prostate cancer:

1. Your risk increases dramatically after age 60.
2. Most men over 80 have it already but will likely die of some other cause.
3. Prostate cancer seems to follow hereditary patterns. If it runs in your family, you are at a much greater risk.

Even with these guidelines, prostate cancer has been elusive simply because it has few early warning signs. Unlike BPH or other prostate problems, cancer offers no significant discomfort, especially in the early stages. Since cancer forms on the outside of the prostate, you do not usually experience the typical problems with urination and inflammation.

Early detection is still the best treatment for prostate cancer. This means that regular prostate exams, especially after the age of 55 or 60, are very important.

The real danger of prostate cancer is not the disease itself but its ability to spread to the bones. Once this has occurred, we are dealing with a much more severe disease condition.

Conventional methods of treating prostate cancer are much the same for all other forms of cancer. Surgery is probably near the top of the list of prostate cancer treatments. Yet, despite this popularity, there is no evidence that the radical prostatectomy is an effective therapy for prostate cancer! Radiation and chemotherapy treatments haven't changed much in decades and their success rate is marginal. Further, these invasive chemical treatments weaken the immune system, which is the reason we get most cancers in the first place.

Mandated radiation and/or chemotherapy should always be promptly followed by an aggressive nutritional supplementation program designed to rebuild the immune system.

I think it is interesting to note that recent data indicates that men 70 years old and older who elected to have the prostatectomy, on average, lived only a month or two longer than men with the same disease who did not have the operation!

Furthermore, the prostatectomy leaves about 85% of its patients impotent and 25% of them incontinent. Due to these serious side effects, a study in the Journal of the American Medical Association (May 1993) concluded that men 75 years of age or older are damaged more by radiation and surgical procedures to the prostate than by simply watching the disease passively. They further concluded that men of this age group were at greater risk from the treatment of their cancer than from doing nothing at all!

What about those prostate tests?

Since we all agree that early detection and careful observation of prostate cancer is important, how can we go about doing that? The most common test performed is a blood test for the presence of a protein produced by the prostate called prostate specific antigen (PSA). Generally speaking, the higher the PSA level in your blood, the greater your chances of having prostate cancer. Normal PSA levels are 0 to 4, while a moderately elevated reading would be somewhere in the 4 to 10 range. Any reading over 10 is considered high.

It is important for you to understand that just because your PSA reading is high, it doesn't necessarily mean you have prostate cancer. Furthermore, the PSA test fails to detect almost one third of all prostate cancers.

Rather than rush hastily into invasive treatments just because of an elevated PSA, we recommend a digital rectal exam, to detect physical changes to the outside of the prostate gland.

If you have prostate cancer, consider using the following recommendations for a few months and then have another exam and PSA test. You may be surprised to find that things are looking much better in that short a time.

Natural Protocol for Prostate Cancer

Following are recommendations of what we routinely use in the prevention and management of prostate cancer. Refer to the protocol section in the back of this book for additional information regarding formulation and product suggestion.

1. If the cancer is isolated in your prostate, you should only consider radiation, chemotherapy and especially surgery under very unique circumstances. These procedures will likely do more harm than good at this stage.

2. Follow the BPH protocol outlined earlier and again in the summary section at the end.

3. Watch your diet. Reduce the amount of animal fats you consume. This does not mean you should avoid quality protein, but be sure to trim fat and eat lean cuts. Add soy protein and soy products such as tofu to your diet. Soy increases the concentration of isoflavonoids in your blood. According to studies published in Lancet

(a highly respected British medical journal), isoflavonoids help regulate hormones in the body; prostate cancer is directly related to hormone balance.

4. Essential fatty acids should be increased to at least 6 capsules per day.

5. Increase your dosage of Serenoa repens to at least 400 mg per day.

6. Vitamin C should be increased to 6 to 12 grams per day.

7. Start a program of shark cartilage. Buy the 750-mg capsules (standard) and take between 8 and 10 capsules per day.

8. Reduce, or eliminate, the consumption of all alcoholic beverages.

Prostate cancer need not strike terror in your heart. Prostate cancer is not a death sentence if it is properly watched and the gland is supported with an aggressive nutrient therapy program. You should consider invasive therapies such as radiation, chemotherapy, and surgery only when absolutely necessary.

Newspapers, magazines, and televised 'special reports' paint a rather dismal picture of prostate problems. Remember, however, that all the horror stories about impotence, retrograde ejaculation, and incontinence ONLY OCCUR WHEN INVASIVE PROCEDURES SUCH AS RADIATION, CHEMOTHERAPY, AND ESPECIALLY SURGERY OCCUR. Remember, too, that prevention is far better than attempting a cure, but if you already have a prostate condition, there is still a great deal you can do to manage and even reverse many of the most common problems.

Find consolation in the fact that you do not have to look forward to impotence or erectile dysfunction in later years of life. The latest global research indicates that you have all the hope in the world for a satisfactory solution to prostate problems.

But, and it is a big BUT... you have to act! You must take responsibility for your condition and aggressively act in a non-invasive manner to provide the body with what it needs.

It is our belief that all disease begins with stress either physical, emotional or most often, both. Stress destroys a tremendous amount of nutrients; nutrients vital to the delicate balance of your internal biochemistry. When that chemistry is out of balance for long periods of time, disease and disorder are the inevitable result.

We all have the ability to return to a healthier and more balanced life. It is an undeniable fact of nature. The decision to make positive lifestyle changes will initiate a metamorphosis within our bodies, enabling us to maintain or regain our optimal health.

Chapter 10
Keeping The Mind As Strong As The Body

Let's face it. On occasion, we all 'forget' something, a regularly scheduled meeting, a birthday or anniversary, or where we left the cordless phone. It's simply a part of being human. However, when we begin to forget things frequently, it's a sign of trouble in the brain. As we age, our memory is frequently not as sharp as when we were younger. Just like the chemical functions in the body, those in the brain require more maintenance as we put more 'miles' on the body. What is the benefit of striving for physical health and well being if our thought process is severely impaired? Aging is inevitable; senility doesn't have to be.

Premature aging of the brain is caused, primarily, by our old enemies, the free radicals. Just as free radicals can attack specific body tissues such as collagen protein, connective tissue, and the muscles of the artery wall, they can also attack brain cells. Over time this free radical proliferation can lead to forgetfulness and senility. It has even been linked to Alzheimer's disease.

We know that there is a direct link between nutritional deficiencies and brain disorders. This direct relationship between malnutrition and dementia is well established. Is it possible to use this information to build a nutritional program that includes 'brain boosting' factors? Not only is it possible, it's a reality!

Factors Affecting Brain Function

The scenario begins very innocently. You find it increasingly difficult to concentrate or your thinking seems 'fuzzy' at times. You forget your appointment or can't remember the address of a close friend or relative. Or you see someone you've known for many years but can't remember his or her name. Are these incidents signs of old age or senility? Maybe, but there is a lot you can still do about it.

This 'annoying forgetfulness' can occur at any age. In younger people it is frequently the result of excess stress. As we age it can be a combination of stress as well as changes in brain chemistry. The latter is brought about by prolonged periods of nutritional deficiencies and the corresponding free radical damage. We know that senility and related brain dysfunction is not the inevitable result of aging since the majority of aging people don't suffer from these conditions. One explanation of the difference in people may be found in the work of Roger J. Williams, Ph.D. In explaining his concept of 'biochemical individuality', Williams reminds us that each one of us is as different on the inside as we are on the outside. This uniqueness makes us individuals. It also makes some of us more susceptible to brain damage from free radicals. Let's examine some of these factors and see how we can minimize their effect on our future.

Stress

Hormones released during prolonged periods of stress can actually impair neurological function in the brain. The nervous system, the center of which is in the brain, is an electrical 'super highway'. Over stimulation is similar to running a strong current through a finer gauge wire. Eventually something burns out. Stress, and stress produced hormones, stimulate the body's nervous system. When it becomes over-excited, access to information stored in our brain becomes restricted. This is why, when we are under excessive stress and pressure, simple facts that we know often escape us. It's not that this information is gone, we just momentarily can't access it.

Once we relax and calm down, this stored information can once again be retrieved. Over time, however, with repeated assaults of excess stress, recovery from temporary memory loss takes longer and longer.

Continuous stress and tension are by-products of our modern life. They wear down our resistance and cause us to be more susceptible to the degenerative forces that lead to chronic disease. Proper nutrition, exercise, and stress management are essential if we hope to preserve the quality of our lives. Since escaping stress is virtually impossible, we need to take positives steps to increase our ability to cope with it.

Managing stress in our lives is essential if we truly want optimal health. Stress can adversely affect so many areas of living that we feel it is truly the cardinal cause of all disease and disorder in the body.

Free Radical Damage

While there are many hypotheses concerning brain aging and function, the cross-linkage theory involving free radical damage to brain tissue is certainly one of the most provable. Free radicals specifically attack neurons and other tissues. Through DNA cross linkage, brain tissue becomes compromised and elasticity is reduced. Cross linkage further shortens protein chains and damages blood vessel walls. Compounds such as aldehydes, sulfur alkylating agents, quinones, and oxidized lipids are all cross-linking agents formed when the body is repeatedly exposed to environmental toxins. Furthermore, in the presence of adrenaline and non-adrenaline stress hormones, free radical formation increases in the bloodstream, thus confirming another connection between stress and brain damage.

Specific antioxidants and other nutrient compounds play a crucial role in preventing or minimizing free radical formation and subsequent cross linkage damage. These substances are essential in retarding physical damage to brain tissue, which is associated with everything from simple memory loss to Alzheimer's disease.

Exercise

One of the most important factors in brain function is exercise. Physical activity oxygenates the brain and also alters the chemistry of brain tissue. Post exercise benefits, especially from cardiovascular type exercise, include an increase in the 'feel good' hormones such as serotonin. Many people notice that they can think clearer and focus better after they take a little break from their work, go for a walk or spend a half hour at the local gym. Exercise is not only important for a strong body but for a strong mind as well.

What You Don't Use, Nature Takes Away

Apathy, indifference, lethargy, and a general lack of interest, enthusiasm, and involvement are among the greatest characteristics and factors adversely affecting brain function. They can lead to memory loss and senility. The brain is like an enormous computer. It stores information away in little library shelves until it is needed. The brain's ability to store and retrieve information depends, to a great extent, on how often the brain is forced to perform these functions.

The old saying, 'what you don't use, nature will take away', has never been truer than in the case of memory. As we age, and especially after we reach retirement, many people tend not to use their cognitive abilities. They spend a great deal of time being entertained in front of the television, which requires virtually no thinking whatsoever. Many older people give up reading, perhaps because of their eyesight. As age advances, many loose interest in the world around them, forming instead, rituals of repetition that require little or no thought process.

Mental dormancy or inactivity causes the brain to literally shut down many of its 'compartments'. This limits 'access' to the information stored in them.

Have you ever noticed that those older people who are sharp and alert are also very active? They participate in hobbies, and frequently partake of mutual interests with friends. They tend to be avid readers and keep up with what's happening around them. Activity breeds activity.

Targeted Nutrition for Brain Function

Recent scientific breakthroughs in brain chemistry research have isolated many nutrients and nutrient compounds, which keep the brain 'tuned up', enabling it to operate at peak efficiency. By adding these specific nutrients to a Full Spectrum dietary supplement program, you can provide an ideal working environment for the brain and allow it to perform at its fullest capacity.

Folic Acid

This B vitamin has been linked with a variety of mental functions. A deficiency of folic acid produces insomnia, forgetfulness, and eventually 'dementia like' symptoms. The good news is that these symptoms all disappear quite quickly after folic acid requirements are once again met.

Vitamin B-12

Another member of the B complex family, vitamin B-12 has long been called the 'nerve' vitamin. This is due to the fact that it has a profound effect on the central and sympathetic nervous system. Studies into the effects of vitamin B-12 deprivation are very revealing. A deficiency of this nutrient can result in both physical and psychological abnormalities. On the physical side, vitamin B-12 deficiencies can result in sore tongues, weakness, irritability, and achlorhydria. On the mental side, these same deficiencies result in a slowing of the mental process, confusion, memory loss, and depression. These mental abnormalities are often so profound that they can be detected by use of an electroencephalograph (an instrument used to analyze brain waves).

Choline

Also a member of the B complex family, choline is one of the oldest memory aids we know of. Students studying for final exams have long known the benefit of taking large doses of choline a few days before the testing. Studies pertaining to the relationship between choline and memory retention continue to support the student's claims that this nutrient does indeed improve the brain's ability to both store and rapidly retrieve information.

Ginkgo Biloba

Herbalists have called Ginkgo biloba one of the most important plant-based medicines in the world. There are over 300 studies demonstrating the positive effect Ginkgo exerts on brain function. It accomplishes this by increasing blood flow to the brain, rapidly improving memory and mental capabilities. Clinical studies show that Ginkgo has restorative effects on the neuronal membrane of the brain, while actually protecting against the ravages of many age-induced cerebral disorders.

Phosphatidyl Serine

Of the many nutrients that affect the brain, Phosphatidyl Serine is one of the most important. Our brain is saturated with fatty acids and phospholipids, a group of fat-like compounds found in lecithin. One of the most important of the phospholipids is phosphatidyl serine. Together with phosphatidylcholine, phosphatidylethanolamine, and phosphatidylinositol, they provide biological maintenance for our brain tissue. Phosphatidyl serine protects brain cell membrane fluid, maintains the solubility of fats, and ensures that brain neurons remain flexible. Through increasing the receptor sites on brain cells, it can directly improve neural communication.

The end result is an improved memory, greater mental energy, and less stress related neurological damage. This powerful nutrient has even shown great benefit in cases of Alzheimer's disease or Parkinson's.

Other related benefits for phosphatidyl serine include the prevention of cellular damage due to stress and alcohol abuse. It also decreased exercise recovery time and is very effective in the management of seasonal depression.

The following nutrients have been shown to be helpful in the prevention and improvement of memory loss, cognitive deficiency, senility, and Alzheimer's disease. A sample formula might include these powerful 'brain nutrients' along with adjunct herbal and nutritional support.

Brain Power Formula

Ginkgo Biloba	150 mg
Vitamin B6	20 mg
Vitamin B12	200 mcg
Choline	500 mg
DHA (Docosahexaenoic acid)	100mg
Huperzia serrata	100 mcg
Phosphatidyl serine	100 – 300 mg
Phosphatidyl choline	50 mg
Phosphatidyl inositol	25 mg
Ginseng Extract (panax)	100 mg
Gotu Kola	500 mg

$\mathscr{C}$hapter 11

Helping Your Body Cope With The Curse Of The 'Civilized' Diet

As science investigates the causes of debilitation and disease, two undeniable facts immediately surface. One, the vast majority of all afflictions today are non-contagious, chronic degenerative diseases. And two, virtually every disease in today's top ten list was rare 100 years ago. For example, if you suffered from heart disease or diabetes in the year 1900, you would likely have to travel hundreds of miles to find a specialist who was capable of diagnosing and treating those relatively obscure problems. Today, heart disease and diabetes are epidemic in proportion. They are so common that almost everyone knows one or more people tormented by them. What has changed so dramatically during this relatively short 'five generation' period to create this literal epidemic of non-contagious diseases?

The answer lies in the only two 'factors of change' profound enough to evoke this type of chronic disease 'explosion'. First is the enormous escalation in the number of toxins entering our environment. Second, and somewhat related, is the evolution of the Standard American Diet (SAD). This unhealthy way of eating has infiltrated every industrialized nation on earth.

In the 1890's and 1900's people ate a simple diet. There were no packaged foods to speak of. Whatever was eaten was 'home cooked' by someone. Refrigeration and other methods of prolonging the life of foods were non-existent, therefore, people ate fresh foods or not at all.

Many people lived in what we might refer to today as a rural environment. They raised their own food. Refined foods, which today constitute the typical diet in industrialized nations, were almost non-existent then..

It was not uncommon to have a sweet baked treat only with Sunday dinner, there simply wasn't time to do all that baking on a daily basis. Today the latest sweet treat, loaded with both refined sugar and flour, is just a short trip away at the convenience store.

In **SelfHealth, Your Complete Guide to Optimal Wellness,** I wrote about choice. Each of us has to make choices when we go to a restaurant, or when we are filling that shopping cart with the week's groceries. The choices we make are continually taking us down the pathway to ever increasing degenerative disorders, stealing precious months and years from our lives. These choices, comprised mostly of over processed, chemically ridden, sugar laden, refined junk, are fueling the greatest worldwide epidemic of disease humanity has ever seen.

There are millions of people all over the world that never eat a healthy meal, except perhaps in a finer restaurant once or twice a week. All three meals come out of bags, boxes, cartons, or metal trays. Each is filled with more substances you can't even pronounce than those you recognize. This has been going on for 3 or 4 generations and today many people don't even know how to cook or how to prepare delicious and nutritious food. Many times I have heard people say, " if it doesn't come in a box or a bag, I don't eat it".

The tragic result of this dead food diet is the compromise of our health. The immune system of the average person is at an all time low. In the environment, poisons and toxins by the thousands compromise the delicate integrity of immune function. With a diet devoid of almost every major and trace nutrient, the immune system doesn't have the raw materials to recover from the first onslaught before the next attack strikes.

This dead lifeless diet we practically worship has been shown to kill every living thing that it is fed to. There are signs at animal parks and zoos warning against feeding the animals 'people food'. Why? Because animal experts know that this type of 'food' will make the animals sick and could possibly even kill them.

In humans, the sugar and sugar-forming foods of the Standard American Diet (SAD), continues to produce hyperinsulinema (excess insulin) in four out of every ten people. Excess insulin has not only been linked to the obvious diseases of hypoglycemia and diabetes, but to heart disease, liver disease, obesity, immune suppression, arthritis, osteoporosis, dental carries, digestive disturbances, and some forms of cancer. Yet we push on, consuming greater quantities of junk, thinking erroneously, that our bodies' have an unlimited capacity to compensate.

Biologically we are very old indeed. These bodies of ours have the greatest ability to adapt to environmental and dietary changes - as long as they are gradual. What has taken place in the human diet in the last 50 or 60 years has overwhelmed the body's ability to cope with the changes. The result is epidemic disease.

This SAD diet consists primarily of calories from refined carbohydrates and is, almost exclusively, comprised of lifeless, dead foods. These foods have been cooked, fried, boiled, baked, dried, canned, frozen, juiced, whipped, mashed, preserved, and otherwise adulterated to the point of being almost unrecognizable.

Digestion of refined foods is often virtually impossible because of the mechanical, chemical, and temperature assaults whole foods are exposed to during the 'refinement' process. In addition, any nutrients remaining are further obliterated by the 'preparation' process. It is common knowledge that heat destroys most vitamins in foods. Certain forms of heating also displace many minerals, leaching them from our dietary intake. Flour, more specifically, wheat flour, is the staple of the American Diet. Through aggressive wheat farming and export, we have converted much of the rest of the world to a wheat-centered diet as well. Since wheat is at the heart of the diet, it is essential that it provide much of the needed nutrients the body requires for health and well being. In its natural state, wheat, whole wheat, provides over 20 nutrients to the human diet. Yet, in its refined state as bleached white flour, the products made from that adulteration carry only a small fraction of the nutrients originally there.

The following chart shows the percentage of loss of both vitamins and minerals when wheat is refined into white flour.

Calcium	60%	Phosphorus	71%
Magnesium	85%	Potassium	77%
Chromium	98%	Manganese	86%
Copper	68%	Zinc	78%
Iron	76%	Selenium	16%
Molybdenum	48%	Vitamin B6	64%
Vitamin E	97%	Folate	32%

You can clearly see that the majority of the nutrients present in the wheat have been destroyed or lost. Keep in mind that the wheat has only been converted to flour. It hasn't been heated yet. The baking and cooking process will further destroy the nutrients to the point that the end result will contain virtually no nutrition whatsoever, merely empty calories. Calories that will turn into pure sugar in the body in as little as 15 minutes after they are eaten. The highly refined nature of white flour products makes their starch molecules break down into simple sugars in a fraction of the time required by their whole grain counterparts.

How Did We Get In This Mess?

How did the SAD diet evolve? There are several factors that have not only contributed to this situation but are also responsible for its perpetuation. First, it's consumer laziness. Instead of demanding quality food and making healthy choices, we can hardly wait for the next junk food to hit the store shelves so we can try something new. The food industry is delighted with our total buy-in because highly refined, preserved foods have a much longer shelf life. This means that the food manufacturers have much less waste and bigger profit margins.

One may ask, "How can the food industry get away with producing thousands of foods which contain little or no nutrition?" This is one of the double-edged swords of living in a relatively free country. People can have the foods they want, as long as there are no recognizably harmful substances in them. David Kessler, former Food and Drug Administration director, initiated the passing of a law requiring that each human food container display a 'Nutrition Facts Box'. The goal of this legislation was to ensure that the consumer knew exactly what they were getting, or not getting, in the food they eat.

Unfortunately, 99 percent of the people who read the nutrition label do not know how to properly interpret it. Through education, primarily perpetuated by the dieticians and their political organizations, the public has been kept 'in the dark' about food facts and correct methods of evaluating such components as fats, calories, proteins, and carbohydrates.

In spite of overwhelming evidence to the contrary, the dieticians are still teaching us that all calories are the same. They hold vehemently to the concept that a calorie of sugar is the same as a calorie derived from a protein source. This of course, is absurd, since the body processes these calories in very different ways. For example, excess carbohydrates are converted to triglycerides and stored in the body as fat. If you have excess insulin production, the majority of carbohydrate foods you consume will ultimately end up around your middle. Proteins and fats, on the other hand, are metabolized quite differently.

Through their stubborn, blind approach to food and diet, the dietetics industry has created recommended eating habits that are 100 percent contrary to the way many people should be eating, resulting in epidemic numbers of cases of diabetes, hypoglycemia, obesity, and heart disease!

For decades the dietetics industry taught and defended the four basic food groups. After years of pressure by nutritionists and scientists alike, they finally agreed to revise this approach. The resultant 'food pyramid' was of little improvement. In fact, Drs. Michael and Mary Dan Eades, authors of the book **Protein Power**, have proven, that for thousands of people, eating the dietetic food pyramid almost upside down, produces a profound sense of health and well being. Other medical doctors, such as Robert Atkins, and to some extent, Barry Sears, have continued to disprove the universal effectiveness of the food pyramid. Yet, in spite of this overwhelming evidence to the contrary, the dietetics industry continues to cling to their antiquated concepts.

Another area of tremendous disservice perpetuated by the dietetics industry is the absurdly low level of recommended daily intake of essential nutrients. The adequacy of the RDA's, as they used to be called, have been disproved through literally tens of thousands of clinical studies conducted in dozens of countries over the last 30 years. In spite of this overwhelming body of evidence against the present recommended nutrient levels, they remain unchanged year after year.

The Dietary Industry's 'Sham of the Century' The Notorious Food Pyramid

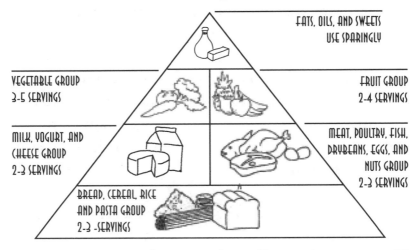

FATS, OILS, AND SWEETS
USE SPARINGLY

VEGETABLE GROUP
3-5 SERVINGS

FRUIT GROUP
2-4 SERVINGS

MILK, YOGURT, AND
CHEESE GROUP
2-3 SERVINGS

MEAT, POULTRY, FISH,
DRYBEANS, EGGS, AND
NUTS GROUP
2-3 SERVINGS

BREAD, CEREAL, RICE
AND PASTA GROUP
2-3 -SERVINGS

In reviewing the preceding illustration, you will note that the dietetics industry recommends that you obtain the majority of your daily diet from foods shown at the base of their 'food pyramid'. However, what they don't tell you is that these foods are the ones that cause many insulin induced chronic diseases. These diseases include hypoglycemia, obesity, and diabetes; they continue to be epidemic in our society. We could eliminate, conservatively, one half of these heath-threatening conditions by increasing our intake of protein, fresh fruits and vegetables, while reducing our intake of starches and sugars. By doing this, we could also prevent untold suffering and save billions of dollars in medical expenses.

However, since politics and hundreds of billions of dollars are involved, the situation is not likely to improve in the near future. The food industry is happy because it can make highly preserved foods with an extended shelf life. These yield a tremendously higher profit percentage than dealing with fresh foods, which can spoil before they are purchased. As long as the public is willing to buy these foods and as long as the dieticians continue to defend such eating habits as healthy, the SAD diet will flourish. As it spreads around the world, it will continue to rob the quality and quantity of life from hundreds of millions of people.

The Dead Food Dilemma

Every food, in fact every plant, animal and human contains chemicals to manage life functions. When that life is over, these chemicals disintegrate the host, returning it to the 'dust of the earth'. Those chemicals are called enzymes and they are the 'stuff' of life.

All foods contain enzymes, that is all fresh, foods in their natural state. When you eat a fresh tomato, it contains the exact enzymes necessary to break itself down once it is eaten. When you cook that tomato, you destroy the enzymes within it, making it dead and lifeless. When this tomato is eaten, the body must go through a great deal of effort in order to manufacture enzymes to replace those missing from the cooked food.

You can easily try an experiment at home for yourself. Take a truly fresh tomato and place it in a small dish. Place this in a window where the sun and light reach it a fair amount of the day. Next to it, in another dish, put some canned stewed tomatoes. After a few days the fresh tomato will become softer and softer. Eventually it will turn completely into liquid inside. The enzymes have digested all of the tomato except the fibrous skin or peel. Take a look at the cooked tomato in the other dish. It will not liquefy; it will develop mold and other parasitic growths. Over time, a long time, these foreign organisms will break the tomato down and return it to its primal essence.

If you were to eat the fresh tomato at any time during its breakdown, it would be completely safe. Oh yes, it may taste sour and unpleasant, due to the high enzyme activity. But it will not make you sick any more than eating a fine imported cheese, which has derived its unique flavor from fermentation and enzyme activity. Should you be foolish enough to eat the cooked tomatoes after they have become even slightly 'hairy' with mold, you could be in for serious trouble. You will suffer from a 'stomach ache' at best, or acquire food poisoning at the worst.

Consuming dead, lifeless foods which are void of enzymes is no different that eating a meal of rotting food. The enzymes formerly in them have been destroyed. Unless the body has the ability to manufacture all those needed enzymes with every meal, the food you eat would not naturally break down for nourishment but rather remain in the digestive system fermenting. This fermentation causes bloating, belching, heartburn, acid reflux, intestinal cramps, flatulence, diarrhea and constipation - the most common health complaints in the world.

The multi-million dollar sales of over-the-counter preparations, consisting of anti-acids, are testimony to the destructive powers of the SAD diet.

Improper digestion of food initially results in annoying complaints and socially embarrassing situations. If left unchecked, it can lead to bacterial and parasitical proliferation within the body. Next, the lack of stomach acid, due to the absence of naturally occurring enzymes, causes an 'over alkaline' digestive tract, preventing the digestion and absorption of protein foods. Subsequent protein deficiencies lead to catabolism (wasting away of lean muscle mass), premature aging, weak and non-responsive immune system, fatigue, nervousness, and other problems.

Further, this over alkaline situation leads to malabsorption of major minerals such as calcium and magnesium, resulting in osteoporosis, arthritis, electrolyte imbalances, cardiac problems and connective tissue disorders to name but a few.

How is it Supposed to Work?

During our lifetime, some 100,000 pounds of food and 60,000 quarts of liquids are processed by our digestive system. Unfortunately, about one out of every three people suffers from some kind of digestive disturbance, which prevents their digestive tract from properly performing this essential life function thoroughly.

The problem is so commonplace that we all know someone who complains of the symptoms of poor digestion. Bad breath, heartburn, belching, bloating, flatulence, abdominal bloat, constipation and diarrhea are all linked to faulty digestion.

Since digestion is the first step in the conversion of food to energy, lack of energy and vitality are also often symptoms of a poor digestive process. Incomplete digestion, usually referred to as indigestion, can further lead to skin problems such as pimples, recurring headaches, muscle deterioration due to lack of protein, and delayed wound healing due to a poorly nourished immune system. Additional problems, which may be caused by, or exacerbated by, poor digestion include anemia, irritable bowel problems, depression, allergies, ulcers, colitis, and diverticulitis.

It may be seen by this extensive list of related problems that it would be a good idea to ensure that our digestive system is functioning at optimal levels. If you are taking dietary supplements and trying to eat a healthy diet, you will only reap the rewards of that discipline if your digestive system is able to break down the foods and supplements and transport them to the individual cells of the body.

The concept of digestion is very simple: Food goes in one end and waste comes out the other. Meanwhile nutrients are separated out, absorbed into the bloodstream and used to provide energy and cellular maintenance.

Except for water, mineral salts, and simple sugars, all foods have to be converted from their complex forms into their basic molecular structures to be used in the body. Carbohydrates become simple sugars, proteins become amino acids and fats eventually turn into fatty acids. These conversions are accomplished by the body's use of over 20 chemicals - acids and enzymes - as the food moves along the digestive tract. If any of these essential acids and enzymes are missing or deficient, digestion becomes impaired.

Enzyme deficiency is one of the first and most common causes of digestive disorder. An imbalance of digestive secretions causes a deficiency of digestive enzymes. Enzymes are highly specialized protein molecules, which act as catalysts, greatly enhancing the rate of specific chemical reactions within the body, in this case, chemical reactions needed to break down food. In milliseconds, they can catalyze complex sequences of reactions that would require days, weeks or even months in a chemical laboratory. Additionally, these reactions have a 100% yield; there are no by-products to slow down further reactions.

Enzymes exist in all living organisms and cannot be reproduced synthetically. They are generally named by their activity, plus the suffix-ase. For example lactase breaks down the milk sugar lactose into glucose and galactose.

There are three types of enzymes: metabolic enzymes, which are responsible for body structure and processes, enzymes found in raw foods, which are designed to break them down, and digestive enzymes, which are formed in a healthy digestive system, in the presence of food.

The digestive enzymes in foods are destroyed when we process the foods. Cooking, in fact any heating, drying, freezing and packaging all destroy these delicate food enzymes. When we eat these 'lifeless' foods, the body must manufacture the needed enzymes missing from the foods, in order to complete digestion. Over time, this exhausts the system and it can no longer produce adequate enzymes to make up for the lack of enzymes in junk foods. This leads to digestive disturbances of all kinds.

Digestive enzymes may be divided into three major groups: proteases, which break down proteins, lipases for fat digestion, and amylases, which break down carbohydrates. The first enzyme to be formed, ptyalin, is found in the saliva of the mouth and helps to break down carbohydrates. This is an important enzyme in the overall digestive process and that's why, when we smell food or even think of it, we often begin to salivate. The body is preparing for the job of digestion.

The pancreas produces the major digestive enzymes. Located behind the stomach, the six-inch long pancreas is famous for its influence on blood sugar levels by the production of insulin. However, the digestive functions of this unique gland are a totally separate, yet equally important function. The pancreas produces enzymes, which are crucial to the digestive process. In fact, the pancreatic juice contains at least four kinds of enzymes: proteases, amylases, lipases, and nucleases. Other enzymes are produced in the stomach as well as the small intestine.

Besides enzymes, there are two other important digestive ingredients necessary to complete the job: hydrochloric acid for proteins and bile for fat emulsification.

The stomach retains food for a couple of hours, longer if it is made up of primarily protein. During this time, it is treated with a bath of hydrochloric acid (HCL). This both sterilizes the food and acidifies it. It also triggers the release of a powerful, potent protease call pepsin. The resulting mixture of acidified food and water is called chyme.

Chyme is released in squirts through a valve, the pyloric valve, between the stomach and small intestine. The presence of the acid chyme in the small intestine stimulates the release of highly alkaline digestive juices from the pancreas, liver, gall bladder and the small intestine itself. These fluids contain many digestive enzymes and neutralize the chyme, leaving it slightly alkaline. The liver and gall bladder work in combination to contribute bile for fat digestion, adding the other non-enzyme digestive factor. The bile emulsifies the fat, which is required before the fat digesting enzymes, the lipases, can do their job. This facilitates not only the use of fatty acids but also the absorption of the fat-soluble vitamins, A, E, D, and K.

With the arrival of chyme from the stomach, bile is emptied into the small intestine along with the pancreatic digestive enzymes. Most of the digestive process and the absorption of nutrients take place in the small intestine. In fact this organ is so important to digestion that if its integrity is preserved, life can be sustained and digestion continued even without the use of the mouth, stomach or colon. However, if we lose the function of the small intestine, the only alternative is intravenous feeding.

At this point in the journey through our digestive system, only about five percent of the food remains to be broken down. This proceeds into the large intestine or colon. There water and electrolytes (mineral salts containing calcium, potassium, sodium, magnesium and others) are extracted and colonies of bacteria, naturally occurring in the colon, feed on the waste, finishing the breakdown process. These bacteria keep any unabsorbed food from causing an autoimmune response by completely breaking it down for elimination.

You now may understand more about the digestive process than you ever did before. But what happens if there is a failure in one or more of the various phases of this digestive process?

If the hydrochloric acid is missing or deficient in the stomach, protein foods cannot be broken down and acidified. This in turn, prevents the stomach enzymes from being formed. This leads to 'heartburn', upper gastrointestinal bloating and belching. When this improperly digested material enters the small intestine, the pH is not acidic enough to stimulate the release of adequate intestinal enzymes. This leads to poor digestion of carbohydrates and subsequent intestinal bloating and flatulence. Are you familiar with these conditions?

If you have been experiencing some or all of these symptoms on a fairly regular basis, you can rest assured that you are not absorbing vital nutrients and calories from your food. Fortunately, improving this situation is not difficult at all.

First of all, a few simple dietary changes may help tremendously. Try to eat, as much as possible, foods in their natural state. Strive to consume foods that have not been adulterated by refining, storage or preparation processes such as cooking, freezing, whipping, juicing, drying and preserving. The food will then be of a much higher quality, making digestion easier.

Enzymes in raw foods contribute significantly to a healthy digestive process; it is vitally important that you preserve their integrity. At temperatures above 118 degrees Fahrenheit, most of these enzymes are destroyed.

As a side note for those of you worried about cholesterol in your food, if you eat your beef rare and your eggs cooked with the yolks still soft, you will preserve the lipase, which is responsible for digesting the fats found in them, including cholesterol.

Examples of raw fruits and vegetables which are very high in natural enzymes include cabbage, carrots, tomatoes, cucumber, endive, avocados, mangos, bananas, apples, oranges, grapefruit, lemons, papayas, pineapples and fresh figs. In fact, most all fresh fruits and vegetables have adequate supplies of enzymes to digest themselves once you eat them - but only if you eat them in their natural state.

Fiber, long known for its ability to keep our bowel movements regular, is also necessary in the formation of natural colon bacteria. These 'friendly' bacteria play a vital role in the final role of digestion. Another note: If you have taken antibiotics for ten days or longer, you need to replace the healthy bacteria in your colon. Since antibiotics kill ALL bacteria, it is essential that you use a comprehensive acidophilus product in order to replenish the 'good' bacteria.

In addition to improving the diet, specific dietary supplements can come to the rescue of those with compromised digestion. We must always begin with the basics. These nutrients include vitamins, major minerals, trace minerals, amino acids, phytonutrients, and antioxidants. These make up the Full Spectrum of known human nutrition. By providing these basic nutrients, we put the vast chemistry of the human body in the best possible position to nurture, repair, maintain and heal itself.

Once the foundation has been ensured, there are some specific supplements that are especially helpful for improving digestion. In fact, these work so well that you can virtually feel the difference in your digestion with the very first use!

Betaine Hydrochloride.

The stomach secretes hydrochloric acid, which is made from chlorides, from the blood and hydrogen. Its presence activates pepsin and together serve as a protein digestive. Since hydrochloric acid production slows down as we age with only about 60 percent of normal present at age 40 and only 15 percent by age 60, we need to consider replacing this primal digestive factor. Many of the symptoms of indigestion such as acid reflux, heartburn, and stomach bloating and belching are not caused by an excess stomach acid, as we are led to believe, but rather a lack of adequate hydrochloric acid. By supplementing the diet with betaine hydrochloride, the natural hydrochloric acid, we can stimulate the stomach to secrete higher levels of acid, normalizing stomach chemistry.

Pancreatin

This is a general term for the digestive essence from the pancreas. It is secreted when chyme begins to enter the small intestine to begin the second phase of digestion. Pancreatin will contain amylase, protease and lipase factors to digest proteins, fats, and carbohydrates. Supplements for enhanced digestion should contain pancreatin as part of their formulation.

Papain and Bromelain

Both of these enzyme ingredients are potent protein dissolving enzymes. Their presence ensures adequate breakdown of proteins from the diet, the essence of the physical body. Proteins are the most important foods we eat. The Greeks first named proteins, a word in their language meaning 'of first importance.'

Bile

Bile is necessary for proper and complete fat digestion. Bile is normally made by the liver and stored by the gall bladder, which modifies it chemically and makes it 10 times more concentrated. When bile is deficient, or there are problems with the gall bladder, taking bile, usually from animal sources, is the best way to stimulate its production and get fat digestion going again. Signs of bile deficiency include indigestion when fatty foods are eaten, light colored stools and constipation.

Without the 'life force' catalysts like enzymes provide, we would be nothing more than a pile of lifeless chemical substances. Every time you suffer from indigestion, it's your body telling you that the food you are eating is not only being poorly digested, but to some extent, it is poisoning your internal environment. This lack of complete digestion leads to increased toxins in the body, which in turn, lead to elevated levels of free radicals. Free radicals, can and do, regularly alter the chemistry of living cells and systems, even going so far as to permanently alter the genetic material of the living cell called the DNA. Once this occurs, the genetic mutation will be passed to every new cell through the altered genetic code.

In order to reduce this downward spiral away from

optimum health, it is essential to address digestive disorders and aggressively take measures to provide the body with what it needs to normalize this life-giving process.

It has been said by many that 'you are what you eat', but if you don't digest and absorb what you eat, you are far less. That ongoing deficiency, over months and years, can lead to fatigue, depression, chronic disease, and premature death.

Something so easy to fix should never go unattended. Do yourself a favor and clean up your digestion first. Everything good you do afterwards will have all that much greater impact.

A Full Spectrum Digestive Formula

Betaine Hydrochloric Acid... 100 mg
Pepsin .... 75 mg
Pancreatin .... 75 mg
Bromelain .... 75 mg
Papain .... 75 mg
Ox Bile .... 75 mg

You should look for a formula that provides these potencies and ingredients in each capsule. Take between two and four capsules per meal. The larger the meal, the more you may need to do the job. Before you know it, you will be enjoying your meals like a twenty-year-old again!

Enzymes & Digestive Agents Produced in the Body

Enzyme	Site Of Production	Action
Ptyalin	Salivary Glands	Begins starch digestion
Pepsin		
Hydrochloric Acid		Protein digestion
Gastric Acid	Stomach	Protein breakdown
Rennin		Protein and fat
(Children Only)		Specific protein
Bile	Liver	
Trypsin, Chymotrypsin,		Emulsify fats
Steapsin, Amylopsin,	Pancreas	Proteins to amino acids

Enzyme Activity and pH Produced During Digestion

Location	Acting Enzyme	Food Class	Product Formed	pH
Mouth	Ptyalin	Starch	Dextrins	Acid
Stomach	Pepsin	Proteins	Proteases	Acid
	Papain		Peptones	
	Rennin	Casein	Fatty Acids	
	Gastric Lipase	Fats	Glycerol	
	Proteins	Trypsin	Polypeptides	
	Fat	Steapsin	Glyceride	Neutral/
			Fatty Acids	Alkaline
			Glycerol	
	Starch			
	Dextrins	Amylopsin		
	Maltose	Maltase	Maltose	
	Sucrose	Sucrase	Glucose	Alkaline

294

Maximizing Absorption through Nature's Way of Eating

If we were to go back in time, deep into our genetic past, we would see that our ancestors ate much differently than we do today. Since there were no methods of food storage, these people ate what was immediately available. As the seasons changed, so did their diet. Protein foods were a high portion of their diet simply because hunting was an option open to them all year long, regardless of the weather. Other foods, such as fruits, vegetables and some grains, were available only seasonally.

Because of these natural restrictions, specific foods were usually eaten alone. For example, when a kill was made, everyone ate that animal until it was gone, since it could not be stored. Likewise, during the late spring and summer, when fruits and vegetables were plentiful, less hunting was done.

What these people of antiquity were doing, because nature dictated it, was to properly separate their foods according to how they are digested. Today, we call this food combining, the art of putting foods that 'fit together', in the same meal. What was nature doing by providing different foods at different times? It was ensuring that the maximum absorption of the essence of each food was achieved through complete digestion.

Today, we are exposed to any and every type of food imaginable. We can have high protein, high fruit & vegetable and high starch and sugar, at the same meal, a situation that could never have occurred in nature. The result of this constant mismatching of foods prevents our digestive system from properly breaking down the foods we eat. This results in the putrifaction of partially digested foods and mal-absorption of the nutrients from those foods. This, combined with the copious amounts of over-processed dead, lifeless foods as discussed above, produces incomplete digestion and multiple nutrient deficiencies, leading to chronic disease.

Proper Food Combining

In order to ensure that we are completely digesting the foods we eat, some attention to which foods we combine with others is necessary. There have been volumes written relative to food combining, some of the programs being so complicated that it can make you to frightened to even eat! For the most part, all of these food-combining rules have their origins in either religious or philosophical roots. They were either products of necessity or belief, and have little basis of science behind them.

There is one basic rule of food combining or rather consuming that is essential if you want to optimize your digestion. The rule is simple and easy to follow. When you follow it, you will be once again eating very much like our ancestors, the way nature intended we eat.

The Rule for Healthful Eating:

Do not consume concentrated carbohydrates and concentrated proteins during the same meal!

While this sounds simple enough, we must truly understand what it means.

Good Food Combinations

Complex Carbohydrates	Concentrated Proteins/Fats
Whole Grains	Meat & Fish
Raw or Steamed Vegetables	Fowl
Real Whole Grain Breads	Eggs & Cheese

Poor Food Combinations

High Sugar/Refined Carbohydrates	Concentrated Proteins/Fats
Cakes, Pies & Pastries	
White Breads	Meat & Fish
White Flour Pasta	Fowl
Fruit	Eggs & Cheese
Fruit Juices	

As you may have guessed, many of our meals do not comply with this essential rule for health. How often do we finish a meal consisting of a steak or some chicken or fish and follow it up with a big sweet dessert? How often do we have white bread with a meat or cheese sandwich? Every time you do, you break the only cardinal rule of food combining. How can we avoid this?

Next time you finish a high protein meal, instead of moving right along to the dessert, get up from the table and take a walk or indulge in some other light physical activity. In three hours, when the protein has had the chance to fully digest, then have the dessert. This will serve two purposes. Firstly, you will not suffer impaired digestion caused by the improper combining of food types. Secondly, if you wait three hours, you are likely not to be in a place where there is any dessert and you will automatically cut down your overall consumption of sugar foods! If you must have sugar foods, you must learn to eat them alone. This, at least from the digestive point of view, is correct.

Why is this all true? At her dining room table, why does Mother Nature separate proteins from refined, concentrated carbohydrates? In order to answer these questions for you, and to help you more fully understand the importance of nature's 'Golden Rule of Health', we must take a look at the inside of your body and see how digestion takes place.

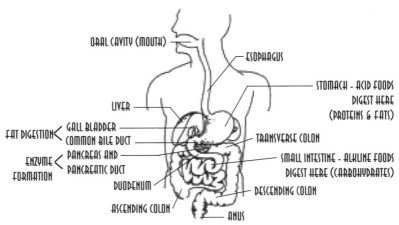

By viewing this diagram, we learn that protein foods, such as meats, dairy products, and fowl, are primarily digested in the stomach. These foods require a very high acidic environment in order to break down properly. The stomach secretes hydrochloric acid, creating a very acidic environment, for the breakdown of proteins.

If we look down to the small intestines, we see that carbohydrates, including all starches and sugars, are digested there. All carbohydrate foods require a very alkaline environment in order to be properly and completely digested. The enzymes secreted into the small intestine produce a very alkaline environment and are specifically designed to break down carbohydrates.

When we mix these two food groups in the same meal, both concentrated proteins and concentrated carbohydrates enter the stomach at the same time. The stomach will automatically begin to secrete hydrochloric acid, stimulated by the presence of the protein foods. In this highly acidic environment, the accompanying carbohydrates cannot be broken down and digested. They merely sit there, for hours, waiting for the protein to be broken down. This prolonged waiting period causes them to begin fermentation due to the high temperature of the body. This fermentation produces the bloating and belching so common after meals. Prolonged abuse of this nature can prevent the stomach from secreting adequate hydrochloric acid. When this occurs, heartburn is frequently the result, due to incomplete protein breakdown. Heartburn, by the way, is rarely caused by excess stomach acid, as we are repeatedly told by the manufacturers of those anti-acids. Rather, it is the lack of adequate stomach acid that leads to this uncomfortable condition.

If this is True, Why Do these Anti-acids Work So Well?

Another look at the preceding digestion diagram will help us answer this question. The stomach is an acidic organ. It secretes hydrochloric acid in the presence of protein foods. Stomach acid levels diminish as proteins are broken down and the protein digestion process nears completion. This allows the pyloric valve (a small valve in the lower part of the stomach) to open. The contents of the stomach then pass into the small intestine. Now let's see what happens when we take a dose of our favorite anti-acid.

The pyloric valve is controlled by the pH of the stomach. When the acid level is high and protein is being digested, the valve stays closed. When the pH of the stomach approaches neutral, the pyloric valve opens releasing the food to the small intestine. When we use powerful, very alkaline, anti-acids, we not only destroy all the natural hydrochloric acid, preventing the digestion of proteins, but by rapidly lowering the pH of the stomach, the pyloric valve opens very prematurely, dumping the undigested proteins into the small intestine. You feel quick relief when you take these products because the pressure in the stomach, caused by bloating from improper digestion, has been eliminated. This dumps the contents into the small intestine. However, as we will now see, our troubles are not over. In fact, they have just begun.

Once this fermented, partially digested protein mixture enters the small intestine where the pH is very alkaline, the protein has virtually no further hope of digestion. The steak, and the sweet dessert, you just ate now sits in an alkaline environment. Digestion of the dessert begins while the partially digested steak sits and begins to ferment in the small intestine. This produces putrefactive bacteria and lower intestinal bloating and gastrointestinal disturbances.

By continually using powerful anti-acid products, you suffer two consequences. You perpetuate protein deficiencies in your body and you replace upper intestinal gas with the much less socially acceptable form, lower intestinal gas!

Another dangerous side effect to over-alkalizing the digestive system is the potential for serious mineral deficiencies. Calcium, one of the most important major minerals in the body, is very difficult to absorb. In its natural state it is frequently found in very alkaline sources. In order for calcium to be absorbed at the cellular level and in order for calcium to be bio-available to rebuild bone, it must be acidified by the digestive system. The constant use of anti-acids prevents the production of hydrochloric acid and hence the necessary acidification of many minerals. Alkaline calcium is either passed out of the body or worse yet, deposited in soft tissues and other sites. This ultimately leads to such problems as calcification of the arteries - leading to heart disease, heal spurs, kidney stones, gallstones and calcium deposits on the spine. An over-alkaline system is also responsible for both initiating and accelerating many forms of arthritis.

Understanding the Acid and Alkaline Balance in the Body

Of all the biochemical activities occurring in the body, one of the most misunderstood is the concept of pH, or the acid/alkaline relationship. Authorities in the nutrition field frequently extol the benefits of alkalizing the body, reminding us that an alkaline state allows the body to cleanse itself. I could not agree more, but these well-meaning experts only have half of the story.

Within each one of us is a chemical sea of life. This ocean is primarily made up of water, with proteins, nutrients and waste matter included. The pH of the body fluctuates slightly from neutral in either the acid or alkaline direction. This fluctuation is called the acid/alkaline tide. This wondrous mechanism is responsible for controlling much of the life process within you, and in order for the body to function perfectly, this acid/alkaline dance must be allowed to take place unimpeded.

During the daylight hours, your overall body, especially your digestive system, should be slightly acidic. In this state, your body is in an absorption mode. This is important in order to extract both calories and nutrients from the foods and supplements you take.

With the setting of the sun, and as you go deeper into the night, your body slowly becomes slightly alkaline. This state of alkalinity is the dumping or detoxification mode. It is during this time that your body gets rid of the waste by-products of digestion and metabolism.

Because a state of alkalinity enables the body to cleanse itself, many people have erroneously sought to perpetuate a state of alkalinity constantly. It can now be seen that this would ultimately result in starvation. We can force the body into a temporary state of extreme alkalinity such as might occur during a controlled fast. This would accelerate the dumping of toxins and the cleansing of tissues. Long-term, however, this state would produce malnutrition and starvation. Conversely, if the body were to be too acid all the time, it would never have the opportunity to properly cleanse itself.

It can be seen that a balance between the absorption state of acidity and the detoxifying state of alkalinity will produce the most optimal state of health.

What is pH?

The term pH is an abbreviation for 'powers of hydrogen', and refers to the degree of either acidity or alkalinity of a substance. The following chart illustrates the pH scale and the location of some of the body organs and body fluids.

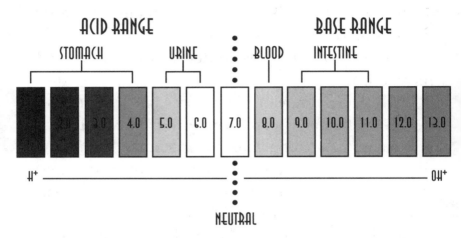

The center of the chart is neutral, neither acid nor alkaline. That point is 7 on the pH scale. It can be seen that anything to the left of neutral 7 is acidic, while anything to the right of the 7 is alkaline.

The stomach, the organ of primary protein digestion, is very acidic due to the production of hydrochloric acid. Its pH should be between 1.0 and 4.0. The intestine, the site of carbohydrate digestion, is slightly alkaline and in a healthy state, should have a pH of between 8.0 and 10.0.

This brings us back to our earlier discussions of both digestion and food combining. You can now see how the human body has been designed to eat according to the table that nature has set for us. Our diets of dead, lifeless, over-processed, 'natural enzyme' deficient food, plus our improper combining of concentrated proteins with concentrated carbohydrates (starches and sugars), have taken its toll. Is it any wonder we find ourselves in such an unhealthy state?

Part III: The Nuts and Bolts

Chapter 12
Choosing A Healthy Diet

The news is full of the 'latest reports' warning us that 'this particular food is bad for you', or 'that food has been adulterated'. All of this can become very confusing especially if you are trying to eat a diet consisting of wholesome, healthy foods. We are told of the horrors of eating red meat, of how it is filled with hormones and other drugs. We are told of the manner in which poultry is handled and how many chemicals are put in the feed. With all this negative information, many are driven to avoiding animal products altogether and choose instead, to become vegetarian. Yet, virtually all of our commercially grown fruits, vegetables and grain products are adulterated with chemical sprays, insecticides, herbicides and fertilizers. Most recently, the food industry has begun altering the genetics of our food. While, on the surface, this seems beneficial in some ways, we really don't know what the long-term results of eating this food will be.

If you were to gather all of the negative stories

about our food and tried to avoid all those with potential problems, you would very likely starve to death! There simply would be nothing left to eat.

It is possible to obtain meat, fowl, and plant foods which have been 'organically raised/grown'. This helps to insure that many of the chemicals typically used in raising/growing these foods have been eliminated. You can also be sure and provide the body with adequate antioxidant nutrients, which will also help protect you from the many chemicals we are exposed to daily, not only from food sources but from the air we breathe, the water we drink and the environments in which we live.

Surrounded by the fears, phobias, myths, and mysteries about the foods we eat, we often pay little attention to ensuring that our bodies are getting a well-rounded diet. While much of the criticism of our food supplies is valid, we must not forget that the body still requires a diet that provides the necessary food sources for energy, rebuilding of the body cells and metabolic functions.

I am frequently asked questions about dietary matters. Common examples include: What is the best diet for health? Is it a balanced diet? What is a balanced diet? Is it a meat and potato approach? Is a vegetarian diet better for us? We can find 'experts' extolling both the necessity and benefits of each one of these diets, making the consumer, who merely wants to eat right, very confused.

The answer is simple, yet complicated. The fact

is, no diet is right for everyone. This applies to diets for good health and maintenance as well as diets for weight control. Roger J. Williams, Ph.D., wrote a pivotal book entitled ***Biochemical Individuality***. In it, he proves that, while we are all members of the same species, we are often vastly different. He proceeds to illustrate that we are as different from each other on the inside as we are on the outside. These differences exhibit themselves in our organs, chemistry, and in how we respond to the world around us. In fact, it might be said that no two people are exactly alike, bio-chemically and internally, any more than no two people share the exact same fingerprints.

The dietetics industry has produced such charts as the four basic food groups, and most recently the food pyramid. They have stubbornly told us that these eating plans are the most ideal for all of us, in spite of our vast biochemical individuality. They cling to the archaic concept that 'a calorie, is a calorie, is a calorie' regardless from where it comes. Our present knowledge in biochemistry has not only long disproved this concept, but we now also know that the way in which people metabolize and utilize calories can vary greatly from one individual to another.

Current mainstream textbooks are touting the perfect balanced diet as being 58% carbohydrate, 30% fat and 12% protein. For most people, nothing could be further from the truth!

First of all, this ratio of basic food groupings provides too little protein for all but the very sedentary.

Secondly, for an ever-increasing multitude, diets containing over 50 percent carbohydrates (the majority of which are highly refined), are contributing to the epidemic of many chronic degenerative diseases. Conditions such as hypoglycemia, diabetes, arthritis, heart disease, and obesity may all be directly linked to the over-consumption of refined carbohydrates.

In spite of the overwhelming evidence linking excess carbohydrate consumption to conditions such as hyperinsulinema, the dietetics industry continues to tell us that 100 calories from sugar are no different than 100 calories from meat, chicken, or fish. Until people become more educated regarding the true nature of food and its varying roles in their bodies, we will continue to follow this outdated rhetoric and march ever closer to the development of degenerative disease.

The first step in building a healthy diet, then, is to learn about each of the 4 food groupings and which selections from each group are the best choices to make. Secondly, once armed with this information, you then need to figure out how your body individually handles various foods and adjust the ratio of the food groupings to your own chemistry.

The Real Food Groups: Protein, Fats, Carbohydrates and Fiber

Every food we eat fits into one of four food groupings. These include proteins, fats, carbohydrates, and fibers. Most foods consumed in their natural state are usually exclusively from one group. Over-processed, adulterated, junk type foods frequently are composed of a combination of foods from different groups, making them much more difficult to digest. This in turn retards absorption and can lead to an im-balanced diet, one which fails to provide adequate amounts of many necessary nutrients. Let's take a look at these four basic groupings individually. By doing so, you will better understand the value of each food group and how to choose the best from each.

Protein

We begin with protein because, for humans, it is the most important food grouping of all. While many people try and tell us that excess protein is harmful, saying that far to many of us get too much protein on a daily basis, the real studies and surveys of people's eating habits, around the world, continue to show that far more people are protein deficient than are in protein excess.

Humankind has known of the importance of protein down through the ages. The ancient Greeks, in their pursuit of athletic and physical perfection of the human form, figured out that when a higher protein diet was consumed, it produced a stronger, well-defined athletic body. While the Greeks did not have the scientific understanding to know why this was the case, their focus on physical ideals made them realize the value of quality protein in their diet. In fact the word 'protein,' is a Greek derivative meaning, 'of first importance.'

Why is this so? Every cell, every organ, every fiber of structural material within your body is built out of protein. Your body consists of approximately 100 trillion cells. Every day billions of these cells die and need to be replaced. They can only be replaced by their individual building blocks called amino acids. Amino acids only come from proteins. Every reaction that takes place within the body, be it nervous, digestive, muscular, or circulatory, is directly dependent upon the presence of quality protein in the body.

Throughout our lives, we need protein for varying tasks. Children require high protein diets in order to meet the demands of explosive cell multiplication brought about by the growth process. Even after the body has formed and grown into adulthood, protein continues to be of primary importance. Living tissue is in a constant state of breaking down, needing to be rebuilt. Amino acids, the building blocks of all living tissue, are constantly being exchanged for new amino acid combinations. We need a continuing supply of amino acids for the repair and replacement of living matter. The body uses protein to carry out the myriad of metabolic reactions that take place within it on a minute by minute basis.

Higher protein diets can have other decided advantages. Candidates for, and those afflicted with, conditions such as hypoglycemia, diabetes, heart disease, and other chronic disorders need to reduce the amount of insulin being produced by their bodies. Presently, the only way in which we can accomplish this is to restrict the consumption of insulin producing foods and replace them, in part, with high protein foods. Proteins do not stimulate the production and release of insulin.

Since the ingestion, digestion, and subsequent conversion of proteins into amino acids is so important to our health, we need to understand how we can not only choose the best quality protein but take measures to ensure that the protein we do eat is properly absorbed and assimilated.

Proteins are among the most complex organic compounds in nature. Digestion of these complex molecules is accomplished in several distinct and important phases. As we discussed in the last chapter, protein digestion begins in the stomach. In fact, the stomach is the primary organ of protein breakdown. Hydrochloric acid, and various proteolytic enzymes secreted from the pancreas, break down the complete molecules of protein into separate amino acids, which are then easily absorbed or assimilated into the body. These individual amino acids eventually enter the blood stream to be carried to the millions of sites where they will be utilized.

Occasionally, because digestion is not complete, whole proteins can enter the blood stream. This is a dangerous situation, since the body will perceive these as foreign proteins and often mount an immune response to their presence, building antibodies in an attempt to destroy them. This process manifests itself to us as allergies or an allergic reaction. In fact, many people suffering from allergies do so because of this very reason.

Because protein is so vital for the building and maintaining of the human body, proper assimilation of proteins, through proper digestion, should be of great importance to us.

After about the age of 35, most people suffer from a significant reduction in the production of hydrochloric acid in the stomach. This occurs primarily because of dietary abuse as discussed in the last chapter. This is the reason why I frequently recommend the use of digestive supplements, which also provide natural hydrochloric acid as outlined previously.

Once protein is properly broken down into individual amino acids, we can classify them into two basic groups, essential and non-essential. Often misleading, these terms refer to whether or not our bodies can manufacture a specific amino acid or not. Essential amino acids cannot be made by the biochemistry of our bodies; therefore, they are 'essential' in the diet. Those amino acids, which can be made by the body, are referred to as non-essential, even though they are vital to human life.

When considering protein requirements for bodily need, it is important to understand that there are two types of protein foods. First what we call complete proteins and secondly the incomplete proteins. Foods that are labeled complete proteins contain all the essential amino acids needed by the body in adequate amounts. These foods may be consumed alone and will provide the body with total amino acid needs. Generally speaking complete proteins are from animal sources. Meat, fowl, dairy, eggs, fish, etc. are all examples of complete proteins.

Examples of incomplete proteins would, generally, be fruits, vegetables, and grains. These foods contain proteins but are missing or deficient in one or more of the essential amino acids. In order to rely on these sources of food for protein, they must be combined in such a manner that all the essential amino acids are present at the same time, in adequate amounts.

There is a biochemical law which states that, unless all the essential amino acids are present at the same time, the amount of protein that can be utilized will be limited to the percent of the lowest essential amino acid. This is called the "All or None Law of Protein Utilization."

This protein limiting law can be understood thusly: There are 8 to 12 essential amino acids, depending on which expert you consult. Let's say for the sake of example that you consumed a meal that provided 100 percent of all those essential amino acids except for 'one'; and that 'one' was present at only 60 percent. The result of this combination of amino acids would be that the body could utilize the total protein present only up to 60 percent, since that is the highest level at which all the essential amino acids are present. Everything past the 60 percent level would be unavailable as protein.

This is never a problem for those consuming protein from animal sources, however vegetarians frequently run into this problem and often suffer from protein deficiency as a result. You can live very well on an all vegetarian diet, but you must be constantly cognizant of the fact that you must combine varying sources of incomplete vegetarian proteins in order to supply the full gamut of essential amino acids.

Essential Amino Acids

Leucine
Isoleucine
Valine
Methionine
Threonine
Lysine
Histidine
Phenylalanine
Tryptophan
Arginine

These amino acids are considered essential either because the body cannot manufacture them at all or not in sufficient amounts to meet ideal needs.

How Much Protein Do We Need?

Our protein requirements vary from one phase of our lives to another. Further, those who are more physically active have greater protein requirements. When we discuss ideal protein intake, we must remember that we are referring to complete proteins.

A good rule to follow, especially if you are reasonable active, is to ensure that your diet provides one gram of protein for every kilogram of your bodyweight. A kilogram is 2.2 pounds so the calculation is an easy one. If you weigh 200 pounds you should be providing that 200-pound body with about 90 grams of protein daily. While women need less protein than most men do, they are also the most protein deficient. Still, there are other factors to consider when attempting to establish protein needs. The following chart may prove helpful.

Protein Requirements Chart

Age and/or Condition	Daily Intake	
Under one year	3.5 grams for every 2.2 lbs.	
One to three years	40	grams
Four to six years	50	grams
Seven to nine years	60	grams
Ten to twelve years	70	grams
Thirteen to twenty years	70 – 100	grams
Male adult, inactive	60 – 70	grams
Male adult, active	70 – 100	grams
Female Adult, inactive	60 – 70	grams
Female Adult, active	60 – 80	grams
Female Adult, Pregnant	85 – 100	grams
Female Adult, Lactating	100 – 200	grams

There has been some controversy generated over the possibility of negative side effects from excess protein consumption. The figures in the preceding chart are certainly not excessive and represent the optimal protein intake for various individuals.

What about protein excess? As long as protein is consumed with adequate amounts of fat (30% of the diet) and as long as sufficient amounts of water and other fluids are ingested, diets consisting of high to even very high amounts of protein have never been shown to be harmful.

A common criticism of the practice of consuming a higher protein diet is that it can cause constipation.

This is often due to the lack of fiber in many protein foods. As long as your diet also contains sufficient fiber, you will not have this concern.

Remember, I am not advising you to eat a diet consisting solely of protein, only that it is essential that you adequately meet your protein needs. Elderly people are frequently the most protein deficient because they often have difficulty in digesting and absorbing protein foods. Rather than avoid these foods, it is far better to fix the digestive deficiencies.

Remember too, that one of the biggest reasons for premature aging is protein deficiency. All the expensive creams and topical lotions you can buy will not replace the collagen protein lost at the sub-dermal levels due to a diet that is not providing the minimum protein needs.

How Do I Know if I Am Protein Deficient?

While many of the effects of prolonged protein deficiency are internal and cannot be seen or even felt until they have progressed to the extreme, the following list includes many of the more obvious signs of protein deficiency.

Dizziness
Nausea
Lowering of hemoglobin levels (depressed immune system)
Increased intra-cellular fluid retention (edema)

Growth retardation in children
Reduced Vitamin A absorption
Loss of liver enzyme activity and liver function
Retarded spermatogenesis
Extreme weakness
Cataracts
Acid and alkaline imbalance
Loss of ability to produce adequate antibodies for defense
Premature aging
Loss of skin tone and elasticity

Fats

Fats are the most concentrated foods we consume. They provide nine calories of energy per gram as opposed to the four calories per gram provided by all other foods. Fats, also referred to as lipids, are the only foods which contain no nitrogen in their structures. This is important, for it places them in a unique category all their own. Our bodies handle fats in a very specialized way, and they are absolutely essential for enhancing bodily functions. In their deficiency or absence, the body cannot carry out many biochemical metabolic functions essential to life. Fats, and their companions, the fatty acids, are responsible for building and maintaining certain specialized cells such as those that insulate every nerve within our body.

In our discussion of proteins, I mentioned that it was important to eat a certain amount of fat as well.

Fats slow down the secretion of hydrochloric acid in the stomach, prolonging the digestion of proteins. This not only helps to ensure that the protein has enough time to completely digest, but for those watching their weight, gives you a longer feeling of fullness after a meal. (One of the side effects to a very low fat diet is constant hunger, making it difficult to remain on those types of diets for extended periods.)

Fats also serve as carriers for the essential fat-soluble vitamins A, D, E, and K. Another negative side effect to the very low fat diet touted by some is it produces a deficiency of these nutrients in the process. By aiding vitamin D absorption, fats help us keep calcium readily available to our bones and teeth.

There are two types of fats in the diet, saturated and unsaturated. The difference in them lies in the types of acids that make up the fat.

Saturated fats are generally solid at room temperature. Examples of saturated fats would include animal fats and several vegetable fats such as coconut and palm oil. Because of their molecular structure, saturated fats are very stable molecules. Saturated fats have what scientists call 'closed bonds' on their molecular chains. This is, in fact, what makes them so dense and solid at room temperature. The closed bonds also prevent them from being oxidized and damaged by the presence of oxygen. Oxidation of any fat produces very high amounts of the free radicals, which attack such tissues as the artery walls, leading to atherosclerosis and heart disease. Since saturated fats are not easily susceptible to oxidation, they do not contribute to this free radical production.

Unsaturated fats, are found mostly in vegetable foods, such as safflower, sunflower, corn, and sesame. These oils are quite different from the saturated varieties. Firstly, they are generally liquid at room temperature and even under refrigeration, remain in a liquid state. The reason for this is that the molecular structure of unsaturated fats or oils is 'open bonded'. This means that the bonds, found along the molecular chain of these fats, contain few carbon atoms. This open weaving, as it were, causes them to be light and liquid. Unfortunately, the open bonds of these fats make them highly susceptible to oxidation damage and subsequent, free radical formation. As I have said previously, it is this particular free radical which attacks the muscle lining of the walls of your arteries, leading to the major cause of heart attack and stroke.

While you may be scratching your head now, what you have read is actually true. Unsaturated fats, the ones we have been told for years are good for us, are actually causing many chronic disease processes within our bodies. Refer back to Chapter 5 on heart disease for further explanation.

Modern science has come up with a third, manmade category of fats. They have been called by many names but the most common is hydrogenated. Fats of this group include solid vegetable shortenings and most margarine. These fats are vegetable oils, solidified by artificial means. All fats are metabolized in the liver. Since these fats are synthetic in their makeup, our livers don't recognize them and cannot metabolize them effectively. All fats, which are artificially altered, should be avoided at all costs.

There is a great deal of controversy over the subject of fats; much more so than with any other food. The low fat diet craze of the past 25 years has not proven helpful or healthful. In that period of time we have witnessed greater increases in heart disease and obesity than at any other time in recorded history.

With the increase of coronary conditions, great focus has been placed upon fats as the possible cause of this epidemic. Cholesterol has been falsely singled out as the culprit. As you can see from our discussion, the true culprits are oxidized concentrated vegetable oils and the free radicals produced by them. They are the actual dietary cause of heart disease.

How did cholesterol get this bad rap?

Of all the nutritional myths perpetuated today, I can think of no greater fiction that the cholesterol scare. Even the subtle mention of the word cholesterol can bring about panic, fear and subsequent guilt for consuming it. When we see a food high in cholesterol, we conjure up images of plugged up arteries, blood clots, heart attacks, and strokes. While these conditions are truly at epidemic incidence, cholesterol in the diet has very little to do with their occurrence and absolutely nothing to do with their cause. (Again, refer to Chapter 5 in order to understand the true cause of heart disease.)

Cholesterol is absolutely essential to your life. In essence, we don't meet our cholesterol needs through diet. In fact, the less cholesterol you eat, the more your body will make in order to fulfill the need. In a healthy person, the more cholesterol you ingest from your diet, subsequently, the less your body will produce. We say 'healthy' person, because many people suffer from elevated cholesterol in their blood, certainly not a healthy condition. This occurs when the regulatory mechanism for cholesterol, located in the liver, fails to do its job. One of the reasons the liver mis-manages cholesterol levels is due to internal liver congestion and the biggest cause of this condition comes from excess toxins in the environment and the ingestion of artificially altered and synthetic fats.

Cholesterol makes up the majority of your brain matter. Cholesterol and fatty acids are responsible for the sheath or insulation around nerves. Cholesterol is so essential to your health that if the levels of cholesterol in your blood fall below 150, you have a ten times greater chance of having a massive stroke.

Fatty Acids

Like amino acids from protein, fatty acids may be classified into two groups essential and non-essential, again for the same reason. Essential fatty acids are those, which the body cannot manufacture internally. There are basically three essential fatty acids that must be supplied by the diet.

Linoleic
Linolenic
Arachidonic

These fatty acids are essential for a variety of reasons:

Resistance to atherosclerosis is directly related to the amount of Arachidonic acid levels in the blood.

Linoenic acid has the ability to reduce clot formations, which are a great risk factor in coronary patients. Clot formations can be greatly reduced in a short period of time with the addition of this essential fatty acid.

Arachidonic acid is responsible for the formation of hormone-like substances called prostaglandins, which support numerous functions in the body.

Digestion of Fats

The old saying that oil and water just don't mix is as true within the body as elsewhere. Since the body is made up of about 70% water, fats and oils in the body do not mix well and enter into solution. Therefore, fats and oils need to be broken down, in order to be absorbed, transported and utilized by the body. So important is this process that the liver produces a powerful substance known as bile, to do the job. After the fats are emulsified by the action of bile upon them, specific enzymes such as lipase, split fat molecules into individual fatty acids and the by-product glycerol.

A Word about Triglycerides

Amidst all the hysteria over cholesterol, another fat molecule, called the triglyceride, is also present in the bloodstream. The triglyceride molecule is one of the largest in the human body. Unlike cholesterol, which is naturally present in the body, triglycerides are formed primarily from excess sugars. The carbohydrate intolerant, the hypoglycemic, and oftentimes the diabetic individual will produce high amounts of triglycerides due to the presence of insulin. One of the functions of insulin is to convert excess glucose into triglycerides, which then are stored in the body's fat cells as excess energy.

Because of both the physical size and the chemical makeup of triglycerides, they are of far greater potential risk in many disease processes, including heart disease and stroke. You may have heard of the terms LDL and HDL when referring to fats. LDL stands for low density lipoproteins and are the 'bad guys.' LDL lipids tend to clump together to form clots and blocks in smaller blood vessels. HDL or High Density Lipoproteins are considered to be the 'good guys', because they actually protect the cardiovascular system. When next you think about all of this or when you hear the next 'cholesterol scare', remember that the greatest concentration of HDL or the good lipids are found in cholesterol!

Choosing the Right Fats

Since fats are very concentrated food sources, a little goes a long way. Just as the very low fat diets have contributed to producing many chronic diseases, so too, can excess fat.

A good general rule to follow would be to allow fats to make up about 30% of your total food intake. These fats should primarily come from two groups, either saturated fats or what we call monounsaturated fats. In fact the monounsaturated fats are, chemically, about half way between saturated and unsaturated fats. They do not have the excessive open bonds of unsaturated fats so hence are not subject to easy oxidation and free radical formation. They contain high amounts of fatty acids, which also makes them ideal. The best monounsaturated fat to use is olive oil. This wonderful oil has been used for many centuries by the people of the Mediterranean. They have enjoyed good health and freedom from heart disease while consuming a diet containing more than three times the amount of fat typically found in the American diet.

Carbohydrates

Carbohydrates make up the largest percentage of most people's diets. There are many different types of foods classified under the general term of carbohydrates and their action on the internal chemistry of the body is quite different. All starch foods such as potatoes, pasta, grains, and root vegetables are concentrated carbohydrates. Green leafy vegetables are also carbohydrates, but provide less grams per serving. All sugars, regardless of their source, are also carbohydrates, we call these simple, concentrated carbohydrates. Regardless of the source, all carbohydrates are eventually broken down by the digestive system into the simplest of sugars, glucose. Glucose is the gasoline or fuel of the body. The primary reason for consuming carbohydrates is to provide energy to the cells of the body.

The modern diet, consisting of high amounts of refined carbohydrates delivers far more 'fuel' to the body than it can possibly utilize. The excess must be stored for later either in the form of glycogen in the muscles or triglycerides in the fat cells.

While carbohydrates, in some quantity, are necessary for a healthy life, most of us consume far too many calories from this food grouping, resulting in the over production of insulin from the pancreas, needed to remove this excess glucose and place it into storage.

The most important point to grasp regarding the carbohydrate group of foods is that the more complex they are, the safer they are to eat. As you might have guessed, like proteins and fats, carbohydrate may be divided into two basic groups, complex carbohydrates and refined or concentrated carbohydrates.

Complex carbohydrates usually have considerable fiber, the fourth food grouping, as part of their make up. This fiber is difficult to break down and slows down the digestion of complex carbohydrates. By slowing down the conversion of complex carbohydrates to glucose, we reduce the risk of producing excess blood sugar and hence invoking an insulin response.

Refined, simple, or concentrated carbohydrates, on the other hand, are digested rapidly and broken down into sugar (glucose) very quickly. Not only are these carbohydrates converted to glucose fast, but they are usually very concentrated, delivering high amounts of sugar all at once. These carbohydrates produce a rapid secretion of insulin in everyone except the endurance athlete during performance.

The repeated ingestion of refined and concentrated carbohydrates over-works the pancreas, forcing it to produce more and more insulin to regulate the excessive levels of blood sugar. Over time, in many individuals, this excess insulin in the blood stream de-sensitizes the sites in the body on which insulin works, eventually producing hypoglycemia and adult onset diabetes. (See Chapter 6 for a complete understanding of this process.)

Starches and grains may be either complex or refined, depending upon if they are consumed in their natural state or if they have been over-processed, or over cooked. Refining of wheat into white flour breaks down the starch molecules into very simple structures. As soon as anything made from these flours is ingested, the body breaks it down into glucose in a few minutes, adding immensely to the overall sugar load of the body.

It is important to remember that you don't have to eat actual sugar to have a high sugar diet. All refined, over-processed carbohydrates convert to sugar within 15 or 20 minutes once inside the digestive system.

Keep in mind that, on food labels, there are many different names for sugar. Sucrose, or common table sugar, is only one of many. Other sugars include fructose, lactose, maltose, corn syrup, molasses, modified food starch, and honey. Add in the refined carbohydrates consumed as white flour and the total consumption of 'sugar-forming' foods and beverages becomes extremely high. If you consider all these different sources of sugar, it is easy to see how the average person, on a refined junk food diet, ingests between 175 and 200 pounds of sugar per year. Is it any wonder that adult onset diabetes is the most rapidly growing epidemic in the world?

The key to consuming carbohydrates safely, without stimulating an insulin response, is to ensure that your choices are complex carbohydrates such as truly whole grains. These carbohydrates can take two to three hours or longer to fully digest and convert into blood sugar. This is long enough for the body to utilize the sugar for fuel without having to produce insulin to remove the excess.

Carbohydrate digestion begins in the mouth. This is why seeds and grains in their whole natural state, should be chewed thoroughly to crack or destroy the fibrous outer covering. This exposes the starchy interior and the ptyalin, an enzyme found in saliva, can go to work, initiating the process of carbohydrate digestion. If you consume foods made from refined flour, for example white bread, chewing it for just a few minutes makes it seem to taste sweeter and sweeter. The ptyalin in the saliva is already converting the simple starches to sugars and you haven't even swallowing it yet!

One last note on carbohydrates. The body's ability to store glucose in the form of glycogen is very limited. Since the only storehouse for glycogen is the liver and the muscles, when they are full, and we keep pouring the sugar and refined carbohydrates down our throats, the body must take further steps and convert the glycogen to triglycerides. As our discussion of fats previously indicated, the triglyceride molecule is stored in the body's fat cells and is the primary cause of being overweight or obese.

As stated before, carbohydrates, more specifically refined and concentrated carbohydrates, make up the bulk of the diet in industrialized nations, yet they are of the least importance to the body. In an emergency, our bodies can convert proteins to glucose for energy, when needed. Carbohydrates on the other hand, can never be converted to proteins.

Fiber

The body has several ways of relieving itself of toxins or poisons. The fastest, most effective way is through the lower digestive tract; specifically the colon, or large intestine, and the bowel area. Most of the body's waste material and potential toxins are passed through this canal. It is imperative therefore, that special care be given to the health and maintenance of these areas to ensure that no infections develop.

Physical discomforts and disorders, common to most people at one time or another, that signal potential problems in the waste elimination system would include constipation, diarrhea, colitis, or diverticulitis. These annoying conditions all signal problems in the colon and bowel that need immediate attention.

Diarrhea is the body's way of removing a potential toxin in a hurry. Water is forced into the lower digestive tract in an attempt to dilute the poison and carry it out of the body as fast as possible. Once cause of repeated diarrhea might be putrefactive bacteria living in the intestinal tract. There are other causes of diarrhea, such as an acid/alkaline imbalance, leading to irritable bowel syndrome, but for the most part, this occurs when waste matter stays too long in the colon, increasing the levels of toxins.

The body also produces many potentially hazardous by-products of metabolism, which, if allowed to remain in the large intestine for prolonged periods of time, may produce cancerous chemicals that act directly upon the walls of the colon.

The tract or transit time of feces is the time it takes for the body to pass the waste products through the colon, into the bowel, and finally eliminate them. The normal healthy transit time for feces is about twenty-four hours. This regularity can be achieved by including enough roughage or fiber in the daily diet.

Modern diets, consisting of over-processed foods and lifeless foods, produce little enzyme activity and contain little or no fibrous material. All of the natural fiber, including grain peels, husks, and hulls, have been removed in the refining stages. Because of this diet, poor in fiber, it is not uncommon to find many people with a feces transit time of forty-eight hours or longer. This additional time of fecal retention sets up the perfect conditions for toxic chemicals to form; the body begins drowning in its own waste.

Constipation is the most common complaint of people today. All sorts of laxative products are available to speed up the transit time through the colon and bowel. None of these however, offer the cleansing abilities that natural fibrous materials in the diet can provide.

Cellulose and hemicellulose are common fibrous materials found in a variety of foods in their natural states. These materials are referred to as insoluble carbohydrates. This type of carbohydrate makes up the majority of the outer coverings of the plant kingdom.

Seeds, nuts, grains, and many fruits and vegetables are protected from their environment by a tough layer of fibrous material known as cellulose. These cells also offer storage sites for the plant's nutrients, hence they are frequently the source of the majority of vitamins and minerals found in these foods.

The human digestive system is unable to digest cellulose because of a lack of specific enzymes. This material is coarse, even rough, and provides a natural cleansing or scraping of the intestinal wall as it passes along the tract.

Scientists have been taking a closer look at the benefits of increased fiber in the diet and the serious side effects that one can experience when insufficient roughage is provided.

Anyone who has ever tried to make wine or beer knows the ability of carbohydrates to ferment. When refined carbohydrates are present in the digestive tract, they increase the fermentation of the whole food mass, therefore, anyone eating a diet consisting of high amounts of refined carbohydrates should pat attention to their bodily processes and note the transit time of their fecal material. Excessive sugar in the diet sets the stage for rapid fermentation in the colon, leading to putrefaction and the formation of toxins.

Problems arise when waste material remains too long in the body. Some of the problems include constipation, leading to more serious conditions such as hemorrhoids, varicose veins, and phlebitis. It is estimated that more than 50% of the population of all industrialized nations over the age of fifty, suffer from one or more of these problems.

The inclusion of dietary fiber in the diet, on a daily basis, can prevent and even correct many of these situations.

Cancer research has shown that a malignancy can be caused when any body tissue comes in contact with a potentially carcinogenic material. This is especially true with the colon. The putrefactive materials that develop in the colon because of slow transit time, are not, of themselves, cancer-causing agents, however, they are susceptible to chemical reactions which do produce carcinogens.

It should be clear that the simple addition of quality fiber to the daily diet would have a host of benefits for the user.

In the next chapter, we will be discussing steps you can take to further detoxify and cleanse your body, both on the systemic and cellular levels.

Building a Healthy Diet – Just For You

Now that you have a basic understanding of the different food groupings that make up everyone's diet, let's see how this information can be utilized in building a dietary program that's best for you.

First of all, it has been said, many times, "You are what you eat". If that were true, then most of us would be French fries! The presence of rampant chronic degenerative disease, premature aging, dental problems, obesity, and stress indicate that our diet of over-processed junk foods has not served us very well.

The first step in building a lifelong dietary habit is to avoid the extremes. It's funny how we humans seem to gravitate to fanatic behavior, first in one direction, then another. It is not uncommon for people to have eaten junk food for twenty years, then the proverbial brick lands on their head and they 'see the light.' Thereafter they eat nothing but 'organic' food and three meals of tofu a day!

We should strive for more of the middle way, especially if we are presently reasonably healthy and would like to stay that way. A good diet doesn't mean you can't enjoy your favorite junk foods, just not at every meal you eat.

If you are in reasonably good health and free from any disease conditions, you should easily build your diet by the following steps.

Building a Healthy Diet for Health Maintenance

1. Fill your protein requirements first (see chart previously shown). Since protein is 'of first importance', it is essential to ensure those needs are met first.
2. Once you have planned your dietary to include adequate protein on a daily basis, you now should address the fat intake. A good rule is to consume enough of the

right kind of fats to make up about 25 – 30 percent of your total calorie intake. This would involve cooking with olive oil, and using butter (in moderation) instead of margarine on your whole grain breads and steamed vegetables.

3. Lastly, fill the balance of your diet in with quality carbohydrates. These would include whole grains and whole grain products, fresh fruits and vegetables.

4. Now the best part of all, the rewards. Choose your favorite snack foods and special treats and decide, consciously, how many times per week you wish to enjoy them. Once or twice may be enough for some, while others are able to splurge a bit more often. Pay attention to how you feel after you eat these foods, are you tired afterwards? Do they upset your system? If so, you may need to consume them a bit more moderately. Do you have a weight problem? If so, this is one area that you may need to show some discipline over.

That's it! If you have no other health concerns, building a truly healthy diet is as simple as that. Now, let's see how our newfound knowledge of the food we eat can be used to modify the diet above for our special needs.

Examples of health challenges that require a modified diet would be arthritis, heart disease and most especially hypoglycemia and diabetes. For a greater detailed discussion of these conditions, refer to the previous chapters covering them. As an example here, we will take hypoglycemia and adult-onset diabetes and show how to modify your food intake if you are living with one of these conditions.

Both hypoglycemia and adult-onset diabetes are disorders of the pancreas, which produces too much of the hormone 'insulin'. The cause of both of these conditions is the over-consumption of refined carbohydrates and sugar foods. In the case of hypoglycemia, excess insulin is produced and drives the blood sugar lower than normal, producing a host of unpleasant side effects. With adult-onset diabetes, the insulin receptor sites have become exhausted and require excessively high amounts of insulin in order to lower blood sugar. In either case, the excess insulin, which is the problem factor, needs to be lowered. The only way we can presently prevent an insulin spike is to remove much of the food that evokes an insulin response, which is the carbohydrate group.

With this in mind let's see how we can modify our basic four step dietary program above, in order to assist the body in managing either hypoglycemia or adult-onset diabetes.

Building a Healthy Diet for Managing Hypoglycemia or Adult Onset Diabetes

1. Begin by reducing the amount of total carbohydrates in your diet to the level recommended for either hypoglycemia or diabetes. (See Chapter 6.)
2. Build the remainder of your daily diet by adding adequate protein to meet your cellular needs according to the preceding chart.
3. Next ensure that your diet is moderate in fat, somewhere between 25 and 30 percent of total calorie intake.
4. Add snacks and treats that do not evoke an insulin response. This means foods that are low in refined carbohydrates and sugars.

You can see by the above example how, armed with a better understanding of the foods you eat, the diet can be modified to meet individual needs.

Further guidelines for those suffering from hypoglycemia would include keeping some food in the system on a regular basis. Lack of food, or fasting, can be very detrimental to the hypoglycemic, especially in the first few weeks of regulation. Snacking is necessary for the hypoglycemic, but snacking on the right foods is essential. Snacks should consist of vegetables or vegetable juices, alone or mixed with a protein powder.

When you first awake in the morning, consider eating a selection from the following list of acceptable fruits. This will assist in normalizing your blood sugar. If you should choose to use fruit juices, remember that they too, are very a concentrated source of carbohydrates and sugars. If you use them, be sure and dilute them at least 50% with water.

Another helpful hint is to consume 6 ounces of either mixed vegetable or tomato juice about 20 minutes before each meal. This will further help to stabilize blood sugar and avoid the spike and fall of insulin.

If you watch your diet and modify your refined carbohydrate and sugar intake, in just 30 days, you can be on the road to managing hypoglycemia. Below are two tables, one for fruits and one for vegetables. They are low in sugars and you may choose from these without drastically upsetting the insulin balance in your blood.

Fruit Listing

Cantaloupe
Rhubarb
Strawberries
Watermelon
Blackberries
Cranberries
Mixed Melons
Raspberries
Oranges

Grapefruit
Plums
Lemons
Limes

Vegetable Listing

Asparagus
Bean Sprouts
Broccoli
Cabbage
Cauliflower
Celery
Cucumber
Lettuce
Mushrooms
Radishes
Sauerkraut
Spinach
Squash
Tomatoes
String Beans
Beets
Brussels Sprouts
Eggplant
Leeks
Onions
Parsley
Red, Yellow, and Green Peppers

Foods to be Avoided by the Hypoglycemic

Beverages: Cordials, sweet wines, sweet cocktails, beer, non-diet soft drinks, coffee & tea, and all other drinks containing caffeine.

Vegetables: Hominy, rice, yams, potatoes, corn, root vegetables, and starchy beans (kidney, garbanzo, pinto, etc.).

Juices: All fruit juices should be avoided unless very highly diluted with water and consumed sparingly.

Processed Foods: White flour, white flour products, white flour pasta, starchy sauces and soups, and high sugar content foods (cookies, pies cakes, etc).

The 'dietary modifications for hypoglycemia' presented in this chapter will result in a truly amazing metabolic metamorphosis for those who religiously follow the protocol. For over 20 years, I have successfully used this 'hypoglycemia management' program on a clinical basis and can attest to the efficacy thereof.

Chapter 13
Cleansing The Toxic Body

When we speak of cleansing the body internally, there are a variety of ways in which to accomplish this. In previous chapters, I have made it clear how toxic our environment actually has become. Over the past 50 years, the shear numbers of toxins present everywhere around us has increased thousands of times. Once these poisons enter the delicate environment of the human body, one of two things happens. One, the body will store these poisons in our soft tissues where they can build to harmful levels. Or two, the body will attempt to break them down for elimination, creating dangerous free radicals in the process. In either case, a toxic internal environment will eventually produce degenerative disease, metabolic disorders and permanent tissue damage.

Since we cannot avoid the majority of our exposure to these substances, finding methods of cleansing and removing these toxins, in a safe and rapid manner, becomes essential.

Depending on concerns and needs, we can cleanse and detoxify the body by using several different approaches. There are two basic concepts of internal cleansing and detoxifying. Systemic Cleansing; This approach targets specific organs and organ systems (the digestive system, the organs of elimination, etc.) when the concerns revolve around isolated or specific areas of the body. Cellular Cleansing; I refer to this approach as cellular cleansing because it is one in which each cell of the body is detoxified and the resulting waste matter is dumped into the blood stream for disposal through the kidneys.

At the Institute, we are frequently asked, "Is detoxifying safe?" The answer is yes, if, like most things in life, it is done properly. Myths are voiced in statements such as "If you detoxify too quickly, it can harm you", or "Removing those toxins from your cells and organs poisons the blood". These allegations are simply untrue. The body has a remarkable capacity for self-cleaning, but it frequently needs help due to the overwhelming amount of poison which must be dealt with.

Systemic Cleansing and Detoxification

Systemic cleansing is valuable in cases where we want to pinpoint or target our efforts to achieve a specific result. The most common application of systemic or system cleansing is with regard to the organs of detoxification and elimination. The liver is the primary organ of detoxification and as such, can become congested and filled with poisons. The colon, kidney, bowel, and bladder all hold waste matter, which will be processed and eventually eliminated from the body if the system is working properly. These organs also need special attention. In addition to ensuring that the diet contains adequate fiber as discussed in the last chapter, an occasional cleanse of the liver and other organs that process waste is prudent. If you have a chronic disease such as arthritis or chronic digestive disturbances, you may wish to cleanse this vital area of your body more often.

The fast I have used since my days in college has proven to be so overwhelmingly responsive that I still recommend it both for general maintenance as well as for therapeutic applications. This fast is relatively easy to do. It requires that you abstain from food of any kind for only three days. (A total fast longer than this should never be conducted by anyone without the express guidance and advice from a qualified health practitioner.) The remainder of the program reintroduces foods into the system slowly in order to maximize the benefits of the fast, while not shocking the body.

The fast utilizes the acid/alkaline concept we discussed in Chapter 11. If you remember, a state of alkalinity produces a dumping of toxins and increases elimination. The first three days of the fast, your body will become very alkaline, accomplishing the cleansing effect we are after. By slowly introducing foods a bit each day, we can slowly bring your digestive system back to its natural acidic state to ensure absorption.

Other factors that make this program so effective include the use of fiber tablets to increase the bulk moving through the colon as well as specific herbs, designed to purge the organs of their toxic residue.

The Liver, Kidney, Colon, Bowel and Bladder Cleanse

Because of the direct role that toxic waste plays in the disease process, it is essential that the body be cleansed of these unwanted poisons if we are to expect to see any real improvement in the condition.

The best way to rapidly, yet safely, remove these toxins from the soft tissues of the body is through a modified fast which causes the liver, kidney, colon, and bowel to dump their stored toxins into the blood stream for eventual elimination via the urine and feces.

Needed:

1. Between 12 and 15 fresh lemons daily for 3 days
2. About 3 quarts of distilled water per day for 3 days
3. A multi-herbal formula which includes the following ingredients. Most herbalists can blend these for you if you are unable to locate an encapsulated form.
   a. Fiber
   b. Quassia Bark (approximately 50 mg)

    c. Black Cohosh Root (approximately 25 mg)

    d. Red Sage (approximately 50 mg)

    e. Golden Seal Root (approximately 10mg)

4. Additional fiber tablets

5. Honey to taste

Day One

Prepare one and one half cups of freshly squeezed lemon juice. Add to two or three quarts of distilled water and mix in a little honey for taste. This will be your total intake of fluid and food of any kind for the entire day. Sip this mixture slowly throughout the day. If you become excessively thirsty or develop a headache this first day, make up another quart of the lemon and honey water and continue sipping it as needed. In addition, take eight (8) fiber tablets in the morning and three (3) capsules of the herbal combination at night. Be sure to consume plenty of the lemon water with both the fiber tablets and the herbal tablets.

Day Two

Continue as on day one. Prepare another fresh batch of the lemon-honey distilled water mixture and sip throughout the day. Take eight (8) fiber tablets in the morning and increase the herbal combination to four (4) capsules in the evening.

Day Three

Prepare another fresh batch of the lemon-honey distilled water mixture. Continue as on previous days, except increase the herbal combination to six (6) capsules in the evening.

Days Four* and Five

Stop using the lemon water mix, but continue taking the fiber tablets. Drink any amount of tomato juice or carrot juice. You may also use white grape juice if diluted with 50% water. DO NOT CONSUME ANY CITRUS JUICES OF ANY KIND. Fresh, non-distilled, spring water may be taken in any quantity. Reduce the herbal capsules to three (3), taken in the evening with plenty of water. *Day four marks the end of the concentrated cleansing program, but continue to follow the outline given for days four and five in order to reap the full benefits of the program and to avoid shocking your body.*

Days Six and Seven

Continue as with days four and five, but you may now add fruits and vegetables. Take the fiber tablets as before in the morning and the three (3) herbal capsules in the evening.

Days Eight and Nine

Add yogurt and/or cottage cheese to your diet. Reduce the dietary fiber to four (4) tablets and stop taking the herbal combination altogether.

Days Ten and Forward

Add whole protein foods such as chicken or fish slowly, for instance, at one meal per day. Gradually return to your normal protein intake over the next few days. You may stop taking the fiber tablets unless you do not get enough on a regular basis. If this is the case, you may wish to continue taking 6 to 8 fiber tablets indefinitely.

This fast is not only safe and easy, but also very effective in removing the buildup of toxins that can contribute to all chronic degenerative diseases, especially arthritis. It is important to remember that you MUST consume the stated amount of the lemon and honey water during the first three days of the program.

Cellular Cleansing

Each of the 100 trillion cells that make up your body are, in reality, individual living systems enveloped in an outer coating called a cell membrane, which keeps the living unit in tact. Cleansing the individual cells of the body requires the use of a substance that is able to not only permeate the membrane of the living cells, but the many other protective barriers the body has in place as well. One of the most difficult barriers to penetrate is the blood/brain barrier. This is designed to prevent harmful substances that have entered the internal environment of the body from being carried by the blood, into the brain. This mechanism will allow only a specific, finite number of substances through. If we want to also cleanse and detoxify the brain tissue, we need to choose a medium that will travel freely throughout the body, to every cell.

There are two substances which fit this description and both exercise a powerful potential cleansing and detoxification mechanism upon both cells and organ systems of the body. The first is a suspension of liquid, bio-electrically active trace minerals from organic sources. These elements, in their organic compounded state, have the ability to chelate or remove heavy metals from living tissue. We will discuss the use and benefits of this later in this chapter. For now, our discussion will focus on the second substance. So important is this element, rightfully called the 'universal detoxifier', we cannot live in its absence for more than a few minutes. The substance is, of course, oxygen.

It's hard to imagine being deficient in oxygen; many of us are and have been, for years. One of the obvious ways in which the body obtains oxygen is through breathing, yet in our sedentary society, very few people have the opportunity to really fill their lungs with oxygen. In fact, if you sit up straight right now and take ten really deep breaths, you may find out just how out of shape your lungs really are! It can be most uncomfortable.

Because of this sedentary lifestyle, the lack of exercise, especially as we age, can provide less than optimal oxygenation of the blood and body tissues.

Oxygen is the universal cleanser. Through the process of oxidation, the thousands of potentially harmful toxins, which enter the body, are broken down or 'rusted' down into their basic elements in readiness for harmless elimination. As the number of toxins in the body rises, so the need for oxygen also increases. This circumstance can easily produce an even greater reduction of available oxygen. Further, the presence of chronic, ongoing disease drains the body of large amounts of oxygen in detoxifying the byproducts of the disorder.

If we wish to cleanse every cell of the body, increasing the oxygen in the blood stream is the single greatest method of accomplishing this. When the blood becomes oxygen rich, it transports the oxygen to every cell of the body, including the brain cells. In the presence of oxygen, cellular waste and toxic buildup are broken down and carried off in the blood stream to the kidneys.

It has been discovered that 'food grade' hydrogen peroxide can be safely introduced, orally or by intravenous infusion, into the body. This effectively raises the blood oxygen levels throughout the entire body and may be the answer to many of our present-day chronic and stubborn infectious diseases.

Hydrogen peroxide is completely natural. In fact, when it breaks down, the residue is simply oxygen and pure water. Under certain circumstances, your body has the ability to produce hydrogen peroxide as a 'natural killer' of pathogens. Use of hydrogen peroxide to increase bodily oxygen is not new.

It has been used around the world since the turn of the 19th Century.

Raising blood oxygen levels is important for many reasons besides its cleansing and detoxifying properties. Most pathogens, viruses and bacteria, which can enter our bodies and ultimately make us sick, have an anaerobic metabolism. In other words, they survive best in an oxygen deficient environment. When we increase the oxygen to the living tissues of the body, these pathogens cannot effectively multiply and in many cases, are destroyed outright. Recent studies have shown that the virus suspected of causing Acquired Immune Deficiency Syndrome (AIDS), as well as herpes, hepatitis, Epstein Barr, and cytomegalovirus, join the group of viruses that are lipid coated. It has also been shown that such lipid-enveloped viruses are destroyed in the presence of concentrated oxygen!

Is Oxygen Cleansing & Detoxification Safe?

Many critics of the use of oxygen therapies claim that since all peroxides are free radicals, there is a serious danger in using hydrogen peroxide internally. While it is true that cellular damage due to free radical invasion is a source of concern, we have learned that not all free radicals are created equal. Oxygen is found in simple compounds such as hydrogen peroxide. When it breaks down they produce the 'free radical' or singlet oxygen. In the case of oral hydrogen peroxide, this breakdown is so rapid that the singlet or free radical oxygen particles pair up with others of a like nature, forming stabilized oxygen once again. This process takes about one ten thousandths of a second. During this incredibly brief period of time, the singlet oxygen particles are unable to effectively produce any free radical damage.

The safety of ingesting an oxygen-donating substance depends completely upon what substance is being used. In the case of hydrogen peroxide, the end results of breakdown produce oxygen and pure water. This is not the case, however, with other forms of oxygen donating substances.

The most common substance used in current retail products sold for oxygen enhancement is chlorine dioxide. Chlorine dioxide is easy to use and remains stable in almost any solution. This is why it is favored over hydrogen peroxide, which is very unstable and almost impossible to suspend in any liquid other than plain water.

The problem with chlorine dioxide however, is that when it breaks down, while it does yield an increase in oxygen, the byproducts are chlorine and oxygen. Chlorine is the stuff we remove from our drinking water because we all know it is a cancer-causing substance! Taking these products is very dangerous and anything containing chlorine dioxide should be completely avoided.

We are therefore left with hydrogen peroxide. What form is best to take? Firstly, any hydrogen peroxide that is to be ingested internally must be of a food grade nature. Food grade hydrogen peroxide has absolutely no impurities, unlike the antiseptic versions sold in pharmacies, which should never be taken internally.

Food grade hydrogen peroxide comes, generally, in a 35 percent solution. This concentration is so strong, it will burn your skin and destroy living tissues. Therefore, it must be diluted down to a tolerable strength.

Mixing, handling and diluting food grade hydrogen peroxide is cumbersome and dangerous. The best way of introducing hydrogen peroxide and subsequently oxygen, into your body is by using a pre-mixed, stabilized form of hydrogen peroxide, buffered by a proprietary process and combined with aloe vera. This product, unlike using the pure food grade hydrogen peroxide in water, is safe and releases the oxygen to the system slowly, over a 15 to 20 minute period, whereas, the pure hydrogen peroxide releases in seconds after swallowing. This rapid release causes much of the beneficial oxygen to be exhaled before it can be absorbed through the stomach wall.

How Does Oxygen Work?

As with all phases of life, there must be a balance, hot and cold, wet and dry, attraction and repulsion. The Oriental philosophies express this two-way flow as the yin and yang.

The human body is no exception to this law of opposites, interacting to form a balance.

These opposites are created through Electro-magnetism.

The four basic elements required for all life, including human life, are oxygen, nitrogen, hydrogen and carbon. Along with minor elements, these are the building blocks of life. In looking at these elements, we find the magic of magnetic polarity at work, creating the push and pull, or yin and yang, of the opposites. The two opposites in all animal life are classified as anabolism and catabolism.

Putting all this together then, we find that hydrogen is anabolic in nature, hence it tends to solidify and concentrate. Oxygen is catabolic, and tends to dissolve and disintegrate. A combination of the two forces is absolutely essential to the continuance of the living organism. It is this disintegrating faculty of oxygen that makes it such as powerful internal cellular cleanser.

As we mentioned earlier, all toxic material, whether natural toxins from cellular activity, or foreign toxins ingested from our environment, must be neutralized rapidly and, in preparation for removal, reduced to harmless substances. Oxygen plays an important part in that process. The average person maintains a venal oxygen level of 60-70 percent. Chronically ill persons can have a depleted oxygen level as low as 55 percent! It has been estimated that a minimum of 50 percent oxygen level is required in order to sustain life. All of these figures are too low in the light of the excessive toxins in our environment. If we examine the blood of any one of several indigenous tribes who have been known for their longevity, we will find the have oxygen levels of 70 percent of the low side, up to as much as 85 percent. Levels of 80 percent or more produce a dramatic increase in cellular activity yielding greater energy and a healthy 'glow' that comes form a physical and mental state of well-being.

While the use of oxygen has many health benefits, the focus of our discussion herein rests with cleansing and detoxifying. The following program, called the 'Oxy Flush', has been used with amazing benefits in cases of extreme toxicity, chronic degenerative illness, acute infectious disease, and under other circumstances. This program will cleanse the body at the cellular level in four weeks. (For further, detailed information on the health benefits of oxygen, I suggest you read my booklet entitled, *Effective Oxygen Therapy for Chronic Conditions,* available through the Institute.)

The Oxy Flush

It is important that you obtain the buffered oxygenated aloe vera mentioned above, for this program. The amounts of product recommended are for this particular product. The use of any other form of oxygen is not to be considered. If you do not have access to oxygenated aloe vera in a buffered suspension, we suggest you write or call The Institute of Nutritional Science for a source.

Week One: Begin by taking one ounce of buffered oxygenated aloe vera two times daily, on an empty stomach*.

Week Two: Take one ounce of buffered oxygenated aloe vera three times per day, on an empty stomach.

Week Three-Six: Take two ounces of buffered oxygenated aloe vera three times per day, on an empty stomach. Stay at this dose for the entire two weeks.

After the six-week program, reduce the intake of buffered oxygenated aloe vera to one ounce twice daily for as long as you feel the need.

After week six, take 10 multi-acidophilus capsules on an empty stomach for 10 days to properly reimplant the healthy bacteria.

*Note: Oxygen products MUST be taken on an empty stomach, <u>a half-hour before or three hours after meals</u>. Taking them with food causes a rapid release of the oxygen and most is lost by exhaling. Further, in the presence of food, oxygen products can cause nausea.

There are many other healthful uses and applications for a high quality, liquid, buffered oxygen product. In Chapter 17, you will find specific protocols for hundreds of health challenges. Oxygen therapy has proven beneficial in many of them and the correct dosages are outlined in each relevant health challenge protocol.

Heavy Metal Removal

Heavy metal poisoning is, sadly, a very common occurrence. Those who live in heavily populated areas need to be worried about such toxic heavy metals as lead, cadmium and aluminum. Those living in rural areas have to be careful of all of these as well as pesticide ingredients such as arsenic and mercury.

Heavy metal poisoning can affect people of all ages, with small children often being the most susceptible. Lead from paint, still present in many buildings, is a common source of juvenile heavy metal poisoning. Mercury from older dental fillings can leak into your system slowly, building up in the soft tissues of the body.

Regardless of how these heavy metals get into our bodies, the results are always the same. Symptoms of heavy metal toxicity can run from minor to complex and devastating. If you suspect that you may have heavy metal poisoning from one or more toxic metals, the most accurate way of determining this comes from the hair mineral analysis. In the United States and many other countries, you cannot get a hair mineral analysis without a script from a health care provider. If you find yourself in this position, the Institute of Nutritional Science offers hair mineral analysis; you may contact the office at the address and telephone number at the end of this book for more information.

Fortunately, there is a relatively easy method for removing most of the troublesome heavy metals from the soft tissues of the body.

All heavy metals build to toxic levels if they are trapped in the soft tissues of the body. These metals carry a positive electrical charge, which is part of the reason the body has difficulty expelling them. When minerals having a negative electrical charge are introduced into the body, they attract the positively charged heavy metal counterparts and remove them from the body. (For a complete explanation of the bioelectrical charge of organic source elemental compounds, see the section on minerals in the next chapter.)

Bioelectrical, organic mineral compounds are available in liquid suspensions as dietary supplements. When purchasing a liquid colloidal mineral product, it is essential that the mineral spectrum be both complete and from plant sources. Many products are not from plant sources but rather from seawater or other solid mineral deposits. These inorganic minerals do not have the chelating effect on heavy metals and can in fact, build up in your body themselves. Still other products, which may or may not be from plant sources, have had certain minerals removed from the mixture. In ignorance, these companies have taken minerals such as lead, arsenic, cadmium and others out of the product, thinking that they are of no value. As long as these minerals come from plant sources, these minerals are very essential to health and wellbeing because they are the same minerals that will remove or chelate their heavy metal counterparts from your body.

Once you have determined that you have the correct source of liquid mineral, follow the program outlined below. Depending upon the amount of heavy metal toxicity you have, this process will effectively remove those heavy metals in three to six months. It is important to remember that initially, the level of heavy metals in hair and blood analysis may increase. This is due not to the liquid minerals themselves, but the fact that they are releasing the heavy metals from the soft tissues, into the blood to be safely carried out of the body via the kidneys.

Begin by taking one ounce of a liquid or ganic trace mineral product once a day. If there are no side effects*, or when the side effects have dissipated, increase the daily dos ages as follows:

Increase intake from one ounce per day to one ounce twice per day.

After a week, increase to one ounce three times per day.

Stay at this level for at least three months. If diarrhea develops, it is a sign of detoxifica tion or the fact that your body has reached saturation and has been cleansed and hence, you no longer need that amount.

*Side effects of any detoxification program can include headache, nausea, diarrhea and vomiting. If any of these symptoms develop, usually early on in the cleansing, simply reduce the amount of 'detox' supplements you are taking until the symptoms disappear. Then, after a few days or a week, slowly increase the daily dosage. As a general rule, those who have higher amounts of toxins in their systems will have the greatest chance of experiencing these temporary side effects.

Once the body has been properly cleansed and any digestive problems addressed, you are then in an ideal situation to absorb vital and essential nutrients from foods and dietary supplements.

In the next chapter, we will discuss essential and non-essential nutrients, their roles in maintaining optimal health, and what happens when they are deficient or missing from your body.

Chapter 14

Dietary Supplementation:
The Hope of the Future

Ask almost any physician or dietitian about taking vitamin and mineral supplements and you will most likely be told that you can get all the nutrients you need from your diet. You will likely hear of the benefits of the 'food pyramid' and how it represents the current scientific thinking regarding the optimal diet, which in turn, provides all the nutrients anyone might need for optimal nutrition. Nothing could be farther from the truth!

As you know from previous chapters of this book, most of what we have learned about healthy eating has been 'taught' by dietetic associations, medical associations and to some extent, the pharmaceutical industry. These groups insist that a healthy diet may be achieved by adherence to the guidelines put forth in the 'food pyramid' or four basic food groups. They promote the philosophy that we do not need to supplement our diets with additional nutrients. These beliefs are hotly contested by virtually all of the leading nutritionists.

Much of the food we eat today is deficient in, or nearly devoid of, many dozens of essential nutrients needed for good health and longevity. There are many reasons for this. The degradation of our food begins on the farm. Farming techniques in place for the last five decades use fertilizers high in nitrogen, forcing the crop to mature faster than normal, enabling the farmer to often squeeze an additional planting in during the growing season. This compromises the quantity of nutrients found in many foods. Minerals, especially trace minerals, have long vanished from our farmlands. For decades we have been planting the same fields with crops that take between 22 and 70 major and trace minerals from the soil. After each planting, the farmer fertilizes the soil with commercial preparations, which replace primarily three minerals. These three minerals are listed on each fertilizer product bag. They are expressed by three letters on the label, N.P.K. These letters represent the minerals nitrogen, phosphorous, and potassium. Each letter is followed by a number which provides the varying combinations and percentages of that mineral. Occasionally, a few other minerals are included in the combination. Typically, dozens of micro trace elements are left out of the mixture. These trace minerals were designed to serve as a catalyst to hundreds of metabolic and biological body functions. After decades of farming practices, which have not included their replacement, they have been almost completely depleted from our soil. You will see, in our following discussion of minerals, just how devastating this has been to both animals and humans.

Harvesting, transportation and storage of food are the next series of steps in the destruction of nutrients contained in food. Most fruits and vegetables are picked green, often weeks before ripening, in order to ensure that they will not spoil before they can be transported and sold at market. Most vitamins do not form in fruits and vegetables until the very last stages of growing. When the produce is severed from the plant prematurely, many of these vitamins do not form at all or only to a small percentage of what they should be.

Our produce is then transported, oftentimes for long distances, from the growing fields to remote locations. Here, the food is kept in large brokerage houses at near freezing temperatures. This keeps the food in suspended animation and allows for long-term storage. When the local market is in need of produce, say oranges, the food broker segregates enough of those round green objects to fill the order and sprays them with special chemicals to ripen them in just a few hours. As an added bonus, he frequently will add a little orange oil to the chemical mix so when you squeeze the oranges in the market, they will smell so 'fresh and delicious.'

This brings us to the last major assault upon our food, often finishing the job of destroying what few nutrients might still be left in the food at this stage. This insult is food processing and cooking.

Fresh food, which is canned, dried or frozen, looses many nutrients in the process. Anyone who has ever done any home canning can tell you that it is essential to ensure that the food to be canned has been sterilized by high heat before the jars are sealed. Failure to do so, could result in the development of potentially fatal bacterial growth inside. Well, in the process of sterilization, most all vitamins are destroyed completely, since they are highly sensitive to heat.

Even when we purchase fresh produce in our markets, the few nutrients that remain are quickly destroyed or displaced in preparation. Cooking of foods, especially the habit of cooking foods until they are nearly disintegrated, effectively destroys any remaining vitamins and leaches out most minerals.

Our love affair with dead foods, which we effectively achieve through premature harvesting, storage, chemical ripening, preserving and over-cooking has been the single biggest cause of epidemic chronic disease, next to elevated toxins in the environment.

If you watch people's eating habits you will see that they are almost frightened of fresh food. They will often choose a can of peaches over fresh ones, even when they are in the height of their season. Any foods that manage to get into the house in their natural state are surely to be destroyed by some means, before anyone eats them.

Other possible factors that can lead to the depletion of nutrients in the human body include malabsorption factors such as toxins and poisons in the body, specific prescription medications and poor digestion.

With all these assaults upon our food, is it any wonder that the majority of us suffer from multiple nutrient deficiencies almost constantly?

Still not convinced? Some people say "I believe the dietitians when they say you get all the nutrition you need from food". Well, consider this.

A group of food researchers conducted a study on the content of vitamin C in oranges. They discovered that when oranges were allowed to ripen on the trees, when they were picked, they yielded an average of 180 mg of vitamin C per orange, that's three times the present DV (RDI) for this nutrient. Oranges picked from the same trees in their usual green pre-ripened state were followed all the way to the mid-west where they were eventually chemically ripened. Upon measuring the vitamin C content of these oranges, it was found that they contained 0 mg per orange. That's right, all of the vitamin C had either been destroyed or was never there in the first place.

If that's not enough to convince you, consider that every medical journal in the world has published hundreds of studies over the past 30 years establishing that the bulk of the population has been and continues to be deficient in multiple nutrients essential to life.

The *Lancet*, the prestigious British medical journal reported in 1998 that "At least 20-30 percent of U.S. adults ingest less than the RDI of 60 mg of vitamin C per day."

"One-third to one-half of all 70 plus year old Caucasian women have lost 25 percent or more of their femoral bone mass and have reached the osteoporotic state, due to calcium deficiency." This was published in *Nutrition and the MD*, in 1997.

According to the *Journal of the American Dietetics Association*, the same organization that tells us we're all getting enough nutrients, published a study in 1997 in which they reported, "Intakes of zinc, calcium, vitamin A, vitamin B-6, and folate were frequently less than two-thirds of the RDA."

Lastly, contained within the pages of the 'Holy Grail' of medicine itself, the *Journal of the American Medical Association*, we find this quote from March 1997… "These prevalence correspond to approximately 700,000 toddlers and 7.8 million women with iron deficiency; of these, approximately 240,000 toddlers and 3.3 million women have iron deficiency anemia…" Keep in mind that this was published in the very Journal of the same medical industry that today, is trying to convince us that we all get too much iron in our diet and that all dietary supplements should now contain no extra iron at all!

In spite of these and hundred of other studies, verifying gross nutrient deficiencies, there are literally thousands of studies, which point to the fact that the established levels of individual nutrients, formerly called the RDI, now referred to as the Daily Value (DV), are dangerously too low. These multitudes of clinical studies repeatedly prove that by increasing the amount of specific nutrients, the body can not only prevent the onset of many diseases but even reverse them in many cases!

This may be illustrated by the following example. The presently recommend amount of vitamin E is set at 30 IU. Back in 1996, a clinical study involving over 2000 participants studied the effects of taking 400-800 IU of vitamin E daily. At the end of the study, researches found that the group taking the vitamin E had a whopping 77 percent decrease in risk of heart attacks and a further 47 percent decrease in all other heart disease occurrences! The placebo group showed no significant decrease in either category.

Evidence indicating that the majority of people of all ages are constantly in a state of multiple nutrient deficiency cannot be denied. The human body needs approximately 120 nutrients on a daily basis. The only truly effective way to meet those needs is to augment your diet with the supplements which provide them. More about choosing and assembling a dietary supplement program in Chapter 15. For now, let's take a look at these essential and non-essential nutrients individually and see what they do inside your body and what happens when they are deficient or absent altogether.

Vitamins

Of all the nutrients essential to optimum health and well being, more of us are familiar with the vitamin group than, perhaps, any other. In fact the term vitamins is frequently used interchangeably with all dietary supplements in day to day conversation.

It all began about a hundred years ago at the turn of the last century, when scientists ushered in a new era in the science of nutrition: the discovery of vitamins. They found that these substances, found in small quantities in foods, were absolutely essential to health. A diet lacking in just one, could cause a whole list of symptoms to develop and ultimately, could lead to death if the deficiency were not solved.

In more recent years, scientists are discovering the power of these nutrients when applied in doses larger than what was previously believed to be sufficient.

Through our research and application of vitamins in the human diet, we have discovered that the old concept of the 'one disease' idea was terribly wrong. In the past, it was thought that a deficiency of one vitamin caused one specific disease or disorder. Today we know that the vitamin family is not only intrinsically linked to each other but to other non-vitamin nutrients as well. This is the concept of Full Spectrum nutrition, and we will explore it fully in the next chapter.

The definition of a vitamin is that it is a catalytic dietary essential that the body is unable to synthesize or manufacture in adequate amounts and therefore, must be taken in from outside sources. The term mega-vitamin therapy is simply the use of higher dosages of vitamins for the betterment of an individual.

Vitamins are absolutely essential for the growth, maintenance and reproduction of the human body. They have been studied in great depth by many biochemists. Vitamins are generally divided into two basic groups, the fat-soluble vitamins and the water-soluble vitamins. We will take a closer look at the vitamin family by starting with the fat-soluble members.

Fat-soluble vitamins include A, D, E, and K. They are found in foods containing fats; people following low or non-fat diets can become very deficient in them.

Vitamins in this grouping are generally stable to temperature changes and are therefore less likely to be affected by freezing or cooking. Fat-soluble vitamins are absorbed from the intestinal tract along with fatty foods. This means that if you have trouble digesting fat from foods, you are also likely not absorbing these vitamins either. Since the fat-soluble vitamins are so important for a multitude of functions, it is important that we ensure adequate supplementation in order to meet individual needs.

Vitamin A

This was the first of the fat-soluble vitamins to be discovered. Vitamin A comes in several forms, natural and synthetic as well as true vitamin A and pro-vitamin A.

As with all the fat-soluble vitamins, vitamin A should NEVER be taken in its synthetic form. The liver, which is responsible for metabolizing all fats in the body, including the fat-soluble vitamins, cannot recognize the synthetic varieties of these nutrients and they can buildup to toxic levels. In fact, every case of vitamin A toxicity ever recorded was in individuals taking high doses of synthetic vitamin A. When you read a label, if it indicates the vitamin A is from fish liver oil, that is the best source of natural vitamin A. It may also be listed by its chemical name, *palmitate*, which also means the natural variety. If your label says vitamin A from *acetate*, avoid it at all cost, as this is the cheap synthetic variety.

Beta-carotene converts to vitamin A in the liver, but only at a specific rate, therefore it is not useful when we need to provide very large doses of vitamin A for specific reasons. For daily use, a combination of natural, pure vitamin A and beta-carotene provides the best of both factors.

I have often said that if I were to be stranded on a desert island and could only have one nutrient with me, it would be vitamin A. This wonderful vitamin is responsible for so many biological functions and serves as a first-line of defense for our immune system. Further, vitamin A deficiency is second only to protein deficiency worldwide!

Vitamin A has been shown to be helpful in preventing and managing skin disorders such as boils, canker sores, acne, athlete's foot, bedsores, burns, dandruff, dermatitis, psoriasis, and shingles.

The primary function of vitamin A is the protection of the mucous membranes, which line all of the openings of the body. This tissue, when properly nourished with vitamin A, has natural antibiotic and antiviral properties, destroying many potential pathogens before they can enter the body.

Other conditions for which vitamin A may be helpful include cystitis, atherosclerosis, mononucleosis, diabetes, colitis, meningitis, ear infections, cataracts, glaucoma, night blindness, cystic fibrosis, prostatitis, swollen glands, sinusitis, arthritis, nephritis, bronchitis, and influenza.

Vitamin A is an important growth factor, especially of the long bones of the body as well as the spacing of the teeth.

Functions of Vitamin A

1. One of the most important functions of this vitamin, and one of particular interest in our text, is that it maintains the health and well-being of the epithelial tissues of the body. These are generally the tissues that line the openings, skin, and mucous membranes. All glands and their duct systems come under the protection of vitamin A. Since these areas are the first potential sites for bodily invasion by outside microbes, we must maintain these sites in optimal health.
2. Vitamin A aids in the growth and repair of body tissues, especially bones.
3. Proper formation and maintenance of

tooth enamel and gums are a vitamin A process.

4. Vitamin A prompts the secretion of gastric juices necessary for proper digestion of proteins.
5. Vitamin A maintains the proper health of sex glands and the uterus.
6. Night vision and the general maintenance of the eye is a function of vitamin A.
7. Vitamin A aids in the synthesis of RNA.

Deficiency Symtoms of Vitamin A

1. The eyes are obvious indicators of vitamin A deficiency. One of the first symptoms is night blindness. Other eye indicators of vitamin A deficiency include dry, itchy, and inflamed eyeballs.
2. Susceptibility to colds, flu, bacterial and viral infections, especially of the respiratory and urinary tract, are indicators of vitamin A deficiency. Sinusitis and abscesses in ears and mouth are also common symptoms, as well as general repeated infections.
3. Acne.
4. Rough, dry, scaly, prematurely aged skin.
5. Sensitivity to light.
6. Reproductive difficulties.

Vitamin D

Vitamin D is often called the 'sunshine' vitamin, because it can be manufactured in the body when sunlight comes in contact with exposed skin. Deficiencies of vitamin D occur when people do not go out of doors, either as a preference or because of inclement whether. This is the reason the FDA mandated that vitamin D be added to milk to prevent a deficiency in children with developing bones. A gross deficiency of vitamin D results in rickets and other deformities of the bones.

As with vitamin A, this nutrient should also never be taken in its synthetic form. My personal favorite form of vitamin D is known as D-3, and comes from animal sources such as may be found in fish oils and eggs. This is the same form of vitamin D as is produced in human skin through the interaction of sunlight.

Like all fat-soluble vitamins, vitamin D is absorbed only in the presence of fat in the diet. Absorption takes place through the intestinal walls by the action of bile. Vitamin D formed in the skin is absorbed directly into the system. Food sources of vitamin D are restricted mostly to the oily fishes such as herring or salmon.

Functions of Vitamin D

1. Vitamin D is necessary for normal growth of children. In its absence, bones and teeth do not calcify. Vitamin D is essential for proper utilization of calcium and phosphorus.
2. Formation of RNA.
3. Formation of certain enzymes.
4. Helps to maintain a stable nervous system, normal heart action, and normal blood clotting.

Deficiency Symtoms of Vitamin D

1. Rickets (bowlegs, knock-knees, enlargement of bones).
2. Poor growth and lack of bone development.
3. Osteomalacia (softening of the bones).
4. Tetany (muscular numbness, tingling, spasm)
5. Thyroid problems (loss of thyroid hormones)
6. Arthritis
7. Fatigue

Vitamin E

Vitamin E belongs to a group of chemical compounds called tocopherols. There are many forms of tocopherols such as alpha, beta, delta, gamma, and zeta.

Alpha-tocopherol is the form commonly referred to as vitamin E and is the most widely distributed form of the vitamin found in nature. Recent studies indicate that some of the other forms of vitamin E, such as gamma-tocopherol, may be responsible for numerous increased benefits to human health. I have always recommended using vitamin E supplements comprised of mixed sources (tocopherols).

Of all the fat-soluble vitamins, it is most critical to avoid consuming synthetic vitamin E. Studies show that not only is the synthetic form far less absorbable, but it can buildup in the liver as well. In order to avoid taking products containing the cheaper synthetic version, you must learn to read labels. If the label says 'd-alpha tocopherol', it is a natural source vitamin E. If however, it reads 'dl-alpha tocopherol', it is artificial and should NEVER be taken! Most manufacturers of the less expensive supplements rely on synthetic vitamin E to keep their cost down. Natural forms of vitamin E often cost the manufacturer several hundred percent more than do synthetic ingredients.

Vitamin E functions primarily as an antioxidant. It protects the body by preventing polyunsaturated fats from forming the specific free radicals, which are known to lead to atherosclerosis and subsequent heart disease. Other antioxidant functions of vitamin E include stabilizing membranes against free radicals, protecting skin, eye, liver, and breast tissues and preserving the integrity of vitamin A.

In the past, vitamin E was associated with sexual

function and even sold as an aphrodisiac. However, there is no connection between the actions of vitamin E within the body and sexual response.

Vitamin E is absorbed, like all other fat-soluble vitamins, in the presence of fat in the diet. You can now begin to see why the super low-fat diet 'craze' of a few years ago was so potentially dangerous. Vitamin E is stored, along with the other fat-soluble nutrients, in the liver.

Functions of Vitamin E

1. Plays an important role in cellular respiration of muscles, most especially the cardiac muscle.
2. Prevents peroxide formation by being an anti-oxidant.
3. Protects all the other fat soluble vitamins against oxidation.
4. Reduces scar tissue formation both internally and externally. This is why creams and ointments containing vitamin E are especially effective.
5. Increases formation of new blood vessels around damaged areas.
6. Stimulates urine secretion, hence has a lowering effect on some instances of blood pressure.
7. Provides protection against poisonous substances such as inhalants and internal by-products of metabolism.

8. Assists in normalizing blood viscosity.
9. Retards muscle degeneration.
10. Protects and ensures permeability of the capillary system.

Deficiency Symptoms of Vitamin E

1. First clinical sign of deficiency is the rupturing of the red blood cells.
2. Faulty absorption of fat and fat soluble vitamins. Evidence shows a link between this condition and the development of cystic fibrosis and inflammation of the pancreas.
3. Retarded growth in children.
4. Nutritional muscular dystrophy.
5. Swelling of the cardiac muscle which can become necrotic.
6. Women severely deficient experience frequent miscarriages, as well as premature births.
7. Angina pectoris
8. Menstrual discomfort and PMS.
9. In males, a reduced mobility of spermatozoa.
10. In females, uterine degeneration, and in some cases, sterility.

Vitamin K

The primary role of vitamin K in the body is as a blood-clotting factor. The vitamin converts to pro-thrombin, the precursor of the blood clotting factor thrombin, in the liver.

A deficiency of vitamin K is rare because it is quite common in many foods and not easily destroyed by heating or other processing.

Recently, vitamin K has been shown to assist in the uptake of calcium and may be beneficial in older people, especially women. Further, it is routinely given to women during pregnancy, since the risk for hemorrhage is greater at that time and vitamin K acts directly to prevent hemorrhage by increasing the bloods clotting ability.

Potential deficiencies of this nutrient might be present when there is a persistent low-grade level of intestinal bacteria in the small intestine. Acidophilus cultures in the form of yogurt, kefir or supplements serve not only as a good food source, but will ensure that sufficient friendly intestinal flora is present for good digestion, health of the intestinal tract, and proper synthesis of vitamin K.

Like the other fat-soluble counterparts, vitamin K is absorbed in the upper intestinal tract along with dietary fat.

Function of Vitamin K

Basic function of vitamin K is to act in the formation of prothrombin, the chemical necessary in the clotting of the blood.

Deficiency Symptoms of Vitamin K

1. Hypoprothrombinemia (loss of blood's ability to clot).
2. Internal hemorrhages, especially in the brain, spinal cord and intestinal tract.
3. Subcutaneous hemorrhage.
4. Nosebleeds.
5. Can be a cofactor in cellular disease and diarrhea.

The Water-Soluble Vitamins

Unlike the fat-soluble vitamins discussed previously, the water-soluble group, consisting of vitamin C and the entire B-complex, are not stored in the body for any length of time. This means that they must be ingested daily in the form of food or dietary supplementation. While they are absorbed much more easily than their fat-soluble associates, they pass out of the body readily with fluids such as urine and perspiration.

The separate and individual members of the B-complex family are also linked because they share many of the same basic functions and work together to perform many of their numerous functions. B Vitamins are cultured from bacteria, yeast, fungi, or mold. Currently, the B-complex group consists of thiamin (B-1), riboflavin (B-2), niacin (B-3), pantothenic acid (B-5), pyridoxine (B-6), cobalamin (B-12), biotin, choline, inositol, folic acid (folacin), Para-Amino Benzoic Acid (PABA), B-13, and B-15.

In general, the B-complex group is responsible for providing energy to the body through direct involvement with the conversion of carbohydrates to glucose. This is especially important for hypoglycemic and diabetic individuals. They are also critical in the metabolism of both fats and proteins.

The proper functioning of the nervous system is also affected by the B-vitamins. Many consider this group of nutrients to be the single most influential factor in the health and maintenance of the nerves.

Vitamin B-1 (Thiamin)

Thiamin is essential in the removal of carbon dioxide or oxidative decarboxylation reactions. This is important in the conversion of foods to energy in the Krebs Cycle. Since thiamin is water-soluble, exercise and alcohol (a diuretic) increases the need for supplementation.

Thiamin is frequently referred to as the 'morale vitamin', since it plays such an important role in the nervous system and subsequently the state of mental health. This vitamin combines with pyruvic acid in the body to form a co-enzyme that is required for the breakdown of carbohydrates into the basic body sugar, glucose.

If your diet is high in carbohydrates and refined sugars, your need for thiamin increases drastically.

This nutrient is also responsible for maintaining muscle tone of internal organs such as the heart, stomach and intestines. Further, thiamin helps to stabilize the appetite by way of improvement in food assimilation.

Thiamin is rapidly absorbed through the small and large intestines. It is carried, via the circulatory system, to the liver and kidneys. There it is combined with other nutrients (mainly minerals) to form specific enzymes.

Functions of Vitamin B-1

1. Assists in conversion of carbohydrates to glucose.
2. Necessary for growth, fertility, and lactation.
3. Controls and feeds nervous system.
4. Stabilizes the appetite.
5. Involved and consumed in the metabolism of alcohol.

Deficiency Symptoms of Vitamin B-1

1. Poor carbohydrate metabolism.
2. Mental instability, forgetfulness, fears, and confusion due to the build up of pyruvic acid in the blood, creating an oxygen deficit.
3. Cardiac malfunctions - palpitations, rapid rhythm, enlarged heart, elevated venous pressure, and myocardial lesions.
4. Loss of ankle and knee reflexes.
5. Muscular weakness progressing to atrophy.
6. Fatigue.
7. Reduced or lost appetite.
8. Inflammation of the optic nerve.

Vitamin B-2 (Riboflavin)

Like thiamin, vitamin B-2 is directly involved in energy metabolism. Enzymes formed in the presence of riboflavin play a role as hydrogen carriers for the oxidation-reduction reactions in the electron transport system in the formation of ATP. Since it too is not stored in any appreciable amounts, we must ensure daily ingestion from foods or supplements.

Riboflavin is a very active substance and may be found as part of many chemical reactions within the body, which are essential to the life process. It combines with many other nutrients to form enzymes and coenzymes.

Riboflavin is essential for normal fatty acid and amino acid synthesis and cellular growth cannot take place when riboflavin is missing.

Riboflavin is absorbed easily through the walls of the small intestine and is rapidly excreted through the kidneys, via the urine.

Functions of Vitamin B-2
1. The respiration of cells.
2. Aids in the conversion of tryptophan to niacin.
3. Critical in the metabolism of carbohydrates, proteins and fats.
4. Needed in the maintenance of skin, nails, and hair.
5. Helps the eyes in adaptation to light.

Deficiency Symptoms of Vitamin B-2
1. Shiny tongue.
2. Eye fatigue - burning, itching, with a sensitivity to bright lights.
3. Capillary congestion in the white area of the eye.
4. Sensation of grit or grinding sand inside eyelids.
5. Lesions of the lips, scaling around the nose, mouth and ears.
6. Difficulty in urination, vaginal itching.
7. Oily skin.

8. Retarded erythrocyte formation resulting in anemia.
9. Cataracts.
10. Pellagra factor.

Vitamin B3 (Niacin or Niacinamide)

Niacin is by far one of the most stable of the B-complex group of nutrients. It is very resistant to both heat and light. Vitamin B-3 comes in two supplement forms, niacin (pure nicotinic acid) and niacinamide. They are virtually identical except niacinamide does not induce peripheral flushing, as does pure niacin. There are times when this flushing is desirable and under those circumstances, pure niacin must be used. Niacinamide is the form of choice in most multiple, broad-spectrum products. Chemically, the difference between the two is that niacin contains an organic acid group as part of its makeup while niacinamide contains an amino acid group in its place. Niacinamide is less likely to produce nausea than is niacin.

Niacin can be formed in the body through a chemical reaction, which converts the amino acid tryptophan into niacin within the body tissues.

Niacin is well absorbed and some may be stored in the liver for short periods of time. Since niacin is not prevalent in most foods, supplementation is often essential unless you regularly consume liver, high amounts of wheat germ, or brewer's yeast. Niacin is also found, to a lesser extent, in meats, poultry, and fish.

Functions of Vitamin B-3

1. Plays the active role in the coenzymes that provide an essential ingredient in tissue oxidations.
2. Necessary for the synthesis of sex hormones.
3. Vital to the activity of the nervous system.
4. Improves circulation and reduces serum cholesterol.

Deficiency Symptoms of Vitamin B-3

1. Pellagra - still a common disease in modern times.
2. Mood swings.
3. Loss of appetite, indigestion.
4. Schizophrenia.
5. Recurring headaches, especially migraine.
6. Canker sores, and other small ulcers.
7. Inflammation and irritability of mucosa linings.
8. Insomnia.

Vitamin B-6 (Pyridoxine)

This member of the B-complex family is very stable except in heat, which makes the possibility of deficiency very real. Many years back, the famous baby food scandal involved gross deficiencies in pyridoxine since all baby food is canned and the process of canning uses enough heat to destroy B-6.

One of pyridoxine's most important functions is as a universal transport mechanism for other nutrients. This is why it is frequently used in conjunction with other nutrient supplements, especially those containing amino acids. Pyridoxine helps to transport individual amino acids across the blood/brain barrier.

Pyridoxine also assists in the formation of specific amino acids, removes sulfur from certain amino acids and metabolizes cysteine to pyruvic acid as well as oxalate to glycine. It can be seen by these examples that pyridoxine is essential in virtually all the activities involving protein, and subsequently, amino acids.

There is a strong connection between long-term pyridoxine deficiencies and both hypoglycemia and diabetes. It has also been shown that people with either of these two conditions almost always have a deficiency of B-6, even when the recommended amount is provided. Thus, higher amounts of B-6 are indicated in persons with glucose metabolism disorders.

Pyridoxine plays an essential role in immune function. Firstly, it is needed for the care and maintenance of the mucous membranes at all points of entry into the body. Secondly, a pyridoxine deficiency causes a definite impairment of thymus-derived lymphocytes (T-cells) mediated immunity. Lack of B-6, over prolonged periods, will decrease the size and weight of the thymus gland. There is further evidence that pyridoxine also demonstrates anti-tumor potential.

Functions of Vitamin B-6

1. Necessary for proper assimilation of Vitamin B-12.
2. Aids in the production of hydrochloric acid.
3. Required in the metabolism of many amino acids.
4. Involved in the metabolism of fats, especially the unsaturated fatty acids.
5. Necessary for the conversion of tryptophan to niacin.
6. Helps to maintain the sodium/potassium balance.
7. Facilitates glycogen conversion to glucose.
8. Must be present for the production of antibodies and red blood cells.
9. Involved in proper synthesis and activity of DNA and RNA.

Deficiency Symptoms of Vitamin B-6

1. Dermatitis.
2. Numbness of hands and feet.
3. Over production of xanthurenic acid (green-colored urine).
4. Low blood sugar and low glucose tolerance.
5. Cramps in the extremities.
6. Dizziness, nausea, vomiting.
7. Kidney stones.
8. Edema.
9. Arthritis during menopause.

Vitamin B-12 (Cobalamin)

Vitamin B-12 is involved in the activation of many amino acids during the formation of proteins within the body. Cobalamin is necessary for the metabolism of most all foods, especially carbohydrates. Impaired fatty acid synthesis is common in prolonged B-12 deficiency and can lead to malformed myelin sheath, the insulation surrounding all nerve cells. This is the reason why B-12 has often been labeled the 'nerve vitamin', since a prolonged deficiency results in hyperactivity and nervous irritability.

Pernicious anemia is another by-product of B-12 deficiency. This condition can develop from either not ingesting enough of the nutrient or may develop as a result of absorption problems. In order for B-12 to be absorbed, it must bind with an intrinsic factor, secreted by the stomach. This, in turn, carries the B-12 to the small intestine.

It is important to note that vitamin B-12 is found only in animal products. Those on a strict vegetarian diet have no choice but to rely on dietary supplements to fill the body's vitamin B-12 needs.

Unlike most of the B-complex family, B-12 is very difficult to absorb. The presence of adequate hydrochloric acid in the stomach facilitates the absorption of cobalamin.

Functions of Vitamin B-12

1. Essential for the functioning of all cells, with emphasis upon bone marrow, nervous tissue, and the gastrointestinal tract.
2. Aids in the synthesis of many other nutrients such as choline.
3. Plays a vital role in the formation of nucleic acids.
4. Because of its connection with bone marrow, it is needed by the body in the formation of the red blood cells.

Deficiency Symptoms of Vitamin B-12

The really serious lasting side effects from a B-12 deficiency can take years to develop.

1. Soreness and tingling of the extremities, indicating the deficiency is affecting the nervous system.
2. Sore tongue, weakness, loss of weight.
3. Brain damage over the long period similar to schizophrenia.
4. Shooting pains, "needles and pins" sensations.
5. Serious apathy.
6. Pernicious anemia (accompanied by degeneration of the spinal cord).
7. Neuritis, menstrual disturbances.
8. Mental deterioration and paralysis.

Folic Acid (Folacin)

The single greatest function of folacin is as a carbon carrier in the formation of heme, which is the iron-containing protein present in hemoglobin. This is necessary for the formation of red blood cells. It is important to note that in the absence of B-12, folic acid becomes trapped in the body as methyl folate and is useless to the body. Therefore, deficiencies of both vitamin B-12 and of folic acid produce identical symptoms.

Folic acid deficiency is another very common vitamin deficiency. The symptoms of which, as we mentioned, are similar to that of B12 and include anemia, irritability, weakness, weight loss, apathy, anorexia, and heart palpitations.

Folic acid is very vulnerable to destruction. If foods are not stored carefully, up to 100 percent of all the folic acid in a given food source may be destroyed.

Folic acid, like many B-complex nutrients, plays an active role in both cellular and humoral immunity.

Folic acid is essential in the prevention of several complications of pregnancy, including serious birth defects. For this reason, high doses of folic acid are now recommended during pregnancy and lactation.

Folic acid is absorbed in the gastrointestinal tract. While some folic acid storage takes place in the liver, it is important to note that many drugs, especially the sulfa drugs, interfere with 'folic acid manufacturing' bacteria in the intestines. Many antibiotics can totally destroy folic acid. Supplementation is now highly recommended for everyone.

Functions for Folic Acid
1. Increases appetite and stimulates HCL production.
2. Enhances liver functions.
3. Necessary for synthesis of nucleic acids.
4. Necessary for some amino acid synthesis.
5. Prevention of macrocytic anemia.

Deficiency Symptoms of Folic Acid
1. Macrocytic anemia (lack of mature red blood cells, or red blood cells that are larger than normal and contain less hemoglobin levels than normal).
2. Smooth, red, tongue.
3. Poor growth, and metabolic disturbances.
4. Graying hair.
5. Possible link to certain types of mental illness.
6. Gastrointestinal disturbances, like diarrhea.
7. Birth deformities; cleft palate.
8. Toxemia of pregnancy, premature birth.

Pantothenic Acid

The primary function of pantothenic acid is in the synthesis of the neurotransmitter acetylcholine as well as in the production of the adrenal hormones. For these reasons, pantothenic acid is vital in ensuring the optimal function of the nervous system. As our nervous system becomes more and more excited and overworked, the need for pantothenic acid rapidly increases. Sad is the fact that the current DV (recommended RDI) of this nutrient is only 10 mg. Under moderate to severe stress, the body can consume as much as 100 mg of pantothenic acid, or more, per hour. When used in large doses, together with B-12, pantothenic acid supports the nervous system and acts like a natural tranquilizer.

Pantothenic acid supports the immune system by promoting antibody formation. A deficiency of this vitamin has been linked to an overall atrophy of the lymphatic system.

Pantothenic acid is required by every cell of the body to fulfill metabolic functions. It is also used in the functioning of the gastrointestinal tract.

Functions for Pantothenic Acid

Pantothenic acid is necessary for the makeup of coenzyme A. This factor is necessary during the intermediary metabolism of carbohydrates, fats, and proteins.

Since this nutrient has an enhancing effect upon the adrenal glands, it becomes an important factor during stressful conditions.

This vitamin is so closely involved with others of the B-group, that the B-complex group of vitamins should always be taken together as a unit. Single dosages of isolated B-vitamins can cause a rapid deficiency in others. Once a balanced combination of all the B-complex group is taken on a daily basis, then mega-doses of isolated B-vitamins can be administered for specific purposes without the fear of creating an imbalance or deficiency.

Deficiency Symptoms of Pantothenic Acid

1. Fatigue, headache, changes in personality.
2. Reduction in metabolic processes.
3. Postural Hypotension, dizziness, rapid heart beat (this is because of the effect of the deficiency on the adrenal glands).
4. Gastric distress, reduction of HCL and Pepsin leading to constipation.
5. Burning sensation of hands and feet.
6. Inclination toward hypoglycemia.
7. Involved in the metabolic breakdown leading to arthritis.

Biotin

Biotin assists in the growth of cells in the body. It is involved in the production of fatty acids as well as in the metabolism of carbohydrates, fats and proteins. Biotin assists the body in utilizing other B-complex nutrients and should always be included in a well-rounded B-complex formula. Biotin is helpful in preventing certain specific types of hair loss in men. Lastly, biotin is necessary for the proper function of sweat glands, nerve tissue, and bone marrow.

Functions for Biotin

1. Acting as a coenzyme, it is essential in the making of fatty acids and in the oxidation of fatty acids as well as the carbohydrates.
2. Required in the formation of glycogen.
3. Required in the synthesis of several of the non-essential amino acids by the body.
4. Aids in the formation of nucleic acids.

Deficiency Symptoms of Biotin

1. Sore tongue and dry skin.
2. Muscular pain; lack of energy.
3. Insomnia.
4. Loss of appetite.
5. Intense depression.

Choline

Sadly, many so-called authorities feel that choline is a rather non-essential nutrient. This is unfortunate since choline is involved in many very important catalytic and metabolic functions. Choline, one of the active constituents of lecithin, is essential in the metabolism of fats and cholesterol. It is used by the liver in cleansing and for the regulation of cholesterol production. Without choline, brain function is impaired, especially memory function. Prolonged absence of adequate choline results in a fatty liver.

Choline is used to support the liver and is very important in such conditions as hepatitis and cirrhosis.

Functions for Choline

1. Aids in the metabolism of fats. (It is for this reason that lecithin has shown sometimes dramatic beneficial results in normalizing cholesterol levels in the blood.)
2. Part of the chemical acetylcholine, which is essential to normal nerve function.
3. Protects the myelin sheaths of the nerves.
4. Regulating effect upon the liver and gallbladder.
5. Assists in the synthesis of hormones such as epinephrine.

Deficiency Symptoms of Choline

1. Fatty degeneration of the liver.
2. Hemorrhaging of the kidneys.
3. High blood pressure.
4. Heart muscle lesions.
5. Atherosclerosis (the single greatest cause of the bypass operation).

Inositol

Inositol is the 'hair' vitamin. It is vital for thick healthy hair. Inositol also helps prevent atherosclerosis. Along with choline, it helps the liver process fat and metabolize cholesterol. Inositol supplementation is especially recommended when liver function is compromised.

Functions for Inositol
1. Plays a great part in the metabolism of fats.
2. Acts as a growth factor.
3. Feeds cells of the brain.
4. Aids hair growth and prevention of thinning and baldness.

Deficiency Symptoms of Inositol
1. Atherosclerosis
2. Eczema
3. Constipation

Para-Amino Benzoic Acid (PABA)

PABA is one of the basic constituents of folic acid and also helps the body utilize pantothenic acid. Once again, we can see the intrinsic relationship between the member compounds that comprise the B-complex group of nutrients. It is an antioxidant and protects against radiation from the sun when taken internally.

Under certain circumstances, PABA may restore color to graying hair, but only if the graying was caused by stress or nutritional deficiency. PABA has been used in successfully treating certain parasitic diseases.

Functions for Para-Amino Benzoic Acid

1. Stimulates intestinal bacteria.
2. Acts in the capacity of a coenzyme in the breakdown of proteins.
3. Assists in the formation of blood cells, primarily red blood cells.
4. Prevents eczema and vitiligo which is a loss of skin pigmentation.
5. Has been shown beneficial in burn pain control.
6. Helps to protect the skin against the harmful effects of overexposure to sunlight.

Deficiency Symptoms of Para-Amino Benzoic Acid

1. Sulfa drugs cause a deficiency of PABA.
2. Gastrointestinal disorders.
3. Irritability and depression.
4. Lupus Erythematosus (mega-doses have shown a positive response in 80% of cases studied).
5. Loss of sex drive.
6. Constipation.

Vitamin C (Ascorbic Acid)

Often referred to as the "King of Vitamins", vitamin C is the most popular vitamin. Most people are familiar with it, and as a supplement, it is used more often than any other single nutrient. This is due, in part, to the work of the late Linus Pauling, and others. While we often associate vitamin C with the prevention of the common cold, this amazing substance has many functions.

Firstly, vitamin C plays a pivotal role in the formation of collagen. Collagen is the intracellular 'cement,' that holds us together. It is also the substance that fills in under the surface layers of skin, giving us our youthful appearance. As we age, this collagen protein becomes depleted and our skin looses its elasticity. Collagen may also be found in intervertebral discs, joint and connective tissue, bones, teeth, tendons, skin and scar tissue. In the capillaries, it is the supporting material that prevents bruising. The symptoms of scurvy, a vitamin C deficiency disease, are due to the failure of sufficient collagen formation.

The discovery that scurvy, a disease once common throughout Europe, was caused by a vitamin C deficiency. This was discovered after it was realized that scurvy particularly afflicted British sailors who were deprived of fresh fruits and vegetables for long periods. Their symptoms of scurvy worsened the longer they were at sea.

Therapeutically, vitamin C may be administered

either orally or intravenously. Most common oral supplements consist of basic ascorbic acid, although many companies are offering buffered forms for those who are sensitive to the acid, especially in higher doses. Intravenously, ascorbic acid must be given in one of two of its salts namely, sodium ascorbate and calcium ascorbate.

While plants need very little ascorbic acid in their metabolism, animals on the other hand often require very high amounts. Interestingly, most all animals, except humans, can manufacture vitamin C in very high amounts and according to needs.

We can get a fairly good idea of how much vitamin C we humans need by comparing ourselves to other animals. For example, the rat has been shown to synthesize up to 26 mg of ascorbic acid per kilogram of body weight per day. If we compare this to the average human, weighing about 70 kilograms (about 154 pounds), that person should then be consuming somewhere between 2500 and 3000 mg of ascorbic acid in an average day.

Ascorbic acid is involved in the synthesis of hormones. During times of excess stress, when these hormones are utilized, the limited storehouses of ascorbic acid in the adrenal glands are quickly depleted.

Ascorbic acid can facilitate in the conversion of tryptophan to 5-hydroxy-tryptophan, producing the powerful neuro-transmitter, serotonin.

Lastly, vitamin C is an antioxidant, which is why it is helpful in preventing and reducing the symptoms of such things as the cold and flu virus. Unlike many other vitamins, vitamin C is actually consumed or utilized as it does its job. This means the more work there has to be done, the greater the body's need for the nutrient. When the body experiences a bacterial or viral infection, or in times of stress, vitamin C can be consumed or utilized at an astonishingly rapid rate. Urine excretion tests have shown that during an attack of a flu virus, a person may ingest as much as 30,000 mg of ascorbic acid in 24 hours with little or no excess spillover in the urine.

Vitamin C is very readily absorbed into the blood stream via the intestines. Absorption is increased during periods of physical or emotional stress. Vitamin C is destroyed by smoking, stress, fever and prolonged ingestion of antibiotics.

Vitamin C is the least stable of all vitamins. It is easily destroyed by exposure to light, heat, and oxygen.

Functions for Vitamin C

1. The most important function of vitamin C in the human body is in the formation of collagen protein. Collagen is the glue for specialized tissues that hold us together, such as skin, cartilage, tendon, and bone.
2. Speeds the healing of wounds.
3. Antihistamine action.
4. Maintains strength in blood vessels.

5. Fights bacterial and viral infections.
6. Promotes formation of hemoglobin.
7. Aids in absorption of iron from intestinal tract.
8. Converts folic acid to folinic acid.
9. Antioxidant action, protecting many other valuable nutrients such as thiamine, riboflavin, vitamins A and E, and pantothenic acid against damage from oxidation.
10. Diuretic action on body cells.
11. Aids in the metabolism of the amino acids, phenylalanine tyrosine, and tryptophan.
12. Helps the adrenals in the secretion of hormones.

Deficiency Symptoms of Vitamin C

1. Skin bruising; bleeding gums.
2. Shortness of breath; impaired digestion.
3. Anemia.
4. Joint pains.
5. Increased healing time of surface wounds.
6. Breaks in capillary walls resulting in clots.
7. Excessive hair loss.
8. Scurvy.

Minerals

Among the types of nutritional supplements consumed (vitamins, major minerals, amino acids, antioxidants, etc.) there seems to be more confusion about minerals, especially trace minerals. Vitamin supplements are available in either natural or synthetic forms. Except for the fat- soluble varieties, most are very similar. That makes it easy to decide which to use. On the other hand, mineral supplements are available in different forms and obtained from different sources. Each form has different characteristics, which determine the body's ability to benefit from them or to be harmed by them. The correct forms will be readily absorbed by the body and serve their numerous roles as catalysts for the human metabolic process. The wrong forms have the potential of building up to toxic levels in the blood and soft tissues of the body. The following information will enable you to make wise choices.

Major minerals are instrumental in forming and maintaining the structure of the human body. Because they are needed in abundance, chelated supplements are the best source of major minerals. The best chelating agents differ with each mineral. For instance, the most absorbable forms of calcium are 'citrate chelates' and 'malate chelates'. Liquid trace mineral products also contain major minerals, but not nearly in the potency needed to meet bodily requirements. These liquid trace mineral supplements serve as the best source of trace minerals, which of necessity must enter the body as part of more complex plant compounds. Let's take a closer look at why.

In order to fully understand what type of trace mineral product you should be taking, a discussion of many factors is necessary. Firstly it is important to establish the fact that the need for trace mineral supplementation is very real. Factors such as soil mineral depletion, due to farming practices and soil erosion is well documented. These factors have reduced the available minerals in farmlands to less than 20 percent of what they were even 100 years ago. The concept of re-fertilizing with NPK (nitrogen, phosphorus and potash or potassium) has been in vogue for decades. There is overwhelming evidence to show that while this nutrient combination produces higher yield per acre, the plants grown on those soils are weak and subject to attack by varieties of pests which then have to be controlled with potentially harmful chemicals. Dr. Weston A. Price, in his pioneer work entitled Nutrition and Physical Degeneration, discussed the issue of NPK fertilization and its dangers to higher forms of animals, including man, that must live off plants produced by such limited nutrients. In the 1940's, Dr. Price established the critical differences between healthy plants and 'NPK' plants. In the 60 years that have passed since then, nothing has been done to address the gross mineral deficiencies in our soils and in the crops raised upon them.

Until the mid 1980's, most people considered good nutrition to be a multiple vitamin with the major minerals and a few isolated trace elements thrown in for good measure. Even though liquid minerals have been produced in limited amounts since the 1920's it wasn't until about 1985 or 1986 that they became popular through the marketing efforts of a very few select companies.

Naturally, as the popularity of these liquid minerals caught on, more and more companies came out with so-called "colloidal minerals" in an attempt to try and capture some of what was rapidly becoming "the latest craze." And understandably so, for the results that users of these liquid minerals were experiencing was nothing less than amazing. It seemed that with the addition of the liquid minerals, people were getting better absorption from the other nutrients they were taking. Furthermore, it appeared that when these liquid minerals were present in the body, the entire biochemistry of the user improved and many aches, pains, and other maladies slowly disappeared. We will explore some of the possible reasons for this phenomenal response shortly, but suffice it to say that with this kind of response, every company in the nutrition industry tried to jump on the bandwagon with a mineral product. Unfortunately, not all of these products are the same, nor to they begin to have the same level of efficacy within the human biochemistry. Many of them have been adulterated in a variety of ways and as we are about to illustrate, this adulteration hampers or destroys the very "life essence" that makes these minerals so valuable to our biochemistry.

Factors That Affect Mineral Uptake & Absorption

Tissue samples from animals and humans have shown that there are between 65 and 75 individual elements present in the 'living system'. Therefore, the first point of concern should be locating a product that provides this 'full spectrum' of elements.

When further evaluating a mineral supplement for human use, several factors come to the surface as being relevant. Such factors as pH, electromagnetic circuitry, particle size and source all determine the final ability for the body to derive benefit from the minerals ingested. The following chart analyzes the three basic types of mineral supplements and shows how they compare in various categories, including absorption.

Type of Mineral	Source	pH	Electromagnetic Charge	Percentage Absorbed
Elemental	Soils & clays	Alkaline	Generally Positive	10-20%
Chelated	Soils & clays	Acidic	Generally Positive	35-60%
Organic Compounds	Plant material	Acidic	Generally Negative	90-98%

Source

Minerals essentially come from one of two sources; inorganic or organic compounds. The former is obtained from rocks, clays, seabed material etc. The latter are minerals obtained from organic compounds derived from plants or plant material after they were processed by the plant's metabolism. This process alters the minerals in subtle and vitally important ways, particularly in regard to the electrical circuitry. For this reason, minerals obtained from plant sources, containing the full spectrum of minerals, is the best source. After all, humans were designed to eat plants, not dirt!

Particle Size

There is a law in physical chemistry that states, the smaller the object or particle, the greater the surface. This is easier understood if, in your mind, you picture a basketball and imagine the amount of surface around the outside of it. Now imagine if that basketball were filled with small marbles. If you measured all of the surfaces around each marble it would be many times greater than that around the big basketball. The amount of surface area of a mineral particle is important since the body breaks it down in preparation for use by attaching microscopic chemicals to its surface. The greater the surface area, the greater the absorption, hence the smaller the particle, the greater the potential for absorption. Colloids are very small particles that suspend in liquids such as water. This means that they neither sink or float, but 'drift' throughout the solution. These particles contribute to overall absorption because their immense surface area makes acidification and subsequent break down easier. Note: Buyer beware! Not all liquid minerals sold as colloidal are necessarily made up of organic compounds. In order to be both safe and effective, they MUST be in the form of organic compounds from plant sources.

pH

pH stands for 'Powers of Hydrogen' and refers to how acidic or alkaline a given substance is. The pH scale runs from 0 through 14. The mid point, number 7, is neutral. Everything lower than 7 is acidic and everything higher than 7 is alkaline. In order for minerals to be properly absorbed, they need to be acidic. When we consume inorganic minerals, which are always quite alkaline, the body must attempt to acidify them for absorption. This is done in several ways, but early acidification of minerals occurs through hydrochloric acid from the stomach. This accounts for why, as we grow older, we have more difficulty absorbing minerals. The natural hydrochloric acid production decreases with age and dietary abuse. Organic colloidal minerals are naturally acidic, about 2.5 to 3.0, and this further contributes to their absorption. (Refer to the section on acid and alkaline balance elsewhere in this book.)

Electromagnetic Circuitry

We have the least data on the final factor that affects mineral absorption. Current research under way at this time will hopefully shed further light upon this mysterious property.

Every element has two charges, an ionic charge, which is either positive or negative and an electromagnetic charge, which is also either positive or negative. They do not necessarily have to be the same. The ionic charge of an element is always the same and never varies regardless of what form the mineral may take. However, the electromagnetic energy, or charge, can vary with each element, depending upon the circuitry within the atoms.

Picture a magnet, for example. While the entire magnet is composed of the same material, one pole has a positive polarity, the other a negative polarity. One attracts while the other repels. The electromagnetic circuitry of so-called 'inorganic minerals' (rocks, clay, etc.) inherently carries a 'positive charge. When a living plant takes these positive minerals up into its internal biochemistry, the electromagnetic circuitry is somehow altered through the biochemical process of photosynthesis, making it negative. This negative electromagnetic energy has been called the "life energy" because it is opposite of the human electromagnetic circuitry, which is positive. Since opposites attract, the negative circuitry is drawn to the body like a magnet!

We can see by this discussion that if a mineral had all of these various factors, in the right order, the absorption potential would be increased by many times. Maximum absorption can only be achieved when the minerals are obtained from organic compounds (plant) compounds. A colloidal size, rather than just ground or powdered rock, a naturally occurring acidic pH, instead of highly alkaline, and negative (attracting) rather than positive (repelling) electromagnetic circuitry are the characteristics of a mineral that is a bioavailable, plant derived (organic) compound. A liquid mineral supplement that possessed all these factors would be almost 100 percent absorbable.

This brings us to a discussion of the many liquid trace mineral products that have recently made their way into the marketplace. Are they all created equal just because they are liquid? What about tablets and capsules that profess to contain bio-available minerals?

Let's begin by addressing the tablet/capsule issue because it is relatively easy to understand. When we refer to colloidal trace minerals, we often use the term "bio-electrical" or "bio-available". The prefix 'bio' means 'life', hence 'life-electrical' refers to an electrical circuitry that supports & nourishes the living system. All life has one thing in common, it needs moisture to survive. This is especially true when we are considering electrical potential. Any physical chemist can tell you that electrochemical reactions occur in the presence of moisture or water. The same holds true for these "life-electrical" minerals. If you totally remove the moisture, the element would lose its bio-electrical charge and revert to the inorganic electromagnetic charge which is positive. At the present time, no practical technique exists which permits the encapsulation of an organic compound without essentially destroying its value as a dietary micro trace element supplement. Several researchers are working on this but so far have failed. The encapsulated/tableted "colloidal minerals" we have tested have not retained their bio-electrical charge.

Not All Liquid Minerals Are Created Equal Either

In looking at a market that has been inundated with liquid mineral supplements, one might wonder if they are all pretty much the same. A closer examination of their makeup shows us that they are not.

The biggest single factor in evaluating a liquid mineral supplement for efficacy is NOT in the quantitative elemental amounts of minerals contained therein as much as it is how much electrical potential the product is able to impart to the living cells of the body.

We live in a society of excesses, where quantity, not quality, is king. When considering the delicate biochemistry of the body, quality is far more important than mere bulk quantity. Organic, colloidal, bio-electrical trace minerals benefit the living system in large part, because of the electrical circuitry, which imparts life force energy to the body cells, making them better able to carry on their individual life functions.

This electrical potential comes from and is generated by the relationship of one element to another. That is why no single mineral can ever hope to have the same benefit alone as it can have in the presence of the full spectrum of all the others. This electrical potential is generated by the interaction of one element with another in the 'synergetic sea of electromagnetic activity' of which organic colloidal solutions are comprised.

This being the case then, the ratios of one mineral to another is of far greater importance that mere quantity alone. The more proportionate the ratios of minerals to one another, the greater the electrical potential and hence the greater the 'life energy' that is imparted to the living system. When these naturally occurring ratios are disturbed, in any way, it reduces the amount of electrical potential that may be passed on to the cells of the body. For example, if a greater quantity of one mineral is added to an already existing 'natural combination' of liquid trace elements, that mineral would then impart a 'greater than normal' electrical charge. In other words, the charge emitted by this mineral would be of a greater charge than one naturally occurring. This, in turn, would suppress the electrical potential of other minerals related to it and ultimately alter the entire electrical circuitry of the aqueous solution. This alteration would make the product far less bio-available than if it had not been altered.

When a liquid mineral product contains an inordinately high amount of certain minerals (calcium, potassium, and others), extra quantities of these minerals have likely been added to the solution in order to boost its elemental quantity. The minerals used to do this are often obtained from inorganic sources. Electromagnetically, these added minerals are positively charged. They typically destroy the delicate, life-giving energies, which were naturally present in the organic compounds originally. One again, buyer beware! We have seen and tested mineral products that, while advocating they contain full spectrum minerals, contain only 20 percent to 40 percent pure mineral water. The remainder of the ingredients included items such as aloe vera, fruit extracts, inorganic added minerals, flavorings, etc. These mineral-poor fillers detract from the true electrical potential of the original minerals, leaving nothing more than an adulterated and incomplete liquid mixture.

If you are using a liquid mineral product that purports to be good for you, read the label. See what else is in the bottle besides minerals! If your liquid mineral product tastes delicious we can guarantee that is has been adulterated in some manner. Pure liquid colloidal organic-source trace minerals are tan to brown in color and are very bitter. Any attempt to mask these characteristics adversely affects both the potency and the electrical charge of the minerals. Once bottled, their quality deteriorates rapidly and even warehousing and shipping times substantially diminishes their value. Know what you are buying!

Non-Toxicity of True Bio-Electrical Colloidal Trace Minerals

Often those who are unfamiliar with liquid trace mineral supplements are under the impression that these liquids contain harmful or toxic minerals. A natural, unadulterated, full spectrum mineral product would contain each of the elements found in nature, including those we have come to believe are toxic.

Minerals such as cadmium, aluminum, arsenic, lead, mercury, and others strike terror in our minds. We have difficulty understanding why they would be present in liquid mineral supplement made for human consumption. Firstly, we must go back to the concept that all minerals are not created equal. In their inorganic rock state, ALL minerals can be potentially toxic because of the body's inability to utilize and break them down. Something as seemingly beneficial as calcium, if very alkaline, can circulate in the blood stream, awaiting acidification. It can contribute to the raw material that occludes the arteries, and forms gallstones, kidney stones, heel spurs and spinal deposits. Yet properly acidified calcium is not only welcomed by the body but absolutely necessary for life.

As our knowledge of human biochemistry proceeds, more and more information will come to light regarding the many micro trace elements and their biological role in the human body. Arsenic, for example, was always thought of as a deadly poison. Indeed, in the inorganic form, is certainly is poisonous. However, recent studies have shown that arsenic is an essential mineral and is even being considered as an addition to the essential nutrient list! As recently as a few years ago, many minerals, including molybdenum, selenium, and chromium, were considered non-essential at best and dangerous at worst. Today, their value is finally being realized. The next decade will undoubtedly bring a much greater understanding of the role of the full spectrum of elements naturally present in the human body tissues.

Toxic-Leaching Benefits of Organic Colloidal Bio-Electric Trace Minerals

In the late 1980's, an interesting experiment was conducted with regard to high levels of potentially toxic inorganic minerals in the body and the ability of their organic bio-electrical counterparts to naturally chelate or remove them safely. The test was conducted, by Gary Price Todd, MD, author of the book <u>Nutrition, Health & Disease</u>. The study involved individuals with a variety of so-called heavy metal poisonings, specifically lead, mercury, cadmium, and aluminum were selected and blood samples were taken to monitor the offending mineral.

Dr. Todd rapidly discovered that blood analyses were not effective in monitoring this process, therefore it was decided that hair analyses would be employed. Prior to the test, base levels of the offending minerals were established via tissue hair sample. Test subjects were then placed on a program of full spectrum bio-available micro trace minerals in proportion to their body weight. In addition they were given a second product which represented the full spectrum of other nutrients such as vitamins, major minerals and amino acids. It is important to note that high amounts of vitamin C were found necessary in order to obtain an optimal response. Vitamin C was administered at 1 to 2 grams per day.

During the study, it was observed that several of the individuals with lower levels of toxic metals on their initial hair analysis, initially experienced a notable rise is those same substances as evidenced by their second hair analysis three months later. (Figure 1.1) This appeared to indicate that there was a mobilization of the stored toxic metals from the body's soft tissues back into solution, which would account for the higher concentration of these substances in the hair.

Repeated hair analysis at six months, and continuing through to sixteen months, the end of the study, demonstrated reduced levels of toxic metal in the hair. The natural chelation process took place and the toxic mineral levels were reduced. (Refer to Figures 1.2 and 1.3 which represent 6 and 16 months average response.)

Physicians and other health care practitioners who wish to use this method on their patients should keep in mind that they will likely experience an initial rise in the offending substances for the first three to even six months depending upon the volume of heavy metal to be removed.

Any professional interested in implementing this procedure in their practice may contact our Institute for a protocol outline. Subsequent results analysis of this pioneering study seem to indicate that there is some type of ionic exchange taking place between the opposite minerals. This would support the theory that organic minerals bear an opposite electromagnetic charge referred to in other studies as the life energies.

Based upon Dr. Todd's findings, those persons suffering from the negative effects of heavy metal contamination should strongly consider the use of bio-electrical colloidal trace minerals as part of their plan to restore their health. Colloidal, organic, bio-electrical minerals cannot be stored in the body for longer than a few hours; they are much like the water soluble vitamins, therefore they cannot build up to toxic levels in the soft tissues. They also assist the body in removing their heavy metal counterparts, which can remain in the body for decades.

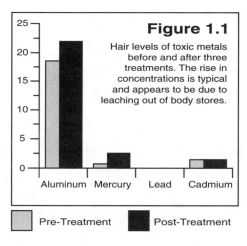

Figure 1.1

Hair levels of toxic metals before and after three treatments. The rise in concentrations is typical and appears to be due to leaching out of body stores.

Pre-Treatment   Post-Treatment

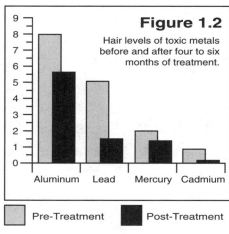

Figure 1.2

Hair levels of toxic metals before and after four to six months of treatment.

Pre-Treatment   Post-Treatment

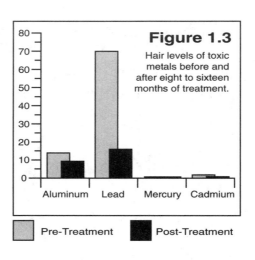

Figure 1.3

Hair levels of toxic metals before and after eight to sixteen months of treatment.

Pre-Treatment   Post-Treatment

Further Reports from European Researchers

Dr. Michael Zimmerman, Chief of Staff of the Specialized Clinic for Chronic Illnesses and Therapy Resistant Patients in Uberlingen, Germany, tested a pure bio-electrical colloidal full spectrum mineral formula as part of his ongoing work with seriously ill patients. His conclusions state that, "This unique mineral formula enhances the de-poisoning ability of the body in a very positive way. It activates and speeds the healing process, especially in the case of chronic illnesses."

Ulrich Sommer, a pharmacist from Burg/ Dittmarschen, Germany, has also used "life minerals" and he goes on to report, "The human body can only stay healthy when it receives the entire spectrum of natural minerals, trace mineral elements, and vitamins in the daily diet. These are the basic building blocks for all life. Vitamins, amino acids, enzymes, hormones and other substances needed by the body to build new cells depend entirely on the influx of mineral elements which especially include the micro amounts of trace elements which are very difficult to get from foods or conventional food supplements."

The Bio-Electronic Test

Biophysicist, Dr. Fritz-Albert Popp of Germany, conducted an extensive study of the bio-electric properties of a true unadulterated liquid colloidal mineral formula. Conclusions and findings of that study are outlined by Gottfried Lange, MD, a toxicologist from Elmshorn, Germany. In essence, Dr. Popp observed that, "All living organisms emit certain electromagnetic waves. If they are in a healthy condition, they emit more. If not, they emit less. This phenomenon is common to all forms of cells. These electromagnetic emissions are called bio-photons."

Any substance that is taken into the internal biochemistry of the body can potentially affect this electromagnetic status either positively, by feeding the cell life force, or negatively, by robbing it of precious energy.

During the test Dr. Popp used a super sensitive organism known as Acetabularia Mediterranean, a certain very sensitive algae from the Mediterranean Sea. This algae is so sensitive to ecological influences that there are scarcely any of these algae left in the Mediterranean. The test, conducted on the liquid colloidal minerals using these organisms, is a highly recognized method of determining whether or not a substance is toxic to the living cell or to what degree the substance might serve to enhance the cell's vital life functions. The following bar graph illustrates the results of Dr. Popp's findings when he exposed the delicate Acetabularia to full spectrum bio-electrical colloidal trace minerals in an unadulterated form. (Figure 2.0)

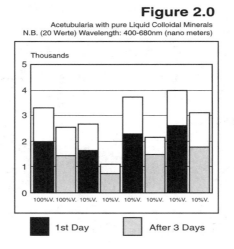

Figure 2.0

Acetubularia with pure Liquid Colloidal Minerals
N.B. (20 Werte) Wavelength: 400-680nm (nano meters)

Charted Photon Emissions of Nutrient Rich and Nutrient Starved Cells

1. The first set of graph bars represents the photon emissions of the cells which had been given the optimum (100%V) vitamin nutrient solution. The black bar measures the photon emission at the start of the test. The following gray bar shows the photon emission after a period of three days without additional nutrients given to them.

2. The second set of two graph bars represents the photon emissions of the cells given a reduced amount (10%V) vitamin nutrient solution. After the three day period, the emissions are so low that the cells are under "great stress", and without further nutrients, would die.

3. The third set of two graph bars represents the photon emissions of cells which had been given a 10%V nutrient solution to which 1.4 micro liters of liquid, organic, bio-electrical trace minerals were added. A significant improvement is shown, even though there was only a 10%V nutrient given. This would indicate that the bio-electrical colloids have an ability to spare nutrients and retain them for longer periods at the cellular level, while making them more easily available to individual cells.

4. The fourth set of two graph bars represents the photon emissions of the cells which had been given a 10%V nutrient solution in which the liquid, organic, bio-electrical trace minerals were reduced to only .14 UL. The improvement was slightly better showing that the benefits to the living cell come not from the quantity of the mineral present, but from the

degree of bio-electrical activity imparted to the cell, thereby increasing the cells' own energy levels.

During the 1930's, studies & applications involving various colloidal minerals, alone and in concert with each other, were common. At the onset of World War II, much of this research ceased, and after the war, the use of colloidal chemistry in health and healing became almost non-existent.

Today we are seeing a resurgence of interest in the full spectrum of micro trace elements. Surfacing thousands of testimonials from people around the world who are experiencing a richer, more healthful life because of the use of these supplements. It has long been a great concern of this writer who, in private practice as a clinical nutritionist, frequently did not observe or obtain expected results with patients by using vitamin, major mineral, and amino acid therapies. Only after we began using the highly absorbable liquid full spectrum, organic, colloidal, bio-electrical trace minerals, did I see a ten-fold increase in desired results. These results and observations have lead to the development of my concept of Full Spectrum Nutrition, which is outlined in detail in the next chapter.

As tests conducted all over the world continue to bear out, the real benefit of liquid colloidal minerals lies in their bio-electrical potential - not just their elemental quantities. Those delicate bio-electrical potentials are generated through the interaction of various minerals with each other - therefore the ratios of those minerals are of supreme importance. Anything that alters or adulterates those bio-electrical potentials, created by nature, robs your living system of the vital life energies that it needs in ever increasing amounts in our polluted, toxic world.

Let's take a closer look at the major and trace minerals and their specific functions in your body.

Major Minerals
Calcium

Calcium reigns as the single most abundant mineral in the body. Bone tissue houses the majority, 99 percent, of the total 1200 grams of calcium in the average human body. Calcium is found together with magnesium, sodium, phosphorus, and strontium and they play an important role in the strengthening of the skeletal tissue. The last one percent of the calcium in the body is used as an electrolyte in nerve transmission, muscle contractions, and blood clotting.

We all know of the importance of calcium in building and maintaining bones and teeth, but as an electrolyte, calcium wears many other hats.

Calcium facilitates the electro-stimulus that flows over our nervous system. A deficiency of calcium produces tetany, a condition of twitching, from the over-stimulation of the nerves. This is the connection between taking calcium before bedtime and getting a better nights rest. When calcium levels are higher in the blood, the neurotransmitters serotonin, acetylcholine, and norepinephrine are affected.

The balance between calcium and magnesium affects the contraction of striated and smooth muscles. Calcium also plays an essential role in the cells by its presence in intercellular fluid.

Calcium is one of the most difficult minerals to absorb. Most sources of calcium, in elemental form, are highly alkaline. In order for this mineral to be absorbed into the body, it must be acidified to a relatively low pH. This is normally accomplished through the action of hydrochloric acid from the stomach. The problem arises in individuals over the age of 35 or 40 who have depleted their production of hydrochloric acid from consuming a diet consisting of dead, lifeless foods.

Nutritional formulators have developed a way of making calcium more absorbable. By binding it with an amino acid or some other acid substance before encapsulating, the absorption rate of calcium can be greatly improved. The most effective combination of calcium chelates presently known is a combination of calcium citrate and calcium malate.

It is important to understand that, under stress and tension, the body can spontaneously dump large amounts of available calcium. As much as 1000 mg of calcium can be lost through fecal excretion during times of worry and stress.

Functions of Calcium

1. Major function is to build bones and teeth.
2. Reduces insomnia.
3. Needed for acid/base balance.
4. Balances potassium and sodium for muscle tone.
5. Aids in regulation of heartbeat.
6. Assists in the clotting of blood.
7. Aids muscle contraction, nerve transmission.

Deficiency Symptoms of Calcium

1. Stunted growth.
2. Calcium tetany – leg cramps.
3. Numbness, tingling in arms and legs.
4. Children, Rickets; Adults, Osteomalacia.
5. Nervousness, heart palpitations, slow pulse.
6. Excessive menstruation - lengthy menstruation.

Phosphorus

As the second most abundant mineral in the body, phosphorus combines with calcium to form calcium phosphate, the material responsible for giving bone and teeth their strength and rigidity. Unlike calcium, phosphorus is involved as a component of all living cells, and is a part of the nucleic acids, making up the genetic code.

Most all of the enzymes in your system, as well as the vitamin group of nutrients, are only activated in the presence of phosphorus.

In spite of these vital functions, phosphorus is rarely found in dietary supplements due to their prevalence in the diet. Meats, in fact all concentrated protein foods, contain very high amounts of phosphorus.

When phosphorus exceeds calcium, as our diets often do, calcium is suppressed, creating potentially serious calcium deficiency symptoms. One source of excess phosphorus is the carbonated beverage. Soft drinks contribute as much as 500 mg of phosphorus, in the form of phosphoric acid, per 12 ounce serving.

The only possible scenario in which a person might be deficient in phosphorus would be those on a low protein diet. Fatigue is the most common symptom.

Functions of Phosphorus

1. Metabolism factor for fats (phospholipids).
2. Required for absorption of niacin and riboflavin.
3. Stimulates muscle contractions, especially the heart.
4. Aids formation of bones and teeth.
5. Serves as a blood buffer to maintain pH.
6. Constituent of all nucleoproteins.
7. Part of enzyme system that oxidizes carbohydrates.

8. Building block for the myelin sheath of nerves.

Deficiency Symptoms of Phosphorus
1. Poor bones and teeth.
2. Arthritis.
3. Pyorrhea.
4. Rickets.
5. Mental and physical fatigue.
6. Loss of appetite.
7. Irregular breathing patterns.
8. Nervous disorders due to breakdown of myelin sheath.

Sodium

Sodium is an essential nutrient found almost exclusively in the body's extracellular fluids, namely vascular fluids within blood vessels, arteries, veins and capillaries. About 50 percent of the body's content of sodium can be found in the extracellular fluids that surround the cells of the body.

Due to over-use of salt (sodium chloride) as a preservative, and seasoning in processed packaged foods, over-consumption of sodium is extremely common.

Like most minerals, which have counterparts in the body, sodium is no exception. Potassium balances sodium, both as powerful electrolytes. When the sodium in the fluids of the body exceeds that of potassium, the typical side effects of excess sodium (edema, elevated blood pressure, etc.) become apparent. These problems are not so much a result of excess sodium as a deficiency of potassium, which is naturally very deficient in the junk food diet. Proper ratios of sodium to potassium should be about 1 part sodium to 2 to 2.5 parts potassium. The person who routinely consumes a diet consisting of over-processed, packaged foods ingests roughly the opposite ratio, resulting in epidemic hypertension and other health complications.

Functions of Sodium
1. Works with potassium to regulate acid/alkali.
2. Works with potassium in the sodium/potassium pump.
3. Nerve stimulations.
4. Aids in digestion.
5. Necessary for hydrochloric acid production.

Deficiency Symptoms of Sodium
1. Dehydration.
2. Indigestion.
3. Indirect relation to arthritis and rheumatism.

Potassium

Sodium is the primary electrolyte in extracellular fluids. Potassium, sodium's counterpart, is the primary cation of intracellular fluids. (Cations are positively charged ions and tend to move toward cathodes in an electrolyzed solution.) In fact, 98 percent of all the potassium in the body is found in the small spaces of intracellular fluid at concentrations up to thirty times greater than in extracellular spaces.

Potassium is the cleansing agent responsible for the removal of the waste products generated as by-products of cellular metabolism.

Through this process, potassium is responsible for maintaining the integrity of living cells as well as internal water balance.

Potassium is primarily found in fresh fruits and vegetables. Since very few of us eat these foods in their raw natural state, and since potassium is easily lost in cooking and heating, a deficiency of this mineral is quite common. To further complicate this problem, potassium is utilized in the metabolism of carbohydrates and sugars. A diet high in these foods will further deplete the potassium stores of the body.

The recommended amount of potassium is 2500 mg to 3500 mg per day. As with all electrolytes, an excess of potassium is not healthy. In fact, it can be fatal.

Potassium is absorbed very rapidly through the small intestine. Potassium, like sodium, is lost through perspiration and via the urine. You are at greater risk of developing a potassium deficiency if you suffer from hypoglycemia or diabetes. These illnesses produce an over-production of aldosterone. This leads to water and sodium retention, which, in turn, displaces potassium.

Functions of Potassium

1. Necessary for normal growth.
2. Stimulates nerve impulses for muscle contractions.
3. Regulates fluids by working with sodium.
4. Stimulates kidneys to eliminate poisonous body wastes.
5. Aids in maintaining healthy skin.
6. Needed for healthy support of the adrenal glands.

Deficiency Symptoms of Potassium

1. Nervous disorders.
2. Insomnia.
3. Slowed, irregular heartbeat.
4. Edema.
5. Acne in adolescents.
7. Dry skin in adults.

Chloride

Chloride is an essential anionic mineral. Between 450 mg and as much as 600 mg of chloride may be found in every 100 ml of blood. While chloride is primarily found in extracellular fluids, it is also present in intracellular fluids as well. Being an electrolyte, chloride is involved in the transport and exchange of materials between these two fluid chambers.

Essentially, chloride is the active ingredient in the all-important natural stomach acid, hydrochloric acid.

As you will recall hydrochloric acid is responsible for protein digestion and mineral acidification.

Further, chloride is essential in helping the body maintain its acid/alkaline balance. It participates in the chloride shift, which transports CO_2 from the body tissues to the lungs for excretion.

Chloride deficiencies are somewhat rare because chloride is found in many foods and is easily absorbed by the intestines. Deficiencies of this mineral can be caused by a rapid loss of chloride due to excessive diarrhea or vomiting, adrenal insufficiency, or metabolic acidosis.

Functions of Chloride
1. Produces hydrochloric acid.
2. Removes CO_2 from tissues.
3. Maintains an acid/alkaline balance.
5. A powerful electrolyte.
6. Facilitates the exchange of materials across cell membranes.

Deficiency Symptoms of Chloride
1. Systemic alkalosis
2. Psychomotor defects
3. Memory loss
4. Growth retardation

Magnesium

In comparison to other major minerals, magnesium is present in the body in the smallest amount. As I mentioned in an earlier discussion, magnesium is primarily needed as a co-factor for calcium. Therefore, the bulk of the body's magnesium supply may be found in the bones. The remainder of the body's magnesium, about one-third, is bound onto various other compounds as part of their chemical makeup.

Magnesium is absolutely essential in energy production and is, therefore, intimately involved in the production of Adenosine Triphosphates (ATP). When magnesium is deficient, it severely impairs the cardiovascular system as well as neuromuscular and renal tissues. Magnesium is so vital to cardiac health that in areas where magnesium deficiency is most common, the rate of heart attacks is appreciably higher. Magnesium and calcium must be present in the proper ratio to ensure a regular heartbeat. The thin filament on the heart muscles known as 'actin', is brought into stimulation by the presence of calcium. In the presence of calcium, the actin tends to contract toward the center of the cells; in contrasting action, magnesium relaxes the muscle cells by a repelling action upon the calcium. For this reason, magnesium supplements are often used in conjunction with other supportive nutrients in the management of various forms of cardiac arrhythmia. (See Chapter 17 for protocols.)

Magnesium is poorly absorbed. Only about 50

percent of what is ingested is absorbed through the intestines. This rate of absorption is governed by the parathyroid hormones, as well as by the amounts of calcium and phosphates present. Magnesium is lost in particularly high rates during periods of excess alcohol consumption.

Functions of Magnesium

1. Generally involved in many metabolic functions.
2. Activates enzyme systems within cells.
3. Necessary for the contraction of muscles.
4. Regulates acid/alkaline balance.
5. Maintains DNA and RNA.
6. Essential for proper utilization of the B vitamins.
7. Involved in the synthesis of certain amino acids.
8. Needed in the conversion of blood sugar to energy.

Deficiency Symptoms of Magnesium

1. Irregular heart beat.
2. Close relation to coronary heart disease.
3. Apprehensiveness and disorientation.
4. Confusion.
5. Irritability of nerves and muscles.
6. Muscle twitching and tremors.
7. Convulsions and seizures.

The Trace Minerals

Trace minerals are present in the body in very small amounts. They are utilized primarily in the chemical reactions of the body rather than the actual physical and structural composition.

At least 65 trace elements have been found within the vast complexity of the human body. While we certainly don't know all of the functions of each one of them at this time, their presence certainly signifies purpose. As research continues, more and more of the functions of these infinitely small minerals will undoubtedly be revealed. Science has already identified biological functions for such obscure minerals as molybdenum, tin, aluminum, lithium, and even arsenic, heretofore believed to be only a poison. Someday we will understand why nature provides all of these trace minerals to both animals and humankind. In the meantime, we can be safe, rather than sorry, by simply providing the body with the total spectrum of micro trace elements from plant-based compounds.

We will now discuss specific trace elements and highlight their functions in the living system.

Iron

Perhaps the best known of the trace elements is iron. Within the body, iron may be found in two forms: Functional forms, including enzymes and hemoglobin (the blood constituent), and Transport and Storage forms, including transferrin and ferritin.

Iron deficiency anemia is still a great concern

worldwide. In the United States, iron deficiency anemia may be found all too often in such populations as the elderly, women of childbearing years, children, and toddlers. It is estimated that one in every four women of college age is seriously deficient in iron.

We often think, erroneously, of iron as being primarily essential only for women, due to their loss of blood during menstruation. This is a dangerous oversight because, chemically, men have equal needs for iron. For example, teenage males require the same amount of iron as women because of significant growth spurts during these developing years.

The recent trend towards removing iron from dietary supplements because of its connection with heart disease and other maladies is, for the most part, absurd. While no one is suggesting that excess iron be consumed, the required amounts for bodily function are still necessary. The increasing numbers of medical patients whose blood tests reveal elevated iron levels likely prompted this absurd trend away from iron supplementation. If you remember our discussion of major minerals and how each one of them has a counter balance, you will have the answer for many of the cases of elevated iron levels in the blood.

Iron requires the trace mineral copper in order to carry it into the cells. In the absence of adequate copper, iron can circulate in the blood but not sufficiently enter the cells. At the Institute of Nutritional Science, we have successfully treated many patients, both male and female, who were diagnosed as having high iron levels by the adding copper to their diets. Once the copper levels were achieved, iron excess was no longer a problem.

Children suffering from iron deficiencies exhibit the same symptoms one might observe in hyperactive cases. Pica, the unusual appetite for strange foods such as ice, clay, chalk, and other non-food items, is often a symptom of iron deficiency.

Functions of Iron

1. A major component of hemoglobin and myoglobin.
2. Promotes oxygenation of tissues and cells.
3. Produces energy.
4. Is a catalyst for enzyme formation.
5. Reduces cellular stress.
6. Participates in completing the Krebs Cycle.
7. Instrumental in collagen synthesis.

Deficiency Symptoms of Iron

1. Anemia (pale skin, abnormal fatigue, etc.)
2. Retarded growth
3. Shortness of breath upon slight exertion
4. Reduced appetite
5. Constipation
6. Hyperactivity and behavioral problems in children
7. Pica (unusual cravings for non-food items)

Zinc

Zinc is the trace mineral most closely associated with immune function. It is a cofactor in at least twenty enzymatic reactions. Zinc is involved in vitamin A absorption and plays a role in alcohol metabolism.

Zinc is a major constituent of insulin, the hormone that regulates blood sugar. Because of its involvement with immunity, it accelerates wound healing, both external and internal. Zinc is frequently recommended as part of a nutrient protocol for acne because it helps to regulate the skin's oil gland production while helping to heal skin eruptions.

This versatile mineral is a main ingredient in the prostate, prostate secretions and in the formation of spermatozoa.

Zinc is the second most prevalent trace mineral. Since cadmium can displace zinc, deficiencies are becoming more and more common. Cadmium, a heavy metal, is found in most combustion generated pollution.

Zinc is readily absorbed in the upper, or small intestine. It is stored in the internal organs of the body. Calcium competes with zinc for absorption, so if you are supplementing with high amounts of calcium, you need to ensure that adequate amounts of zinc is also provided.

Functions of Zinc

1. Necessary for proper absorption of the B vitamins.
2. Integral part of at least 25 enzymes related to metabolism
   and digestion.
3. Healing of wounds and burns.
4. Proper prostate function.
5. A vital component of insulin.
6. Growth and development of sex organs.
7. Recent studies show a connection to the synthesis of DNA.

Deficiency Symptoms of Zinc

1. Increased fatigue.
2. Decreased alertness.
3. Susceptibility to infections.
4. Slow healing of surface wounds.
5. Prostatitis, sterility.
6. Poor appetite.
7. Loss of sense of taste.
8. Stretch marks on skin.
9. White spots on fingernails.
10. Possible diabetes.

Iodine

In the body, iodine's main functions are regulating cellular oxidation and serving as a compound of the thyroid hormone. The concentrations of iodine in the thyroid gland are 1000 times greater than found anywhere else in the body.

Supplemental iodine is frequently taken to stimulate a sluggish thyroid. This is very safe, under most conditions, as long as iodine from plant sources is used. The best source of iodine supplementation is not iodized salt, but rather kelp tablets. The organic compounds surrounding the iodine in kelp buffer it and prevent it from building up to toxic levels in the body.

The production of thyroxin in the thyroid gland is essential to the well-being of the body. Thyroxin is directly involved in the metabolism of converting foods to fuel. It also establishes the basic metabolic rate at which the body burns calories.

Iodine is rapidly absorbed from the gastrointestinal tract and then carried to the thyroid gland where it is stored and used in the production of specific hormones.

A slow metabolism often signifies insufficient functioning of the thyroid gland. This can be measured by taking your temperature upon first waking in the morning. Shake down a common mercury thermometer before you go to bed at night and set it next to your bed. Upon awakening in the morning put the thermometer under your arm and lay quietly for ten minutes. Read the temperature on the thermometer. If it is consistently lower than 98 degrees Fahrenheit, you can suspect a sluggish thyroid. The addition of extra iodine from kelp is a safe way of boosting thyroid function.

Functions of Iodine
1. Production of the hormone, thyroxine.
2. Regulates production of body energy.
3. Promotes growth and development.
4. Thyroxine aids in the synthesis of cholesterol.

Deficiency Symptoms of Iodine
1. Goiter.
2. Sluggish metabolism.
3. Dry hair.
4. Rapid pulse, heart palpitations.
5. Nervousness, restlessness, and irritability.
6. Slowed mental reaction time.

Manganese

Manganese is an essential trace mineral about which little is known. We do know that it plays an important part in activating many enzymes. Manganese also enhances the utilization and functions of choline, biotin, thiamin, and ascorbic acid.

Manganese is essential in the absorption of calcium into bone tissues. It also is involved in collagen and urea formation, fatty acid synthesis, and the digestion of proteins.

Manganese is very poorly absorbed by the body. Since it is a trace element, little is needed. The body only stores about 20 mg and it may be found in bones, the liver and pancreas. Persons who have hypoglycemia or diabetes often need extra amounts of this mineral.

Functions of Manganese
1. Utilization of glucose.
2. Synthesis of fatty acids and cholesterol.
3. Pancreas function.
4. Feeds the nerves and brain tissues.
5. Retards the onset of sterility.

Deficiency Symptoms of Manganese
1. Poor glucose tolerance.
2. Weakness of ligaments and tendons.
3. Paralysis, convulsions and blindness in children.
4. Dizziness, and loss of hearing in adults.
5. A possible connection to multiple sclerosis and myasthenia gravis.

Copper

Until recently, a deficiency of copper in the diet was somewhat rare. Recently, more and more symptoms of copper deficiencies are manifesting in greater segments of the population. This is likely due to the fact that the primary source of copper is from vegetation grown on copper rich soils. As the overall trace mineral stores are being depleted from over-used farmlands, multiple trace mineral deficiencies are occurring in higher numbers.

Copper is necessary for the absorption of iron at the cellular level. Zinc and copper compete for intestinal absorption so it is important that both minerals are equally represented in supplementation and diet.

Like most trace elements, copper participates as a co-factor in enzyme production systems and serves as a catalyst in the synthesis of hemoglobin.

Copper, in the right form, is relatively easy for the body to absorb. In organic compounds, it is more readily used and retained. Inorganic sources of copper are only about 30 percent absorbable. The greatest concentration of copper may be found in the brain and liver.

Functions of Copper

1. Essential part of many enzymes.
2. Protein metabolism and with zinc for healing.
3. Formation of the myelin sheath of the nerves.
4. Aids in conversion of tyrosine into skin & hair pigment.
5. Assists the body in oxidizing vitamin C.
6. Necessary for the production of RNA.

Deficiency Symptoms of Copper

1. Possible link to schizophrenia.
2. Loss of mental alertness.
3. Anemia

4. Impaired respiration.
5. Skin sores.

Chromium

Chromium is most widely known for its involvement in the Glucose Tolerance Factor (GTF), necessary for blood sugar regulation. A hundred years ago, chromium deficiencies were rare. Food was eaten in its more natural state and chromium in the diet was adequate. Today, the best source of chromium (grains), are refined into white flour, destroying up to 98 percent of all the chromium.

As our diet increased in sugar and refined carbohydrates, the demand for additional chromium increased. These increased needs have not been met. This, in part, contributes to the epidemic of adult onset diabetes we have seen in the U.S. during the last 40 years.

Chromium is beneficial in lowering cholesterol levels due to its involvement with niacin. Chromium works together with another trace mineral, vanadium, and together their action on blood glucose normalization is much more potent that with either mineral individually.

Chromium is very difficult to absorb. By the addition of chromium from organic plant compounds, overall chromium absorption is enhanced dramatically. Estimates show that less than three percent of ingested chromium is absorbed into the body tissues.

Functions of Chromium

1. Stimulates enzyme activity.
2. Glucose metabolism.
3. Synthesis of fatty acids.
4. Possible link to protein synthesis via RNA.

Deficiency Symptoms of Chromium

1. Glucose intolerance.
2. Diabetes.
3. Poor amino acid metabolism.
4. Link to atherosclerosis. (The addition of chromium to the diet seems to reverse atherosclerosis. The mechanism for this is still not clearly known. Research continues along these lines.)

Selenium

This trace mineral leads the pack as a powerful anti-oxidant. In fact, selenium has been shown to be one of the most powerful anti-oxidants known. Some reports indicate it may be as much as 100 times more powerful than vitamin E!

As with most trace elements, the amount ingested and the prevalence of deficiency are directly related to selenium content in soils as well as the manner in which food is prepared. Selenium is rapidly leached out of foods when they are heated.

Selenium deficiency in both water and food sources has resulted in a marked increase in cardiomyopathy and myocardial deaths. Keshan cardiomyopathy in China is prevented solely by the use of selenium supplements.

Because of selenium's powerful antioxidant properties, a deficiency of this element has resulted in an increase of cancer incidence.

Selenium is absorbed rather poorly and is best taken bound together with plant proteins in the form of an organic based supplement.

Functions of Selenium
1. Selenium's major function is as an antioxidant.
2. Prevents some forms of cancer especially male cancers.
3. Protects against toxic effects of other metals such as
   lead and cadmium.

Deficiency Symptoms of Selenium
1. Premature aging.
2. Cancer (due to free radical damage).
3. Atherosclerosis (due to free radical damage).

Vanadium

This trace element is involved in the regulation and metabolism of glucose. When combined with chromium, it has been successfully used to manage and even reverse adult-onset diabetes.

We also know that vanadium plays a part in the natural circulatory regulating system of the body. The presence of it in brain tissues seems to retard cholesterol formation in blood vessels. In fact, vanadium exercises a positive regulating effect on many types of lipids in the body.

Molybdenum

This trace mineral is the component of several essential enzymes. Two of the most important include the catalytic role of xanthine oxidase in uric acid formation and the aldehyde oxidase role in the oxidation of various aldehydes. These functions are important in electron transport systems.

While no specific deficiencies have been recognized in humans, molybdenum has recently been added to the absolutely essential list.

Nickel

Nickel is prevalent in larger amounts than most of the micro trace elements. We know that it is involved in the formation of RNA, the genetic transfer material. Further, nickel is a catalyst involved in the hydrogenation of certain edible vegetable oils. Nickel is linked to specific gland secretions and hormone synthesis of the thyroid and adrenal glands.

Nickel is found in seafood as well as in unrefined, unprocessed grains. Nickel seems to play a protective role in regard to the liver. The mechanism for this is still not fully understood.

Aluminum

Aluminum is one of the minerals we associate with toxicity. And, in its metallic, non-organic, state is certainly is. Dangerous forms of aluminum are becoming more widespread in our diet. Many of the food additives used in processing and refining foods contain metallic aluminum. Cosmetics and some chemicals are also additional sources.

Aluminum does play and essential role in cellular replication and metabolism. It is also involved in stimulating and regulating growth. One of the most important functions of aluminum is in the detoxification of the body from a variety of toxins.

In order to ensure that inorganic metallic aluminum is kept at a minimum in your body, consider taking a plant-based mineral product that provides high amounts of aluminum in the form of organic compounds. Aluminum in this form is not only harmless but it will assist in removing the 'heavy metal' aluminum from soft tissues.

Cadmium

This is yet another mineral, when ingested in the wrong form, can rapidly poison the living system of the body. Yet in the organic compound state, cadmium, like most micro trace minerals, has both biological function and essentiality.

Clinical studies recently have begun to identify the role of cadmium in the human biochemistry. Body function activities in which it is involved include growth regulation, birth weight, weight gain, and the activation of several enzymes at the cellular level.

Tin

Tin is another mineral involved cellular maintenance and growth of the human body. Lack of adequate tin in the body can contribute to certain specific types of hair thinning or hair loss.

Deficiencies of tin, bromine, lead, and molybdenum has been linked to diminished trace mineral absorption and a decreased life expectancy.

Lithium

This mineral has gained widespread attention in recent years, due to its application in the management of certain forms of mental illness. Sadly, physicians are using the heavy metallic form of lithium and need to constantly watch for signs of toxicity and poisoning. Side effects from treatment are also considerable in some people.

The use of organic compounded lithium from plant sources would greatly reduce the incidence of side effects and prevent sensitive issues of toxicity from becoming a problem.

Lithium has also been helpful in treating depression and mood swings.

Lithium is a simple element and belongs to the alkaline group of metals, which include sodium and potassium. Studies have shown lithium to be helpful in the treatment of alcoholism, and perhaps it may be of some use on other types of chemical dependency.

Other benefits of the use of this valuable nutrient include its ability to dissolve urate deposits, hence it is useful in conditions of gout, rheumatism and some forms of arthritis.

Arsenic

This is another of the feared elements. Most of us associate arsenic with the poisonings that took place in old black and white movie plots. Yet, in spite of the toxicity of arsenic in its metallic state, in organic compounds, it does have metabolic function in the body.

Lead

Yes, even this mineral performs biological functions in the body. We have heard so much about lead poisoning, especially among children. This is justified, as it has been, and continues to be, a major cause of illness.

This does not change the fact that lead is necessary in the human body. But again, and I cannot stress this too strongly, it must be in the form that nature intended for us to ingest, namely as part of more complex organic plant compounds.

So what does lead do in the body? Clinical studies have now identified lead as a factor in iron metabolism. In fact, when bio-available lead levels are depressed in the body, iron levels also become depleted.

As we have said previously, little is known about the majority of the micro trace elements consistently found within the human body. It would be absurd to say they have no biological functions simply because we do not yet know there individual functions.

It is better not to second-guess nature. Until quite recently, we didn't know the function of many vitamins. Did that make them any less important to human health and longevity? Of course not.

What is important is to ensure that your source of these micro trace minerals comes from a product completely derived from plant-based organic compounds, with no additives or other minerals added.

Following is a listing of all the minerals presently identified in the human biochemistry.

Known Essential Minerals for People

Major Minerals

Calcium	Magnesium	Potassium
Chlorine	Phosphorus	Sodium
Sulfur		

Trace & Micro Trace Minerals

Aluminum	Hafnium	Ruthenium
Antimony	Holmium	Samarium
Arsenic	Indium	Scandium
Barium	Iodine	Selenium
Beryllium	Iridium	Silicon
Bismuth	Iron	Silver
Boron	Lanthanum	Strontium
Bromine	Lead	Tantalum
Cadmium	Lithium	Tellurium
Cerium	Lutetium	Terbium
Cesium	Manganese	Thallium
Chromium	Molybdenum	Thorium
Cobalt	Neodymium	Thulium
Copper	Nickel	Tin
Dysprosium	Niobium	Titanium
Erbium	Osmium	Tungston
Europium	Palladium	Vanadium
Flourine	Platinum	Ytterbium
Gadolinium	Praeseodymium	Yttrium
Gallium	Rhenium	Zinc
Germanium	Rhodium	Zirconium
Gold	Rubidium	

This brings to a close our discussion of individual vitamins and minerals. There is one overriding concept that you must understand when thinking in terms of these all-important nutrients. You must NOT take them alone! If you recall, throughout our discussion of these individual vitamins and minerals, I was continually linking and cross-referencing a nutrient to one or more others. This is because these 'chemicals of life' must act in concert with one another. Only after the base line of all 100 to 120 essential nutrients has been met is it safe to add individual nutrients in higher amounts for specific purposes.

In the next chapter, we will discuss my concept of Full Spectrum Nutrition and show you how to put this information together. Further, we will discuss how you can now customize your nutrient program to ensure your specific needs are being met.

*C*hapter 15

Full Spectrum Nutrition:
The Concept of Totality

Now that we have seen the power and purpose of the many members in the family of essential nutrients, what do we do with this information? How can we best utilize these nutrients, major minerals, trace minerals, amino acids, antioxidants, and phytonutrients? What is the best way to choose and use supplements needed for optimal health? How do I know what to take and how much to take?

These and other questions concerning dietary supplements have plagued both researchers and consumers alike.

In my more than 27 years in the health and nutrition industry, I have seen many changes. Being part of one of the most rapidly unfolding areas of science has been both stimulating and rewarding. During that time, I have seen our industry change, mostly for the better. Some of these changes were hard coming because once a belief is accepted, change comes with reluctance.

In the earlier days of nutrition as a science, nutritionists looked for guidance as to how to approach the practical implementation of nutrition principles in the lives of their clients and customers. The industry turned to the only source of inspiration and guidance that existed, and that was the medical profession. Do you remember our discussion of the standard medical model from chapter one? Well, nutritionists adopted much of this same model in the practice of nutrition.

Upon evaluating a client, if the nutritionist felt that their symptoms reflected a specific nutrient or group of nutrients were in deficiency, they often recommended the addition of those nutrients and those nutrients only. What they didn't realize fully in those early days was that fragmenting nutrition by the introduction of high amounts of certain nutrients, in the absence of others, often resulted in the development of other symptoms as a result of the imbalance created in the internal body chemistry.

An example of this flawed thinking at work may be illustrated through the use of vitamin C. In years past, if a client were to present with a depressed immune system, perhaps getting more than their fair share of colds and flu during the year, the nutritionist would often recommend supplementing the diet with high doses of vitamin C. Rightfully so, since the work of the late Linus Pauling and others have demonstrated that the antioxidant and immune properties of vitamin C can, in fact, prevent and even shorten a bout with the cold and flu virus.

What these early nutritionists failed to consider was the fact that vitamin C is a diuretic, and in high doses, flushes out not only toxins, which is a good thing, but also all the other water-soluble nutrients such as the B-complex and many minerals. As a result, the individual felt better initially. Their cold went away much quicker and they didn't get a second one this year either. But as time went on, this person began to develop other symptoms as a result of B-complex vitamin deficiency as well as a lack of such important minerals as calcium, magnesium and others.

The individual would continue their quest for health by consulting other nutritionists and health care providers who would add more nutrients in the attempt to balance the body.

What we have learned since those earlier days is that you cannot fragment nutrition and expect optimal results. If you review our discussion of the many vitamins and minerals in the previous chapter, you will see that virtually every single one of them is related to at least one or two others.

With this fact in hand, it should be easy to see that supplementing with only a few nutrients, in the absence of others, can do nothing but create more deficiency-related complications. There must be a better way.

Enter the concept of totality. If each of these nutrients is indeed, a part of a much larger picture within the vast complexity of the human biochemistry, than does it not make sense to ensure that all the players in this infinite 'chemical dance of life' are present at the same time?

With the concept of totality taking hold, nutritionists tried to find ways in which they could combine as many nutrients as possible into tablets and later on, into capsules. The problems with this were ones of capacity and chemistry.

Today we recognize the presence of about 100 essential nutrients. If you consider the environment in which we live, the addition of at least another 8 to 12 heavy hitting antioxidants should also be added. Finally, since few people ever eat a sufficient amount of fresh fruits and vegetables, the complex chemical compounds found in these foods are rarely supplied to the body's chemistry. Therefore, if we want to really round out the program, we must consider adding phytochemicals, from plants, to our list of necessary nutrients and nutrient compounds. This brings the total of players to about 120 or more.

In order to obtain all 120 of these substances on a daily basis, consumers were confronted with buying and taking many multiple products. Often this resulted in a ritual of opening and counting the contents of as many as 15 or more products. The cost and inconvenience of this practice soon caused all but the most dedicated to abandon the program. These people frequently settled instead for the best multi-vitamin/mineral product they could find. While this is certainly better than nothing, the previous chapter's discussion of the many dozens of micro trace elements reminds us that it is necessary for ALL nutrients to be together, at the same time. Only then can we achieve biochemical synergy. What was the answer?

About seven or eight years ago, I began toying with the idea of putting all the essential nutrients in one bottle. If this could be accomplished, it would eliminate many of the objections to taking so many individual nutrients. Consumers would not have to purchase so many different products, saving them a considerable amount of money. They would not have to spend so much time counting and carrying around so many tablets and capsules. But how to achieve this goal???

Enter Full Spectrum Nutrition

From the very beginning, my mind was set on trying to find a way to fulfill the concept of Full Spectrum Nutrition in a liquid medium. Liquids possess the ability to deliver nutrients in a much more bioavailable form while allowing for maximum absorption.

In reviewing and analyzing the existing liquid products on the market, I quickly realized that the potency of these products was minimal and the spectrum of nutrients they contained was equally limited. Once I began experimenting with the liquid concept for myself, it became apparent why this was the case.

When we deal with tablets or capsules, many varying ingredients may be combined and compressed together. Liquids however presented an entirely different set of rules. Water is the universal catalyst. Chemical reactions that normally take place very slowly or in most cases, not at all in a dry environment, react explosively in the presence of water.

I can remember, in the early days of formulation of my Full Spectrum liquid products, bottles would literally 'explode', sending the thick, less than attractive contents all over the room. Later, I had to deal with the 'ionic exchange' going on between specific major electrolytes. When suspended in water, these elements reacted powerfully with each other, releasing gases, which would bloat the bottles to the point that they would literally roll off the shelf, their bottoms were so inflated!

After over eight months of trial and lots and lots of error, my dream of creating a Full Spectrum product containing adequate potencies of vitamins, minerals, trace minerals, amino acids, phytonutrients, and the very latest in high tech antioxidants became a reality.

With that reality came the ability for anyone, regardless of age or physical condition, to provide their body's with the full gamut of ALL the necessary nutrients in a formula that was convenient, complete and economical.

In the course of this development, I was able to prove another of my long-time concepts, that being "ratio is equally important as potency when it comes to supplying the body with what it needs for health and longevity."

In the science of nutrition, the trend to develop products with higher potencies in an attempt to 'force' the predicted results of supplementation seems somehow wrong to me. While potency is important, another key is absorption. Without adequate numbers of nutrients present, body chemistry cannot function properly.

In the early days, if we observed an individual who was not absorbing say, calcium, perhaps due to poor pH, lack of enzyme activity, etc., we would just give them more and more calcium until their symptoms of deficiency disappeared. Today we know that, in order for calcium to be absorbed, not only into the cells of soft tissue, but back to bone tissue as well, it needs a variety of co-factors. Magnesium, manganese, boron, zinc, copper, vitamin D, and natural hydrochloric acid must all be present *at the same time,* in order for the body to maximize calcium uptake. Once these nutrients are combined in the right amounts, in relationship to each other, much less calcium is needed in order to meet bodily need. We must never forget that it is not how much of a nutrient we ingest, but how much we absorb and retain.

Keeping these myriads of interrelationships in mind, I designed the Full Spectrum liquid nutritional formulation to ensure that each nutrient complimented the others.

The final step was to prevent ongoing chemical reactions in the formula, which may be brought about by temperature rise and time itself. In order to help prevent this, and to extend the shelf life of the formula, I had to 'insulate' some nutrients and compounds from others. The end result was the birth of a whole new concept in delivering nutrients to the cells of the body, where they are needed most.

With Full Spectrum nutrition, in a bio-available liquid form, now a reality, the people I worked with, even those who had been taking some form of dietary supplement for years, began to almost immediately 'feel' the difference when they first consumed it. When we gave it to new clients at The Institute, the response was truly amazing. When Full Spectrum Nutrition was applied, aches, pains, and other complaints seemed to just slowly disappear, as if by magic. Often for the first time in years, their bodies were receiving ALL the nutrients in a balanced potency that delivered these raw materials to the chemical laboratory of the body.

When I wrote my first book, **SelfHealth: Your Complete Guide to Optimal Wellness**, I put forth a concept I learned many years ago. Simply stated, it was "Only the Body Can Heal." This is one of the most profound concepts in understanding human health. If you think about it, there really is very little any doctor or other health practitioner can do to restore health to the body. You can be drugged, cut open, mended, manipulated, massaged and loved, but when it's all said and done, your body has to recover and get well.

By providing the body with all the raw materials it needs, *at the same time*, its internal intuitive instinct to 'self heal' can move into high gear. It is no accident that I keep stressing 'at the same time.' Since the inter-relationship of nutrients to each other is practically unlimited, second- guessing seems futile. Clients of the various offices of our Institute of Nutritional Science experience first hand the power of 'the body healing' through the use of Full Spectrum Nutrition.

The Next Step

Once the body has been given the Full Spectrum of nutrients that it needs and begins to respond accordingly, we can then turn our attention to specializing or customizing an individual's nutritional program. Ever since biochemist Roger Williams put forth the concept of 'biochemical individuality', I have tried to view those who came to our offices as individuals rather than merely 'stock models.'

One of the greatest challenges in nutrition has always been addressing the specific needs of one person vs. another. The big question was "How could we accurately determine individual needs, over and above what was being met through base-line Full Spectrum supplementation?" Born of a need to fulfill this void, The Institute of Nutritional Science developed a variety of clinical testing procedures to determine what each individual body may require in the way of specialized nutrition in order to meet its own biochemical need. Through these tests, we are able to very accurately pinpoint a person's special requirements.

The Nutrient Evaluation Test

After someone has been taking Full Spectrum nutrition for 30 to 90 days, it's a good time to reevaluate the overall status of that person's health. After this time, the synergy of Full Spectrum Nutrition will have begun to work its magic. Any leftover symptoms may likely require special nutrient combinations, often in higher dosages.

In order to determine both need and dosage, we use a computerized nutrient evaluation test. Consisting of about 250 yes or no questions, sometimes combined with a food intake analysis, this test accurately tells us how the body is reacting, based upon 'symptomatology'. When you have symptoms, such as aches or pains, headaches, frequent diarrhea, constipation, insomnia, indigestion, and hundreds of other 'complaints', these are really your body trying to tell you of an imbalance in the 'chemistry of life'. Instead of paying attention to these signs, we all too often take some drug to cover them up and temporarily take them away. Following this practice brings immediate relief and result but, in most cases, does nothing to correct the problem that caused the annoying symptom in the first place.

So many people go through life just 'learning to live with it.' Since everyone they know seems to have similar or identical problems, they rationalize that it must be 'normal.' As a biochemist and nutritionist, I view these symptoms in a much different light. 'Symptomatology', or the language of the body, can tell us much about not only what is taking place in the biochemistry of the body today, but what we can likely expect, in the future, if we do not correct existing problems today.

Each one of these symptoms may be traced back to one or a multiple of nutrient deficiencies. Since we are all unique in our body chemistry, our need for specific nutrients can vary greatly. Through the application of The Nutrient Evaluation Test, my staff of trained nutritionists can often quickly identify specific nutrient deficiencies beyond what a base line Full Spectrum program can meet and we can subsequently provide those nutrients on top of their foundation program.

Another test we routinely use at the Institute is a hair mineral analysis. It is used primarily to determine the presence of heavy metal toxicity in the body and to ascertain overall mineral levels and ratios. This test is not only valuable in determining heavy metal presence but in monitoring the removal of these poisons while we are utilizing either oral or intravenous chelation.

Still another test we frequently use is the pH test. It determines whether or not an individual has a proper acid/alkaline balance. If not, we can take measures to insure that their acid/alkaline tide rolls in and out in a manner conducive to good health.

By the use of a diagnostic urinalysis test, we can detect the level of free radical activity in the body. This activity is directly responsible for premature aging, genetic damage, and most disease processes. On an individual basis, we can use this information to regulate the type and amount of antioxidant nutrients each person might need.

Once this information is gathered, we are in an excellent position to customize a lifetime nutrition program, which will meet both the general requirements as well as your own specific needs.

In the next chapter, we will look at disease in relationship to specific nutrient deficiencies and show how targeted mega-dose nutrition can often bring about a startling and positive metamorphosis in a person's life.

Chapter 16
When Full Spectrum
Is Not Enough

Throughout the previous chapter, the concept of Full Spectrum Nutrition was described in detail. When the body is simultaneously provided with the correct ratios and potencies of all available nutrients, phenomenal results occur. In fact, through the daily use of a Full Spectrum Nutrition regimen, most people achieve a significant improvement in their overall health. After a short transitional period of one to three months, they discover that their bodies are able to function much more effectively.

In order to understand how nutritional supplementation works, it is important that you grasp the concept of balance or equilibrium. All chemical activity within the body is regulated by a complex system of checks and balances. This ensures that powerful chemical reactions, necessary for life but devastating when out of control, remain in balance. Nutrients, vitamins, minerals plus other compounds are directly responsible for multitudes of chemical activities. These elements play a vital role in disease-free living by supporting the body's chemical 'checks and balances' function.

Delicate 'checks and balances' in human metabolic systems are often upset or destroyed by a seemingly innocent practice. Well intentioned individuals often will resort to 'fragmented nutritional supplementation' in an attempt to improve or prevent chronic disease. They will frequently ingest dosages of specific nutrients while omitting all of the others. This agenda, simply referred to as 'fragmented nutrition', is usually ineffective at best and devastating at worst. In an earlier chapter, the excess intake of isolated vitamin C was used to illustrate the shortcomings of this type of supplementation program.

We can, however, utilize the power of what has been called mega-doses of specific nutrients, providing we apply them properly. When we take extra vitamin C for the prevention of colds and the flu, or when we take extra calcium in an attempt to stave off osteoporosis, we are, in essence, fragmenting nutrition! This can be done safely providing that the Full Spectrum of nutrients has been provided *first*. Once we have ensured completeness and balance, we can then introduce high doses of selected nutrients to nurture and assist the body. I have coined the phrase 'targeted nutrition to describe this concept of specialized nutrient use. When combined with a daily Full Spectrum nutritional program, 'targeted nutrition' programs can be a powerful tool in resetting the internal equilibrium of the body.

How Does Targeted Nutrition Work?

Disease is an extreme. It is the end result of months or years of health compromises, which have culminated in a malfunction the internal biochemistry. When disease, especially chronic disease, manifests itself as symptoms, this is the *end process, the final stages of biochemical imbalance.* This is why we call disease a state of the extreme. Let's use arthritis, for example. It is irrelevant whether you have just recently noticed the symptoms or have suffered from them for years. Relevant is the fact that they are the result of long term chemical imbalances and nutrient deficiencies.

Keeping this in mind then, we can picture the disease process as a pendulum. Optimal health would be when the pendulum is perfectly centered and the body chemistry is allowed to carry on the life process unimpeded. As the pendulum swings in either direction, ripples of discord reverberate through the living system. Fortunately, the body has the ability to re-balance or re-center itself from the myriad of little deviations caused by the act of simply living. In fact, these fluctuations in balance are actually important, for they create the need for response, keeping the many systems of the body functioning and not becoming stagnant.

As this pendulum swings farther and farther away from the center however, the body finds itself in an increasingly difficult position of bringing it back to center or balance. As the pendulum swings still further from center, the body exhibits symptoms of discomfort. Digestive problems, aches and pains, insomnia, water retention, stiff joints, and thousands of other 'little complaints' are the body's way of telling us that the pendulum is swinging farther out of balance than our internal body chemistry can effectively re-balance.

Over months or even years of constant biochemical imbalances within the delicate chemistry, the pendulum can swing so far that it cannot be brought back to center on its own. Once the chemistry of the body stays in this extreme state for prolonged periods, permanent or semi-permanent damage to both the structure and functionality of the body can occur. It is in this state we are diagnosed with disease.

In this advanced disease state, with the pendulum shifted far from center, a Full Spectrum nutritional program may not be enough to bring the body back into balance. In those situations, we can benefit tremendously by adding an appropriate 'targeted' megadose nutritional program to the base-line Full Spectrum regimen.

In order to see how large, targeted doses of specific nutrients can assist the body in its journey back to balance, picture the pendulum in your mind, or picture a large heavy concrete ball. The farther this ball is away from where you want it, the more force is initially needed to move it there. Your body often works in the same manner. The farther away from balance your body chemistry becomes, the more 'force' or potency of nutrients it takes to return it to where you want it to be. Hence, the use of very high doses of specific nutrients, for short periods of time, can often accelerate the body's ability to heal itself.

This 'targeted nutrition' concept of achieving internal harmony through temporary extreme compromises the fundamental principles of the many nutritional protocols offered in the next chapter.

Utilizing 'targeted nutrition' to achieve specific results by augmenting a Full Spectrum program is entirely different than fragmenting with isolated nutrients. Each of the protocols in the next chapter are meant to be used in conjunction with a Full Spectrum program providing the 100 to 120 nutrients we have been talking about throughout this book. Once those are present, the often high doses of specific nutrients recommended in the various protocols are not only effective but safe as well.

Before we move on to health-restoring recipes, let's take a look at some of the popular nutrients recently featured in the news and discuss how they might be applied to specific 'targeted nutrition' programs. In the next chapter, you will likely see many of these nutrients appearing in the protocols for health.

We are in a nutrition revolution. In fact, science has been able to so completely demonstrate the power of all-natural substances in helping the body to heal, that many of us now refer to these nutrients as 'nutraceuticals', or substances that are natural, yet serve pharmacological functions.

At the Institute of Nutritional Science, we see

miracles every day. Adult-onset diabetics, with moderate to severe degenerative symptoms, are improving or reversing their condition regularly. Arthritics, whose quality of life had been destroyed by intense pain, reduced mobility, and disfigurement, are now joining local gyms, exercising, and enjoying their lives once again. Individuals, disabled by advanced heart disease to the point that they can no longer walk even a few blocks, are once again pursuing their lives with the fullness of activity. Other individuals who suffer from severe asthma are once again able to participate in athletics. Women, loosing precious bone by the day, are once again increasing their bone density and moving away from osteoporosis. Men, set for surgical procedures on their prostate glands are now free from the annoying and potentially dangerous symptoms of benign prostatic hypertrophy.

Where does it end? The potential for the human body to heal itself, *under the right circumstances*, is almost limitless. These seeming miracles are the gifts of nature when we follow her rules of living. Disease and premature death are often the results of disobeying. In my youth, I was fortunate enough to learn from this greatest of all teachers. The vast wisdom of Nature, from which our physical bodies have come, gives to us a home in which to live that is incredibly agile, potentially smart, and amazingly resilient. Yet, when we disobey the laws under which our bodies were created, the toll can be considerable.

The beauty of the human body is that no matter how terribly you may have abused it in the past, or no matter what your health history or your genetic potential, you can start to change the course upon which you are traveling at any time. The best news is that the results of these efforts are visible almost immediately.

Through unhealthy practices, primarily involving poor diets and the lack of exercise, many people unknowingly abuse their bodies. After years or decades of unhealthy living, they become afflicted with every disease imaginable. Over the years, I have personally helped thousands of them return to vibrant health and I have witnessed the amazing metamorphosis which can take place. These changes were not accomplished through use of drugs or surgery, but with lifestyle changes. In every instance, their return to optimal health was accomplished with only three simple modifications. They improved their diets by including fresh, 'living' foods, incorporated exercise into their lifestyles, and added the daily use of a Full Spectrum nutritional program with added 'targeted' nutritional support when needed. Through the use of base-line nutrients such as vitamins, minerals, essential fatty acids and amino acids, accompanied by the additional application of specific herbs, phytochemicals, and antioxidants, virtually anyone can build a road that will carry them to better health and greater longevity. Several of my personal favorite 'wonder substances' are described as follows.

Black Cohosh

Throughout the ages, tribal peoples have recognized the effectiveness of black cohosh in the life cycles of women. It is estimated that one out of every three women of childbearing age suffers from some degree of premenstrual syndrome. For many women these symptoms can be so severe that they are crippling.

While there are certainly many factors that can contribute to PMS, out of control hormones are a major factor. Enter black cohosh. This wonder herb has the ability to positively affect a woman throughout her entire life. It can ease the discomfort from PMS, decrease the difficulty of child birth and help to ease a woman through menopause.

Coenzyme Q10

Mentioned in many places throughout this book, CoQ10 is both an oxygenating factor as well as the 'spark' in the mitochondria production of energy. CoQ10 is also a powerful antioxidant, protecting delicate internal structures of cells from oxidative damage and mutation.

Because CoQ10 is ubiquitous, it is of benefit in virtually every site of your body. CoQ10 has been influential in improved heart health due to its positive affect upon everything from angina to advanced coronary artery disease. It is involved in helping the body to regulate blood sugar in cases of diabetes. Studies have shown its positive affect upon blood pressure, athletic performance, chronic obstructive pulmonary disease and cholesterol regulation. As an antioxidant, CoQ10 is one of our most powerful weapons available to fight the debilitating effects of asthma.

Genistein

Derived from soy, genistein is a powerful plant hormone that can be very helpful to humans, especially women. Through its hormone regulating effects, genistein can reduce the risk of breast cancer, lower the risk of heart disease in women, ease the symptoms of menopause, slow down the progression of osteoporosis, and increase the thyroid gland's production of thyroxin.

The soy family of nutrients continues to prove its incredible worth in the arena or women's health. Genistein is one of the newest additions.

Ginkgo Biloba

Blood flow is essential to life. Through this highway of the body all nutrition must flow to each of the more than 100 trillion individual cells. Oxygenated blood feeds every cell and organ system. This cardiovascular tree may be likened to highways upon which vehicles travel. In order to ensure adequate circulation, ginkgo biloba comes to the rescue.

Because of its profound effect on circulation, ginkgo can become involved at many levels of health. Studies have shown that ginkgo can protect specific brain tissue from oxidative damage. Further, by increasing blood flow to the brain, the cells can benefit from increased oxygen. It is the oxygenating effect of ginkgo biloba that makes it important to the heart muscle.

Any condition, in which oxygen deprivation may be involved, such as respiratory conditions including asthma, may be helped by the introduction of ginkgo biloba. Since blood flow is critical in male sexual performance, ginkgo biloba has enabled over 50 percent of men who use it to regain their sexual potency.

Glutamine

Over 30 percent of your immune system is located in and around the intestines. The health of the intestinal tract ensures that nutrients and calories are properly extracted from the foods and supplements we ingest. The natural bacteria present in the intestines are responsible for proper digestion and elimination. These bacteria depend on glutamine for health and maintenance.

Since immune function is related to glutamine, this nutrient can enhance immune response in such cases as severe infections and the trauma associated with burns or surgical invasion. Glutamine is critical in treating colitis and other colon and bowel diseases such as Crohn's disease.

Food allergies are often relieved with the supplementation of glutamine, since foods are more completely broken down, reducing the possibility of whole proteins entering the blood stream. Glutamine increases natural growth hormone so it is an important factor in muscle strength and growth as well as in anti-aging.

Kava

Anxiety is the most common complaint among members of our society. In fact, more people suffer from some form of anxiety than any other health problem. It is estimated that over 40 million people, worldwide, suffer from severe anxiety, which is debilitating and often requires powerful drug therapy. Most of us live with low levels of anxiety and have done so for so long, that we deem it 'normal.'

Having spent much of my time in the South Pacific, I have been familiar with kava for many years. Piper methysticum, or kava kava, as it is called in the islands, is a powerful substitute for many of the anxiety drugs. It is highly effective and does not produce the annoying side effects of drugs. Captain James Cook first introduced kava to the Western world in 1768.

In addition to the calming effects, kava has been used successfully to eliminate a variety of infections.

While kava is considered a sacred plant in the South Pacific and is used in a variety of ceremonies, it is a lifesaver to the anxious Western world. Stress produces both anxiety and depression if left unchecked. So devastating is unmanaged stress that I have frequently referred to it as the "cardinal cause of all disease". Through the use of such natural herbs as kava and valerian, we can gain control over the debilitating effects of anxiety and stress out of control.

Lutein

This member of the carotenoid family has burst onto the nutritional scene and has been a lifesaver for those suffering from eye disorders. A powerful antixoidant, lutein protects the delicate eye tissues from free radical damage from sources such as sunlight, smoking, heart disease, heredity and age itself.

Lutein is concentrated in the retina of the healthy eye and when present, protects against and prevents macular degeneration. This is good news since there are no conventional medical processes or procedures that prevent or reverse this disease.

Lutein also serves a powerful anti-cancer factor due to its antioxidant effect. Studies show that it is especially important in breast cancer as well as lung cancer.

Milk Thistle

As I have emphasized elsewhere in this book, we are all being poisoned daily by literally tens of thousands of toxins found in our food, water, air, and environment. The liver, the grand chemist of the body, must process each one of these toxins. Over time, the liver can become congested and thereby loose the ability to perform many of its biochemical processes.

Glutathione, essential for protecting the liver, may be effectively increased through the herb silymarin or milk thistle. This herb should also be considered in cases of liver disease such as hepatitis, cirrhosis, and in treating the infectious disease mononucleosis.

If you smoke, live with someone who smokes, work in an environment of fumes or pollution, drink excessive amounts of alcohol, take prescription drugs, eat fatty fried foods, or work around toxic substances, you need to nourish and support your liver function. Milk thistle comes to the rescue.

N-acetyl Cysteine

One of the most powerful antioxidants presently known, N-acetyl Cysteine or NAC, is almost the universal antioxidant since it affects so many areas of free radical prevention and scavenging.

NAC is often associated with the lungs and breathing. Rightfully so, because NAC can clear out lungs, lower lung inflammation and purge the tissues of free radical damage.

Other benefits of NAC include the elimination of cold and flu symptoms, the relaxation of blood vessels, lowering of blood pressure, and the prevention of colon conditions such as colitis, diverticulitis, and irritable bowel syndrome. In one study, NAC eliminated the symptoms of asthma in 76 percent of the people involved.

Together with milk thistle, NAC raises vital glutathione levels in the liver, assisting the organ in its role of detoxification. One of the most important functions of NAC is the prevention of genetic damage and subsequent mutation.

Phosphatidylserine

What an injustice it would be if we managed to keep our body healthy so that we could enjoy our golden years of retirement only to end up suffering because we are no longer able to remember simple things. Keeping the mind or brain healthy is just as important in quality aging is maintaining the physical aspects of the body. Phosphatidylserine, together with many other factors found in lecithin, can ensure that our cognitive abilities remain as functional as the rest of our body.

Thoughts are nothing more than the activation of nerve cells in the brain. Neurons, firing electrochemical messages to each other, create thoughts from nothing. These signals are fed by specific fatty acids and binding chemicals. Of the many members of this group, phosphatidylserine is the leader.

Dementia and Alzheimer's disease are on the rise. As more and more people successfully cross over past age 50, this will continue. Phosphatidylserine is the most powerful weapon we have against these crippling conditions.

Quercetin

Over 20 million people in America alone suffer from a condition called allergic rhinitis. This outcome of allergies to environmental factors such as dust, pollen, molds, and plants, can often become chronic, staying with the sufferer for months at a time.

Quercetin, another powerful antioxidant, has been shown to be very effective in the management of airborne allergies. Quercetin acts as a natural antihistamine and anti-inflammatory, preventing the causes of allergy symptoms, often before they can develop.

Quercetin is also helpful in preventing oxidation of fats within the body, especially the oxidation of cholesterol.

In one landmark study, quercetin was shown to prevent the proliferation of both breast and colon cancer cells.

Saw Palmetto

We started with a discussion of black cohosh, the woman's best herbal friend. We end off our discussion of specialized nutrients with saw palmetto, the man's best herbal friend.

Long recognized as a preventive and treatment for prostate inflammation and cancer, saw palmetto is helpful in many areas of male health. Regular consumption of saw palmetto can enhance libido in males as well as prevent sexual impotence.

Benign Prostatic Hypertrophy, or BPH, is the

single greatest reason why men over the age of 50 visit a medical doctor. Saw palmetto can reduce the incidence of BPH to less than 10 percent of its present level.

These are just some of the shinning stars within the spectrum of nutrients and nutritional compounds. Each one can play an important role in the health, maintenance and well being of our human family. The key is knowing when and how to use them properly for maximum benefit.

Through combining the right nutrients together with a broad-based Full Spectrum of nutrition, thousands of people are slowly working their way back to health and happiness.

Today, we are poised at the edge of an era where the average life span will likely jump to over 100 years. What will be the value of these added years if they must be spent in a state of physical and mental compromise?

There are hundreds of ailments and conditions, both large and small, which can steal life's quantity and quality from you. In the next chapter, I offer my protocols for the management and reversal of these conditions. Countless others have benefited immensely from the programs I have outlined. Through the proper implementation of the following protocols, you too can help your body heal itself, thereby enabling you to remain healthy throughout your lifetime.

Chapter 17
The Nutraceutical Pharmacopoeia

I n my first book, **SelfHealth: Your Complete Guide to Optimal Wellness**, I put forth two pivotal concepts, which I feel are essential when addressing the issue of either prevention or reversal of any disease condition. They are of such importance that stating them here would not be redundant.

The first concept is that "Microbes, in and of themselves, do not cause disease. Disease and disorder occur only when the body's internal chemistry becomes im-balanced."

This means that by the time you catch that winter cold or flu, your body's immune system was weakened and compromised for perhaps weeks or months before. While it seems almost normal to blame the 'little bugs' for our distress, these little bugs are with us almost constantly and we are all exposed to them, yet only a few of us actually get sick from them. Whether we will come down with the flu in the presence of the flu virus or not, depends entirely upon how rapidly our immune system can respond to the invading pathogen and build the necessary antibodies to destroy it. If the response is rapid, as it should be, then it is unlikely that we will feel the presence of the virus at all.

When addressing infectious conditions with the protocols that follow remember this point. While we can help the body respond better to these invading pathogens through mega-dose nutrition, our ultimate goal should be to strengthen the immune system so that it is prepared for the next invading pathogen.

"Only the body can heal", is the second concept that you must understand before we proceed with the protocols in this chapter. If you think about this statement for just a moment it makes more and more sense.

If you have an illness, you can visit a doctor. He may give you medications or perform surgery, but when they are finished doing all that they can, you are the one that must go home, get well, and recover.

The truth is that there is not a medical doctor, chiropractor, drug, nutritionist, or nutritional supplement that can cure you of anything, including the health conditions contained in this chapter. Only your body can heal itself.

The following nutrient combinations will provide the body with the high doses of 'raw materials' it needs to heal itself. Remember our discussion of the disease pendulum in the last chapter? The following protocols often take advantage of the temporary extreme concept. High doses of specific nutrients for periods of time in order to accelerate the body's ability to rebalance itself and more rapidly return the disease pendulum to center. It is in this center, or balanced state, that we can live free of disease and disorder.

Don't Forget Full Spectrum

Each of the protocols that follow offer targeted nutrition through the application of specific nutrients and compounds, which have been shown in clinical studies, to aid the body in its management of and recovery from specific conditions. It must be understood, however, that these targeted nutritional recommendations are fragmented nutrition and should not be taken alone! In each of the protocols, you MUST also ensure that you are taking the Full Spectrum of base line nutrition in addition to the specific recommendations. In Chapter 15, we discussed the dangers of fragmenting nutrition and possibly throwing the delicate chemistry of the body out of balance. Many of these protocols, if taken in the absence of a Full Spectrum program, run the risk of just such an occurrence.

This being the case, do not follow my protocols without including the Full Spectrum nutrition concept, unless you are specifically told to do so for a given condition.

What follows, is one of the most current and complete Nutraceutical Pharmacopoeia currently available. The recommendations given for each condition have been carefully researched and are, in many cases, the result of years of personal successful application with individuals just like you.

When reading through specific conditions, you may wonder why certain recommendations you may have read about are missing. In many cases, it is because I could not find sufficient clinical data to support their use. I have tried to include only those recommendations for which there are clinical studies, trials or usage. By so doing, I can assure you that the suggestions made are both safe and effective. Over time of course, as science progresses, there will be legitimate additions to these protocols and they will appear in subsequent editions of this book.

The protocols that follow are in alphabetical order, making them easy to access and refer to. Interpreting the Protocols

The protocols that follow MUST be taken with a Full Spectrum nutrition program as outlined in previous chapters. The supplementary recommendations are to taken *in addition* to a base-line Full Spectrum nutritional program.

A Full Spectrum Nutritional Program

- A Broad Spectrum Liquid or Capsule providing 16 vitamins, 8 –12 amino acids, 7 major minerals, 65+ trace minerals and phytonutrients from plants.
- A Liquid Organic Source, bio-electrical trace mineral supplement.
- Essential Fatty Acids in airtight gel caps.

Reference Range

In many instances, you will see a range of potency for a specific nutrient (i.e. vitamin C- 2 to 4 grams). This represents the range of dosage used in clinical studies for a specific condition. You should start with the *lowest dose* and work upwards until the desired response is achieved.

I have provided this reference range so that you will know what the minimum effective level is as well as the maximum safe upper dose.

Abscess

An abscess is a localized infection that has become encapsulated. They are frequently treated with antibiotics and occasionally they need to be opened or removed surgically. The use of antibiotics destroys B vitamins and the natural bacteria in the gut This bacteria must be replaced to maintain digestive system health. Emphasis should also be placed upon immune enhancement to ensure that these localized infections are minimized in the future.

> **Full Spectrum nutrition**
> **Immune Enhancing Factors**
> Collostrum Concentrate 100mg
> Mushroom Mycelial Biomass200 mg
> Beta- 1,3-D Glucan .... 50 mg
> Echinacea Purpurea Leaf Ext. 25 mg
> Astragalus Ext. .... 50 mg
> Pau D'Arco Ext. .... 50 mg

The Immune Enhancing combination may be given every two hours for several days during acute infection.

> Zinc Gluconate .... 60 mg per day
> Vitamin C .... 1-3 grams per day

If antibiotics are used add multi-acidophilus capsules in order to replenish the 'good' bacteria throughout the digestive system:

> Multi-acidophilus ....
> ..... 10 capsules per day for 10 days

Acidosis

A condition of excess acidity in the body, acidosis may be caused by the presence of kidney, liver, or adrenal disorders. Improper diet, obesity, stress, fever, and excess acidic vitamins can cause a temporary state of acidosis. Diabetics are also at risk if they are uncontrolled.

To determine if your acid/alkaline range, consider taking the pH test offered by The Institute of Nutritional Science. Our contact information may be found in the Resources section at the end of this book. Also review the section on acid and alkaline balance in Chapter 11.

Acidosis is not nearly as common as a condition of excess alkalinity, if you have this problem, it needs to be addressed quickly.

Full Spectrum Nutrition
Kelp......................... 10 tablets daily
Potassium .... 100 mg/ twice daily
B-complex .... 100 mg/ twice daily

Increase consumption of raw fruits and vegetables and reduce consumption of protein foods temporarily until your pH has been balanced.

Acne

Labeled the curse of youth, acne strikes over 80 percent of those between the ages of 12 and 25. During this period of time, hormone acceleration depletes the body of much of its zinc supply. This mineral is essential in preventing the bacterial infection, which develops in the sebaceous glands in hair follicles. The extra rush of hormones accelerates the production of oils, especially on the face, chest, and back. This situation, combined with multiple nutrient deficiencies, leads to skin infection. Other factors that can cause acne, or make it worse, include heredity, excessively oily skin, allergies, oral contraceptives, stress, and high amounts of junk foods containing unnatural fats.

This condition is addressed both topically and through supplementation internally. It is important to keep the skin clean. Use an alcohol-free cleanser and apply a hypo-allergenic cream containing zinc stearate to promote healing.

Full Spectrum Nutrition

Zinc Stearate Cream (15%) .... Use topically twice daily

Zinc Gluconate/chelate .... 20 mg 2-3 times per day

Chromium Chelate .... 200 mcg per day

Vitamin A (natural only)................... .... 50,000 – 100, 000 IU per day

Reduce vitamin A once improvement is seen to 25,000 IU per day

Essential Fatty Acids .... 4-6 capsules per day

Lecithin Granules........................... .... 1 tablespoon per day

Acne Rosacea

Follow the preceding outlined program but add the following...

> Niacin (as Niacinamide) ....
> .... 200 mg 3 times per day
> High potency Stress Formula
> B-Complex ....
> .... as directed
> Multi-Enzyme with Hydrochloric acid
> ....2-4 per meal

Acquired Immune Deficiency Syndrome (AIDS)
Also see Immunodepression

A devastating destruction of the immune system, believed to be caused by a virus, AIDS rarely kills anyone in and of itself. The secondary infections within the body develop as a result of severe immune suppression and rampant free radical formation and subsequent damage.

Combine the protocols under immunodepression while adding high amounts of the antioxidant N-acetyl L-cysteine.

Addison's Disease - See Adrenal Disorders

Adrenal Disorders

The adrenal glands are responsible for producing powerful hormones, many of which are involved in the stress response. Through increased stress and tension these glands can become exhausted, leading to the over-production of the hormones responsible for the 'fight or flight' syndrome. This can result in exhaustion, anxiety, mood swings, and even depression.

Long term use of drugs such as cortisone can cause the adrenal glands to atrophy. Diseases such as pituitary disorders and tuberculosis can cause outright adrenal failure.

Stress management is an all-important factor in restoring good adrenal function. Fortunately, there are several nutrients which nourish the adrenal glands, thereby helping to prevent excessive exhaustion.

Full Spectrum Nutrition

High potency Stress Supplement
.... 4-8 capsules per day
Pantothenic Acid ....
.. 500 – 1000 mg /2-3 times per day
Vitamin B12....................................
.... 200 mcg/ 2 times per day
Raw Adrenal Extract ....
.... 6-12 per day
Vitamin C ....
.... To bowel tolerance

Age Spots

Those flat brown spots, sometimes called 'liver spots' are most often caused by radiation damage to the skin from free radicals. While the spots themselves are benign, they do indicate that the body is overloaded with internal toxins. This waste is steadily destroying living cells within the body, including brain and liver cells. These spots are most often caused by excess sun exposure, the consumption of vegetable oils, lack of exercise, or a toxic liver.

Full Spectrum Nutrition

Follow the systemic liver, kidney, bowel, bladder, and colon cleanse found in Chapter 13.

Multi- Antioxidants ....
.... 400-800 mg per day
Bioflavonoids ....
.... 2,000 mg per day
Vitamin A (natural only) ....
.... 10,000 IU

AIDS – See Acquired Immune Deficiency Syndrome

Alcoholism

Alcohol is a classic example of a substance that can have beneficial effects in moderation but can become a relentless executioner when taken in excess. Alcoholism is a chronic disease wherein the victim must have alcohol on a regular basis. It is not necessarily based upon quantity, although with time, more and more usually is needed. Excess alcohol causes massive destruction within the body. It is an immune suppressant and generates massive amounts of free radicals. Prolonged misuse results in damage to virtually every cell of the body.

While abstinence is essential with most alcoholics, achieving this goal may be impossible without the help and support of a professional clinic or organization equipped to deal with addiction. During recovery, the following nutrients will prove helpful by both protecting the body from the ravages of alcohol and easing the cravings.

Full Spectrum Nutrition
B-Complex Stress Nutrients ....
.... 4-8 capsules per day
Vitamin B1 ....
.... 200 mg 3 times per day

Fatty Acids ....
.... 3 grams per day
Pantethine ....
.... 300 mg 2-3 times per day
Selenium ....
.... 100 mcg
L-Glutamine ....
.... 1 gram 2 times daily

Heavy Hitting Antioxidants including
N-acetyl L- Cysteine, Milk Thistle,
Coenzyme Q10, Grape Seed Extract,
and Quercetin ....
.... 400 –1200 mg per day

To lesson the cravings for alcohol:

Evening Primrose Oil ....
.... 1 gram 3 times per day
Taurine........ 1 gram 3 times per day

Alkalosis

The opposite of acidosis, and far more common
in its mild form, alkalosis occurs when too many alkaline forming foods are ingested or when the natural
production of the stomach's hydrochloric acid is depleted. Symptoms of alkalosis include poor digestion,
heartburn, sore muscles, creaking joints, bone spurs,
drowsiness, hypertension, hypothermia (or being cold

all the time), edema, night cramps, asthma, constipation, and burning, itching skin.

Emphasis must be placed on fixing first the hydrochloric acid levels in the stomach. In addition to the specific supplements listed below, the diet should be adjusted to include more protein foods such as meat, fish, and fowl. You can test your acid and alkaline balance quite easily by obtaining a pH test kit from The Institute of Nutritional Science. (See Resources at the end of this book.)

> ### *Full Spectrum Nutrition*
> Betaine Hydrochloric Acid..............
> .... 2-4 capsules with each meal
> Multi purpose enzyme formula........
> .... 2-4 capsules with each meal
> Apple Cider Vinegar ....
> .... 2 Tbl 2 or 3 times per day

Allergic Rhinitis – See Hay Fever

Allergies

All allergies are an autoimmune response to either food or environmental factors, which are normally innocuous to the human body. These hyper-sensitivities can be genetic in origin, like most autoimmune disorders, or they can be the outcome of excess toxicity within the body for prolonged periods of time.

Food allergies are best dealt with by either avoiding the offending foods or rotating them so they are not consumed more than once every five days.

Airborne allergies are much more difficult to deal with, since they cannot be avoided. Mold, pollen, dust, animal dander, and chemical sensitivities present the greatest challenges.

While avoidance, as much as possible, is still the best way to deal with multiple allergies, the following nutrients may lesson the symptoms.

Full Spectrum Nutrition

High potency Stress Formula..........
.... 4-8 capsules per day
Pantethine ....
.... 600 – 900 mg per day
Quercetin ....
.... 1000 mg per day
Vitamin C ....
.... 3-5 grams per day
Fatty Acids ....
.... 1000 mg daily
Licorice extract.............................
.... 1-3 capsules
Niacin (a natural antihistamine) ....
..........50-100 mg 2 or 3 times daily

Alopecia – See Hair Loss

Aluminum Toxicity – See Heavy Metal Poisoning

Alzheimer's Disease (see also Memory Improvement)

This debilitating disease is estimated to affect over 2.5 million people. As the mean population exceeds age 50, this condition will likely become more and more prevalent. Simple forgetfulness should not be confused with Alzheimer's disease. (see memory improvement) Dementia, a symptom of Alzheimer's, is also a symptom of many disorders and can be induced by the presence of many diseases and nutritional deficiencies.

True Alzheimer's is difficult to diagnose, but we approach it nutritionally from many angles, which include modalities for dementia and other memory-related conditions.

Antioxidants are likely to be our biggest natural weapon against these types of disorders.

Full Spectrum Nutrition
High Potency Antioxidants: Coenzyme Q10, Superoxide Dismutase, Grape Seed Extract, Quercetin and N-Acetyl Cysteine .... 400 mg 3 times per day

> Ginkgo biloba ....
> .... 50 mg 3 times per day

Amyotrophic Lateral Sclerosis – See Neuromuscular Degeneration

Anemia

Anemia is a condition that reduces the amount of oxygen that the blood is able to transport. This reduces the amount of red blood cells resulting in weakness, dizziness, irritability, depression, pale complextion, and loss of menstruation. Early symptoms of anemia include loss of appetite, headaches, constipation, irritability, and lack of concentration.

Iron deficiency is the most common cause of anemia. Any condition that causes regular or prolonged loss of blood can induce temporary anemia.

Note: Iron deficiency can be caused by a lack of copper in the diet, which prevents available iron from being absorbed into the cells.

Full Spectrum Nutrition
Folic Acid.......................................
.... 800 mcg twice daily
High Potency B-Complex
.... As indicated on label
Iron Gluconate ....
.... As determined by doctor
Raw Liver Extract.............................

.... 500 mg 2 or 3 times per day
Copper Chelate .... 2-6 mg daily
Zinc .... 20 mg daily
Raw Spleen Extract ....
.... 100 mg 2 –3 times daily
Vitamin B12 .... 100 mcg for 30 days
Digestive Enzymes w/ Hcl
...................................2-4 per meal
Selenium .... 500 mcg per day

Angina

Excessive pain in the upper torso, specifically the center of the chest to the left shoulder and arm. There are many causes, but generally it is a lack of oxygen to the heart muscle, which is most often caused by the narrowing of the arteries around the heart.

Oral Chelation Formula
(instead of regular Full Spectrum) ...
.... 6-9 per day
Bio-electrical Trace Minerals ....
.... 1 ounce twice per day
Calcium/Magnesium ....
.... 1500 mg per day
Essential Fatty Acids ....
.... 3 grams per day
Arginine .... 4-8 grams per day
L-Carnitine .... 2 – 3 grams per day
CoQ10 .... 100 – 200 mg per day

In severe, acute cases, consider the immediate use of intravenous chelation treatments from a trained chelation therapist or doctor. Follow up this treatment with a tested oral chelation formula for prevention.

Ankylosing Spondylitis

Exercise is very important in reducing the degree of permanent damage that can result from this condition. Emphasis should be upon flexibility exercises. A program of exercise done under water, in an exercise pool, is frequently tolerated best especially in the beginning.

Full Spectrum Nutrition
Vitamin B6 .... 50 mg per day
Chondroiton Sulfate ....
.... 200 – 400 mg per day
Glucosamine Sulfate ....
.... 200- 400 mg per day
MSM .... 100 mg per day

Natural Pain Relief
dl-Phenylalanine* ....
.... 250 mg 2 or 3 times per day
*Note: do not take if you have uncontrolled high blood pressure.

Anorexia

This eating disorder, which primarily affects females, was often thought to be solely psychological. While there is no doubt that emotional ties exist, nutrition may be very helpful for those suffering from this condition. Of special importance would be liquid nutritional products, since their absorption rate is much higher than capsules or tablets.

Even though the individuals are frequently of ideal weight or even underweight, they become obsessed with the concept that they are fat. This results in such dangerous practices as vomiting up meals, taking laxatives, or simply starving. While this condition should not be addressed without including psychological counseling, the following nutrients will help to keep the body nourished and replace those specific nutrients lost through the use of laxatives or the practice of regular vomiting.

Full Spectrum Liquid Nutrition

Calcium .... 1000mg per day
Magnesium .... 500 mg per day
Potassium ..... 100 mg twice per day
Zinc .... 50 mg per day
Additional Liquid Trace Minerals ......
.... 1 ounce per day
Acidophilus ... 5 capsules per day on empty stomach

Multi Enzyme Product ....
.... 2-4 with each meal
B-Complex Stress Formula ....
.... As indicated on product label

Anxiety

Stress has become a way of life in our society. With everyone trying to fit 90 minutes of work into every hour, it's no wonder than stress-related health problems are escalating. Of all the leading prescription drugs, over half of them are for either anxiety or depression. Prolonged unmanaged stress overworks the adrenal glands, which are the 'fight or flight' system of the body. This results in anxiety due to the constant presence of powerful adrenal hormones in the blood stream. Following are nutrient recommendations for helping your body to deal with stress by nourishing the adrenal response system. Also listed is my all-natural tranquilizer replacement formula, which may be used for short periods of excess stress.

Full Spectrum Nutrition
Calcium .... 800 mg per day
Magnesium .... 400 mg per day
Essential Fatty Acids ....
.... 500 mg extra per day
B-Complex Stress Formula ....
.....................As per label directions

Valerian Root Extract ....
.... 2 Capsules at bedtime
Kava Root Extract ....
.... 100 mg 2 or 3 times per day

Natural Tranquilizer Replacement
Take the following combination every
four hours:
Calcium .... 400 mg
Magnesium .... 100 mg
Vitamin B6 .... 50 mg
5- Hydroxy Tryptophan (5-HTP) ....
.... 200 mg
Kava Root Extract .... 100 mg
B-Complex Stress Formula ....
.... 1 capsule
Vitamin B12 .... 500 mcg

Appetite Problems

Many health challenges can result in a compromised appetite. Chronic diseases, infections, and digestive disorders can lead to poor eating habits. This is especially true with older people, because as we age our digestive processes become less and less effective. The following program may help in correcting digestive problems and may improve appetite.

Full Spectrum Nutrition

Multi-Enzyme Formula with Hcl ....
..................................2-4 per meal
Acidophilus ....
...........5 per day on empty stomach
B-Complex Stress Formula.............
....as indicated until appetite returns
Zinc Gluconate ....50 mg per day

Aphthous Stomatitus (Canker Sores)

Ulcerations inside the mouth, the canker sore manifests itself as a small white ulcer like sore. These sores can take as long as two weeks or more to heal. There are several factors that contribute to the canker sore such as acid/alkaline imbalance, allergies to chocolate, stress, immune suppression, and a bacterial imbalance in the mouth. Diabetics often have problems with this condition due to metabolic acidosis.

Full Spectrum Nutrition

Multi-Acidophilus ....
......................3-6 capsules per day
Betaine Hydrochloride (Hcl) ....
.... 1 –3 capsules per meal
Zinc Gluconate ....
.....50 –100 mg per day (short term)
Folic Acid....................1 mg per day
Vitamin B12.....................................
.... 1000 mcg twice per day

> Licorice Root Gargle......................
> .... 3 –4 times per day
> Acidophilus ....
> .... 3-5 capsules per day

Arrhythmia - See Cardiac Arrhythmia

Arteriosclerosis (Atherosclerosis)

These conditions are really one and the same. Arteriosclerosis is the thickening of the artery wall due to calcium deposits and is also referred to as calcification of the arteries. Atherosclerosis, a similar condition, is when fatty deposits also line the interior of the artery wall. Both these conditions have the same basic cause, which is free radical damage to the muscle wall of the artery, primarily through the over-consumption of vegetable oils in the diet. (See Chapter 5 for a complete discussion of this condition.)

> Oral Chelation Formula
> (Instead of regular Full Spectrum) ...
> .... as directed on product label
> Liquid Plant Derived Minerals ....
> .... 1 ounce twice per day
> Vitamin E .... 400 –800 IU per day
> Lecithin Granules........ 2 Tbl per day
> Garlic Concentrate ....
> .... 4 –8 capsules per day

Multi-Digestive Enzymes.................
.... 2 – 4 with each meal
Folic Acid....... 1 mg 3 times per day
Niacin .... 100 mg 3 times per day
Taurine.................. 1000 mg per day
Essential Fatty Acids ....
.... 4-6 grams per day
Multi-Antioxidant Compound containing Coenzyme Q10, Grape Seed Extract, Bilberry Extract, Quercetin, Silybum Marianum and N-Acetyl Cysteine .... 400 –800 mg per day

Note: If the condition is acute, the above protocol will work too slowly for you to benefit from. Consider taking intravenous chelation therapy from a professional trained in this procedure. After the initial crisis has passed, follow up with this protocol for prevention and maintenance.

Arthralgia – See Rheumatism

Arthritis (See also Rheumatoid Arthritis)

There are several forms of arthritis. The most common is osteo-arthritis, which is characterized by inflammation and pain in a joint or several joints. Arthritis is a condition caused by the proliferation of free radicals within the body. Once developed, arthritis produces multiple toxins, which increase both the inflammation and pain as well as the actual progression of the disease. Therefore, any program addressing arthritis, must also address detoxification of the body. (See Chapter 7 for a complete discussion of arthritis and Chapter 13 for a cleansing and detoxifying program.)

Full Spectrum Nutrition

Essential Fatty Acids .... 4-6 grams per day

Liquid Organic Trace Minerals .... 2-3 ounces per day

Calcium/ Magnesium/ trace minerals .... 4-8 capsules per day

Vitamin C .... 2- 4 grams per day

B-Complex Stress Formula............. ..... as indicated on label for 30 days

Arthritis Combination Including:

Vitamin B6 .... 50 – 100 mg/day

Quercetin .... 100 mg/day

Evening Primrose Oil ... 100 mg/day

Glucosamine Sulfate ... 500 mg/day

Chondroitin Sulfate ...... 500 mg/day

Cetylmyristoleate .... 150 mg/day

Nettle Leaf Extract....... 400 mg/day

Niacin (as Niacinamide) . 40 mg/day

Detoxification Program Chapter 13

Multi Enzymes with Hydrochloric acid .... 2 –4 with each meal

If pain is considerable, consider the following:

dl-Phenylalanine* ....
.....................500 mg twice per day
*Note: do not take if you have uncontrolled high blood pressure

Liquid Oxygen...............................
...........1 ounce three times per day

Asthma

A severe form of allergic response, asthma is a series of spasms in the muscles surrounding the small air passages in the lungs. Symptoms of asthma include coughing, wheezing, tight constricting feeling in the chest, and difficulty in breathing. Asthma can be a very acute, life threatening condition and must be handled aggressively. When histamine forms as a result of the allergic response mucus fills the lungs and bronchi.

Full Spectrum Nutrition
Vitamin A (natural only)..................
.... 25,000 IU per day
B-Complex Stress formula.............
..........as indicated on product label
Multi-Digestive Enzymes...............
.....................2-4 with each meal

Essential Fatty Acids ....
.... 2 grams per day
Pantethine .... 600 – 1000 mg/day
Antioxidant Combination Including:
Coenzyme Q10, Quercetin and espe-
cially N-Acetyl Cysteine ....
.... 800 mg per day
Calcium .... 1000 mg per day
Magnesium............. 600 mg per day
Vitamin C .... 2 grams daily
Ma huang .... 15 mg twice per day
DHEA .... 25 – 50 mg per day
Ginkgo biloba .... 40 mg per day

Atopic Dermatitis – See Eczema

Atherosclerosis – See Arteriosclerosis

Athlete's Foot

This fungal infection can be very virulent and difficult to control once it sets in. The environment of
the feet is ideal for the proliferation of fungal growth.
Like most fungus in the body, this is also controlled
by the presence of healthy bacteria in the gut. When
these bacteria are destroyed, the fungus is free to spread
very rapidly.

> ### Full Spectrum Nutrition
> Multi-Acidophilus ....
> .... 5 Capsules twice per day
> Garlic Extract ..... 5 capsules per day
> Liquid Oxygen ....
> .... 1 ounce three times per day

You may soak your feet in a solution of 35 percent food grade hydrogen peroxide and water. Make this by adding one ounce of pure 35 percent hydrogen peroxide to a gallon of water. Soak feet twice a day for 20 minutes.

Atrial Fibrillaton – See Cardiac Arrhythmia

Attention Deficit Disorder (ADD)

Severe learning disabilities can lead to the inability to focus and concentrate and are becoming more common. The theory is that it is caused by a combination of genetic mutation from the parents and exposure to toxic chemicals in the children. Research done at The Institute of Nutritional Science, has proven that radical treatment with powerful drugs are not only unnecessary for this condition but may cause more harm than good in the long run. Nutrient deficiency is most assuredly at the heart of these problems. There are also several adjunct factors, which if present, can contribute to the overall problem.

Full Spectrum Liquid Nutrition
1 tsp. per 20 pounds of bodyweight
Or for children age 10 and older .....
.... 1 ounce per one hundred lbs.
bodyweight
Essential Fatty Acids ....
.... 2 –3 capsules per day
Calcium Citrate/Malate
Ages 2 –5 .... 200 mg per day
Ages 6 + ... 500 – 1000 mg per day

Stress-Related Nutrients
Children under 45 pounds:
Niacin (as Niacinamide) ....
....25 mg up to 100 mg max per day
Vitamin C ....
.... 50 mg up to bowel tolerance

Children over 45 pounds:
Niacin (as Niacinamide) ....
.... 50 – 200 mg
Vitamin C .... to bowel tolerance
Pyridoxine................... 50 – 400 mg
Riboflavin................... 50 – 200 mg
Calcium Pantothenate ....
.... 100 – 800 mg
Magnesium................... 50-200 mg
Zinc .... 5 – 30 mg

If excessive hyperactivity is a factor, test for heavy metal poisoning such as mercury, lead or cadmium and add:

Caffeine .... 100 mg per day

If the child craves sweets, suspect carbohydrate intolerance, and add:

Chromium .... 100 mcg
Vanadium .... 500 mcg
Aspartic Acid .... 300 mg
Bilberry Extract .... 20 mg

If short-term memory is affected consider adding the following:

Phosphatidylserine ....
.... 100-200 mg per day
Phosphatidylcholine ....
.... 100-200 mg per day

Finally, many individuals displaying attention deficit symptoms suffer from multiple allergies. I suggest you take the RAST test (a blood test) which will determine all airborne and food allergies. If food allergies are detected, it will be necessary to either eliminate those foods or rotate them, eating them no more often than once every five days.

Those dealing with attention deficits may want

more information. I suggest my booklet entitled, *Drug Free Answers to Correcting Learning Disabilities*, available from The Institute.

Autism – Attention Deficit Disorders

Auto-Immune Disorders

Auto-immune conditions come about due to a genetic mutation, which causes the immune system to view harmless substances as toxic. Allergies, Crohn's Disease, and Rheumatoid Arthritis are typical examples. The body sees substances such as dust, mold, pollens, and certain foods as toxins and builds antibodies against them. This produces histamine and the classic allergic response. In the case of rheumatoid arthritis, the body sees its own cartilage and connective tissue as foreign and builds antibodies to attack and destroy it.

Anyone suffering from any auto-immune condition should NOT take immune stimulating substances without the express supervision of the trained professional. In many cases these ingredients accelerate the activity of the immune system and can accelerate the auto-immune disorder thereby making it much worse.

Full Spectrum Nutrition
Vitamin C .... To Bowel Tolerance
Vitamin E .... 400 IU Extra per day
Selenium .... 100 mcg per day

Backache

Most aches and pains in the lower back are due to weak muscles, which can no longer hold the spine in proper alignment. Exercises to strengthen these muscles are often essential. Calcium and magnesium deficiencies can contribute to low back pain as well.

Full Spectrum Nutrition
Calcium/Magnesium/ trace minerals
.... 4 –8 capsules per day
Horsetail Extract ....
.... As indicated on product label

If arthritis is the cause of the lower back pain, see the arthritis protocol.

Baldness – See Hair Loss

Bed Wetting

While the cause of this condition is unknown, it is believed to be a combination of psychological and nutritional factors. Factors that can contribute to this problem physically include, food allergies, small or weak bladders, and urinary tract infections. It is believed that protein deficiency can also cause this problem.

Full Spectrum Nutrition
Protein Powder Drink ....
.... 10 –25 grams protein per day
Calcium .... 500 mg per day
Magnesium............. 250 mg per day
Zinc .... 10 mg per day

Take the RAST blood test to determine possible allergies.

Bee Sting

For the most part, bee stings are annoying and a little uncomfortable, but for some they can be life-threatening. If you have a severe allergy to bee stings, you must carry the appropriate medications to avoid possible anaphylactic shock. If you don't have an allergy to the venom, simply remove the stinger carefully with tweezers and apply liquid minerals to the bite two or three times per day.

Full Spectrum Nutrition
Pantothenic Acid (natural Antihistamine) .... 500 mg per day

> Drink Yellow Dock Tea and apply topically to sting area

Bells Palsy

A neurological condition, usually of the face, which can come on quite suddenly and last for several days or even weeks. It causes a drooping of one side of the face due to an inflammation of the nerves.

Full Spectrum Nutrition
Vitamin B-12 .... 1000 mcg per day
Calcium .... 1000 mg per day
Magnesium .... 500 mg per day
Essential Fatty Acids ....
.... 1000 mg per day
Valerian Root Extract ....
.... As indicated on product label

Benign Breast Cysts

While this is a relatively harmless condition, it can be frightening to a woman who feels lumps in her breasts. Naturally, she will assume the worst and think it is evidence of cancer. Most of the time these lumps are blocked ducts, or in some cases, benign cysts, which form as a result of fat metabolism irregularities stemming from the liver. By cleansing the liver and providing nutrients to help the liver process fats, we can virtually eliminate the occurrence of these benign cysts in breast tissue.

> ### Full Spectrum Nutrition
> Lipotropics Choline/Inositol/
> Methionine ....
> .... 1000 mg 2 to 3 times per day
> Vitamin A....................................
> .... 10,000 – 25,000 IU per day
> Vitamin E .... 400 IU per day
> Kelp (iodine) .... 6-10 tablets per day
> Essential Fatty Acids ....
> .... 1500 mg 2 times per day

Benign Prostatic Hyperplasia

The most common reason why men over age 50 visit a doctor, chronic prostate inflammation is not only annoying but potentially problematic as well. When the inflammation is sufficient to prevent the voiding of the bladder, waste material remains for prolonged periods, greatly increasing the risk of urinary tract and bladder infections. (See Chapter 9 for a complete discussion of this condition.)

> ### Full Spectrum Nutrition
> Serenoa repens (saw palmetto) ......
> ....150 –500 mg per day
> Pygeum africanum (70:1) ....
> .... 100 – 200 mg per day

Glycine
L-Glutamic Acid
Alanine .... 200 – 300 mg per day
L-Lysine .... 200mg per day
Pumpkin Seed Powder ....
.... 100-200 mg per day
Stinging Nettle Leaf (Urtica dioica)
100 mg per day
Selenium .... 100 mcg per day
Zinc .... 25 mg per day extra
Essential Fatty Acids ....
.... 1000 mg per day

Note: It is important to rule out cadmium toxicity, which can produce the same prostate symptoms. A hair mineral analysis will reveal the presence of any heavy metals in soft tissues.

Beriberi

This is a nutrient deficiency disease caused by a gross deficiency of the B-complex vitamins, especially B1 (thiamin).

Full Spectrum Nutrition
High potency B-complex 50 mg ......
.... 1 twice daily
Vitamin C .... 2-4 grams daily

Bladder Infection (Cystitis)

A bacterial infection and inflammation of the organ responsible for holding urine until voiding. If left unchecked this condition can result in cystitis. Oftentimes, antibiotic therapy is necessary to arrest a long-term infection, however the following protocol can prevent reoccurrence.

Full Spectrum Nutrition
Cranberry Juice ....
.......12 ounces 4 or 5 times per day
Vitamin C .... 4 –5 grams per day
Multi-Acidophilus ....
.... 3 capsules three times per day
L-Cysteine ....
 500 mg twice per day until infection
subsides
Zinc Gluconate ....
.... 25 mg extra per day

Bleeding Gums

This condition is frequently the result of multiple nutrient deficiencies or the presence of bacterial gum disease. In either case, the following protocol has been instrumental in saving the teeth of many thousand of clients who have visited The Institute over the years.

Blood Lipid Elevations

While it is my position that elevated lipids play only a very small role in the progression of cardiovascular disease (see Chapter 5), I do not believe that elevated or imbalanced lipids are a healthy situation either. When we discuss lipids in the blood, we are referring to three basic things, cholesterol/ cholesterol ratio, triglycerides, and elevated lipoproteins. Elevated cholesterol is caused by the liver's inability to effectively regulate the body's production of cholesterol. Elevated triglyceride is a result of excess carbohydrate and refined sugar consumption.

Lecithin Granules ....
.... 2-3 tablespoons daily
Essential Fatty Acids ....
.... 1000 – 2000 mg per day
Vitamin C .... To Bowel Tolerance
Garlic .... 2 – 4 grams per day
Vitamin E ....
.... 200- 400 IU extra per day
Beta Carotene .... 25,000 IU per day

Consider adding more fiber to your diet – up to 10 grams per day.

High Triglycerides
Full Spectrum Nutrition

L-Carnitine .... 2 – 3 grams per day
Essential Oils from Fish (EPA/DHA)
.... 1 – 2 grams per day
Chromium ...... 400-800 mcg per day
Vanadium .... 500 mcg per day

Reduce consumption of refined carbohydrates and sugars and increase exercise level.

High Lipoprotein (a)
Full Spectrum Nutrition

N-Acetyl Cysteine ....
.... 2 –4 grams per day
Vitamin C .... 4-8 grams per day

Lipotropic Formula
(choline, inositol & methionine) ....
.... 1000 mg twice per day
Gamma Oryzanol ....
.... 500 – 1000 mg per day
Lysine .... 500 mg per day
Proline .... 500 – 1000 mg per day

Boils

Localized infections on the skin, which are usually filled with pus. Boils are a result of excessive toxicity in the system, especially the blood. This situation may be brought on by excessive consumption of junk foods, oxidized vegetable oils, food allergies, stress, poor hygiene, toxic bowels, or bloodstream. Emphasis must be ultimately placed upon removing the cause of the toxins and cleansing the blood and the organs of elimination.

Full Spectrum Nutrition
Chlorophyll . 1 tbsp. 3 times per day
Garlic extract ....
.... 2 capsules 3 times per day
Vitamin C .... To bowel tolerance

Detoxification Fast ....
.... See Chapter 13
Liquid Oxygen ....
.... 1 ounce twice per day

Bone Spur – See Heal Spur

Breast Cancer – See Cancer

Breast Cysts – See Benign Breast Cysts

Breastfeeding Difficulty

Frequently, a mother wishing to breastfeed a newborn may have problems either producing milk or producing an adequate supply of milk for baby's needs. These problems are often caused by stress or a protein deficiency.

> ### Full Spectrum Nutrition (1/2 dose)
> Protein Powder Drink ....
> ...... 50 grams protein twice per day
> Multi-Acidophilus ....
> .... 2 – 4 capsules per day
> Calcium .... 1500 mg per day
> Magnesium............. 500 mg per day

Bright's Disease – See Kidney & Bladder Problems

Broken Bones

The healing time for broken bones can be reduced considerably through the use of aggressive nutrition, especially from plant derived liquid bio-electrical trace minerals. These minerals accelerate the positive/negative knitting of bone tissue and reduce the healing time.

Full Spectrum Nutrition
Calcium .... 1200 mg per day
Magnesium .... 600 mg per day
Bio-electrical organic trace Minerals
1 ounce 3 or 4 times per day
Vitamin C .... 3 –5 grams per day

Bronchial Asthma – See Asthma

Bronchitis – See Asthma

Bruises

A condition where the small blood vessels under the skin rupture and fill the surrounding tissue with blood, bruises can be very painful and quite unattractive. While it is normal to bruise after a blow to the skin, when bruising occurs on only slight contact, it is usually a sign of bioflavonoid deficiency.

Full Spectrum Nutrition
Vitamin C .... 2 –4 grams per day
Citrus Bioflavonoids ....
.... 3 –6 grams per day
Alfalfa tablets ...5–10 tablets per day
Vitamin E .... 200 IU extra per day

Bruxism

The clinical name for tooth grinding. Bruxism is usually the result of un-managed stress, which manifests itself during sleep as the grinding of teeth. The best way to approach this matter is through managing the underlying stress. Elevating specific nutrients to reduce stress may also be helpful.

Full Spectrum Nutrition
Calcium .... 1500 mg per day
Magnesium .... 750 mg per day
Stress B-Complex formula ....
As per the label instructions
Vitamin C .... 3 grams per day
Zinc .... 25 mg per day

Bulimia – See Anorexia

Burns

The following protocol will help heal any degree of burn and reduce the scaring.

Full Spectrum Nutrition
Potassium ..... 100 mg twice per day
Protein Powder Drink ....
.... 25 – 50 mg extra protein per day
Vitamin C .... 2 – 4 grams per day
Vitamin E .... 400 IU extra

Vitamin E Cream...........................
..... Apply topically to healing wound
Liquid bio-electrical Trace Minerals..
..... Apply topically to healing wound
Bromelain Cream...........................
Apply topically after burn has healed
to prevent scaring

Bursitis

This painful condition is the result of an inflammation of the bursae, the small fluid sacs around joints, muscles, tendons, and bones. While the most common cause is over-straining and injury, this condition can also be caused by allergies or calcium deposits from an over-alkaline system.

Full Spectrum Nutrition
Calcium .... 1500 mg per day
Magnesium............. 750 mg per day
Multi-Enzyme ....
.... 2 –4 capsules per meal
Hydrochloric Acid (Betaine) 2-4 capsules per meal
Vitamin C .... 2 grams per day
Bioflavinoids .... 2 – 4 grams per day
Quercetin & N-Acetyl Cysteine ....
.... 400 mg per day

Anti-inflammatory herbs: Bilberry,

Cadmium Poisoning – See Heavy Metal Poisoning

Cancer

The treatment modalities for cancer are almost as extensive as the number of cases. There are certain specific treatments for specific types of cancer. Sadly, many of the most effective alternative treatments for cancer are not available in the United States. The following nutrient recommendations are divided into two groups, the prevention of cancer and the more aggressive program for those with existing cancer. Since cancer, of all types, is the result of a faulty immune response, it is imperative that stress in your life either be eliminated or effectively managed.

Full Spectrum Nutrition

Bio-electric Organic Trace Minerals
.... 2 oz extra per day
High B-Complex Stress formula......
.... Per the label instructions
Antioxidants: Coenzyme Q10, Lycopene Quercetin, Milk Thistle and
N-Acetyl Cysteine ....
.... 800 – 1200 mg per day

Essential Fatty Acids ....
.... 2000 mg per day
Folic Acid............. 1 – 3 mg per day
Zinc .... 25 mg per day
Mushroom Extract .. 300 mg per day

Existing Cancer: In addition to all of
the above add:

Shark Cartilage 750 mg capsules ...
.... 10 per day
Liquid Oxygen................................
.... 1 ounce 3 times per day
Increase Folic Acid ... 10 mg per day

Candidiasis

The candida albicans organism is a naturally occurring entity within our gastrointestinal tract and has
important function. It is kept in balance by the presence of acidophilus. When acidophilus is destroyed
by poor diet, antibiotics, birth control medications,
or disease, the candida albicans can explosively multiply. If left unchecked, it can become systemic, taking
up residence in various sites of the body, including the
brain. The most common site for systemic candidiasis
proliferation in males is in the lungs.

Full Spectrum Nutrition
Liquid Oxygen Flush ....
.... See Chapter 13

Multi-Acidophilus ....
..... 10 capsules per day for 10 days
After the above oxygen flush.
Multi – enzymes ....2-4 per meal
Betain Hydrochloride (Hcl) ....
.... 1 – 3 per meal
Essential Fatty Acids ....
............................500 mg per day

Canker Sores – See Apthous Stomatitis

Capillary Fragility

When the walls of the capillaries become thin due to nutrient deficiencies, they can rupture (see Bruises) and produce unattractive spider-like veins. This is primarily due to a citrus bioflavinoid deficiency.

Full Spectrum Nutrition
Vitamin C ....2-4 grams per day
Citrus Bioflavinoids ....
...........................2-4 grams per day
Vitamin E ....400 IU extra
Zinc ....25 mg extra

Capillary Hyperpermeability – See Edema

Cardiac Arrhythmia

Cardiac arrhythmias are electrical disturbances,

which cause the heart to beat out of natural rhythm. While there are potentially many causes, the most recent research shows that most all arrhythmias are linked to an imbalance of electrolytes, especially magnesium.

Full Spectrum Nutrition

Magnesium Chelate...................... 1000 mg per day
L-Carnitine .... 1000 mg per day
CoEnzyme Q10 .... 100 – 200 mg per day
Essential Fatty Acids .... 1000 mg per day
Garlic Extract .... 2 capsules 3 times per day
Taurine........ 1000 mg twice per day
Hawthorne Berry .... 250 – 500 mg per day
Vitamin B1 .... 100-200 mg extra per day
Liquid Bio-electrical Trace Minerals . 1 –2 ounces extra per day

Cardiomyopathy

A condition of the heart, which produces enlargement and ineffective cardiac performance. Cardiomyopathy may be caused by a variety of adjunct factors. Nutritionally, this condition has been linked back to a selenium deficiency. In fact, in China, Cardiomyopathy is treated very effectively with high doses of selenium. If you have Cardiomyopathy, which is accompanied by congestive heart failure, please see our further recommendations listed elsewhere under that heading.

Full Spectrum Nutrition
Selenium Chelate .... 1 – 10 mg per day
Vitamin E . 400-800 IU extra per day
Hawthorn Berry .... 300-500 mg per day
Vitamin B1 .... 100-200 mg per day
Magnesium.... 600-1000 mg per day

Cardiovascular Disease – See specific condition

Carpal Tunnel Syndrome

This debilitating condition is related to the process of arthritis and is likely caused by prolonged nutrient deficiencies and specific joint stress.

Full Spectrum Nutrition
Vitamin B6.............. 100 mg per day
Pantothenic Acid .... 500 mg per day
Calcium .... 1000 mg per day
Magnesium............. 500 mg per day
Zinc .... 25 mg per day

Glucosamine Sulfate ....
.... 500 mg per day
Chondroitin Sulfate ....
.... 500 mg per day
Essential Fatty Acids ....
.... 1000 mg per day

B-Complex Stress Formula .. As indicated on product label (take for three
months)

Cataracts

The lens of the eye, like all tissue, is made up of a variety of specialized proteins. The protein structure of the eye lens is unique in its transparency. As protein cells are broken down, they need to be replaced. This is accomplished by the breakdown of dietary protein into individual amino acids and reassembling them into the thousands of specific proteins needed by the body. Enzymes are essential for this process and the enzyme involved in the formation of lens protein is glutathione. We can raise the glutathione levels of the body by stimulating its production in the liver through the use of specific antioxidant nutrients.

Full Spectrum Nutrition
Vitamin C .... 2-3 grams per day
Zinc .... 30 mg per day

Liquid Oxygen ....
.... 1 ounce twice per day
Alpha Lipoic Acid ....
.... 100 –300 mg per day
Bilberry Extract ....
.... 250 – 500 mg per day
N- Acetyl Cysteine ....
.... 500 –1000 mg per day
Riboflavin .... 10-15 mg per day
Folic Acid .... 1 – 3 mg daily
Vitamin A (natural only) ....
.... 25,000 IU per day
Citrus Bioflavonoids ....
.... 1- 3 grams per day

Celiac Disease

This rare disorder is thought to be an autoimmune response to gluten in foods and can be very debilitating. Grains containing gluten such as wheat, barley, rye, and oats must be completely avoided. Symptoms of the condition such as abdominal swelling, irregular bowel movements, anemia, skin rash, and joint pain, become worse when these foods are eaten. Over time the intestinal lining can become damaged and nutrient absorption is compromised. Liquid nutritional products, therefore, are of utmost importance in this situation.

Full Spectrum Liquid Nutrition Protein Powder Supplement

From rice or soy ....
.... 25 – 35 grams per day
Extra B-Complex....... 50 mg per day
Vitamin K...
.... As directed on product label
Zinc .... 25 mg per day
Essential Fatty Acids ....
.... 2-4 grams per day
Vitamin C ....
.... 1 –2 grams extra per day

Cerebrovascular Disease – See Atherosclerosis and High Blood Pressure

Cervical Dysplasia

The term dysplasia indicates an abnormal cell development and in this case involves the lining of the uterus. This condition is considered to be one of pre-cancer and aggressive treatment is necessary to ensure that the condition does not progress.

Full Spectrum Nutrition

Folic Acid.......... 15 – 30 mg per day
Beta Carotene .... 50,000 IU per day
Vitamin A...
.... 25,000 – 100,000 IU per day

Vitamin C .... 1 – 3 grams
Selenium .... 200 – 400 mcg per day
Vitamin B12 .... 1 –5 mg per day
Gotu Kola (standardized) ....
.... 1-3 capsules per day
Grape Seed Extract ....
.... 200-300 mg per day

Chemical Allergies – See Allergies

Chemical Poisoning – Heavy Metal Poisoning

Chicken Pox

This disease, like many infectious conditions may be improved and recovery time reduced by stimulating the immune system. In addition to Full Spectrum nutrition, follow the protocol outlined under immunodepression

Chlamydia – See Immunodepression

Cholecystitis – See Gallbladder Disease

Choleithiasis – See Gallbladder Disease

Cholesterol Elevation

While elevated cholesterol is constantly implicated

in heart disease, the fact remains that cholesterol, at any level, has never caused one case of heart disease. This is not to say that elevated cholesterol does not complicate the situation once heart disease has advanced. Elevated cholesterol is a sign of poor liver function and when the liver is cleansed and properly nourished, cholesterol usually normalizes in a few months. (See Chapter 5 for cleansing program.)

Full Spectrum Nutrition
Extra Liquid Trace Minerals ....
.... 1 – 2 ounces per day
Vitamin C .... 3 grams per day
Lecithin Granules (not liquid) ....
.... 1 Tbl 3 times per day
Essential Fatty Acids ....
.... 1000 mg per day
Lipotropics
Choline
Inositol
Methionine ....
.... 1000 mg once or twice per day

Chronic Fatigue Syndrome/ Epstein Barr
These recently identified conditions are thought to be related to a low- grade chronic viral infection. This being the case, we should approach these conditions in much the same manner as with any invading pathogen and utilize immune stimulation while providing adjunct nutrients.

Full Spectrum Nutrition
Liquid Oxygen Flush ....
.... See Chapter 13
Multi-Acidophilus ....
.... 10 capsules per day on empty
stomach after the oxy flush
After the flush add:

Take a combination of the following 3
to 4 times per day

Colostrum Concentrate 100mg
Beta- 1,3 Glucan .... 25 mg
Mushroom Mycelial Biomass ....
.... 200 mg
Echinacea Purpurea leaf........ 25 mg
Astragalus extract .... 50 mg
Pau D'Arco Extract .... 50 mg
Antioxidant combination of Coen-
zyme Q10, N-Acetyl Cysteine, Quer-
cetin, and Grape Seed Extract ....
.... 400-800 mg per day

Cirrhosis of the Liver

The liver has an unbelievable ability to heal and
regenerate itself, but through constant and prolonged
abuse deterioration can become chronic and a diagnosis of cirrhosis is appropriate. This degenerative,
inflammatory disease results in the hardening of liver

cells, producing scar tissue, which eventually takes over the entire organ causing liver failure.

> ### *Full Spectrum Nutrition*
> Lipotropics (non-stimulating)
> Choline, Inositol & Methionine ....
> . 1000 mg combination 3 times/ day
> High Potency B-Complex Stress Formula .. As indicated on product label
> Garlic ....
> ....2 –4 capsules with each meal
> L Cysteine ....500 mg per day
> Lecithin Granules...........................
> .... 1 Tbl twice per day
> Heavy Hitting Antioxidants
> CoQ10, N-Acetyl Cysteine,
> Quercetin, Milk Thistle ....
> .... 400 mg 3 times per day

Cold – See Common Cold

Cold Sores – See Herpes

Colitis

An acute inflammation and irritation of the colon, which may become chronic if left unchecked. Colitis can strike at almost any age. There are many types of colitis, some cases mild and others quite debilitating. Causes of this condition range from allergies to foods, bad eating habits, excess stress, and intestinal bacteria imbalance. Once all food allergies have been eliminated consider the following:

Full Spectrum Nutrition

Increase Fiber ....
.... 8 – 10 grams per day
Multi-Acidophilus ....
.... 10 capsules daily
Liquid Oxygen..... 1 oz twice per day
Liquid Aloe Vera Concentrate ....
.... 2 oz 3 times per day
Multi-Enzymes with Hcl.................
.... 2 –4 with each meal

Common Cold

In spite of miraculous advances in conquering bacterial infections, the virus that causes the common cold has managed to escape the vast wisdom of medical science. An occasional cold is not only normal, but is actually beneficial to the immune system. However, colds should be very infrequent and should never last more than 72 hours. If you get more than one cold per year and it lasts and lasts, it's a sign that your immune system is weakened and unable to respond quickly with antibody production.

Full Spectrum Nutrition

Take a combination of the following nutrients

Every two hours for two days...

Colostrum Concentrate ...... 100 mg

Beta-1,3-D Glucan .... 25 mg

Mushroom Mycelial Biomass ....
.... 200 mg

Echinacea Purpurea leaf .... 25 mg

Astragalus Extract .... 50 mg

Pau D'Arco Extract .... 50 mg

Vitamin C ....
.... 1,000 mg every two hours

Vitamin A (natural only) ....
.... 25,000 IU per day

Zinc Lozenges ....
.... 1 every 4 hours

Congestive Heart Failure

A symptom, more than a condition of its own, congestive heart failure occurs most often after prolonged periods of high blood pressure , which results in heart damage. As the heart struggles to meet bodily demands, it often becomes enlarged and cannot function fully. This results in a buildup of water in the lungs and the lower extremities of the body. The treatment of this condition should begin with finding the cause and correcting it. The following nutrients will help strengthen the heartbeat.

Constipation

Constipation is a condition of sluggish bowels brought about by waste material exiting too slowly. As a result of constipation, the sufferer can develop gas, insomnia, bad breath, varicose veins, indigestion, diverticulitis, bowel cance, and hemorrhoids. The most common cause of constipation is a lack of adequate fiber and fluids in the diet. Some medications can also cause constipation. It is important that the bowels move at least once per day to avoid reabsorbing potentially toxic substances from the feces.

Take a combination of the following herbs twice a day:

Cascara Extract	2 mg
Rhubarb Root	10 mg
Bukthorn Berry	10 mg
Elderberry	10 mg
Licorice Root Extract	50 mg
Garlic	50 mg
Quassia Bark	50 mg
Red Sage Root	50 mg
Increase Fiber	10 grams per day
Increase Water	8 – 10 glasses per day
Multi Acidophilus	5 capsules per day
Multi Enzymes	2 – 4 with each meal

Copper Toxicity – See Heavy Metal Poisoning

Crohn's Disease

An autoimmune condition, Crohn's disease can be very dangerous if not properly controlled. Attention to diet and dietary restrictions are a must. Eliminate all possibility of allergies by testing and avoiding all offending foods. Crohn's disease often strikes at a fairly young age, usually in the 20's. Since this disease causes malnutrition and absorption difficulties, liquid nutritional supplements are essential.

Full Spectrum Nutrition

Fiber .... 10 grams per day
Multi-Acidophilus ....
.... 8-10 capsules per day
Aloe Vera Juice ....
.... 6 ounces 3 times per day
Folic Acid.............. 2 – 5 mg per day
Vitamin B12 (sublingual) ....
.... 500 mcg 4 times per day
Calcium .... 1000 mg extra
Magnesium .... 500 mg extra
Zinc Gluconate .... 50 mg per day

Cystic Fibrosis

This hereditary disease involves both the endocrine and exocrine glandular systems and is characterized by repeated lung infections and poor nutrient
absorption. Again, for this condition, liquid nutritional
formulas are an absolute must.

Full Spectrum Nutrition

Multi-Enzyme Formula....................
.... 2- 4 capsules with each meal
Whole Food Enzymes ....
.... 2 – 4 capsules with each meal
B-Complex Stress Formula............
.... As indicated on label
Vitamin C .... 3-6 grams per day
Vitamin K.............. 4 tablets per day

Zinc Gluconate ....50 mg per day
Protein Powder Drink
from rice or soy ... 25 grams per day

Cystitis

A severe, often chronic infection of the bladder, cystitis must be handled aggressively.

Full Spectrum Nutrition
Vitamin C .... To bowel tolerance
Cranberry Juice ....
.... 8 ox 3-6 times per day
Liquid Oxygen................................
.... 1 ounce 3 times per day
Multi-Acidophilus ....
.... 4 capsules twice per day
Bromelain .. 200 mg 3 times per day

Follow immune protocol under Immunodepression heading.

Dandruff

Dandruff, those embarrassing white flakes of skin that appear in the hair and on your clothes, is a product of dysfunctional sebaceous glands in the scalp, which have probably been damaged through free radical activity.

Full Spectrum Nutrition

Kelp Tablets .... 5 – 10 per day
Essential Fatty Acids ....
.... 2 grams per day
Vitamin E .... 400 IU extra
Zinc Gluconate .... 25 mg per day
Vitamin A (natural only) ....
.... 25,000 IU per day

DDT Poisoning – See Heavy Metal Poisoning

Dementia (Senility)

Age often brings with it many symptoms due to the deterioration of bodily function. As the brain ages, deterioration can take place as well. While one of the best proven remedies for dementia is 'exercising' your brain in a challenging manner. The following nutrients have been shown to increase cognition and improve short-term memory.

Full Spectrum Nutrition

Folic Acid...
.... 5 – 10 mg daily for 1 week
Niacin .... 100 mg 3 times/ day for 1 week

Vitamin B12 (sublingual) ....
.... 1000 mcg per day for 1 week

Follow-up after 1 week with:
Folic Acid .... 1 mg per day
Thiamin ...... 100 mg 3 times per day
Vitamin B12 .... 500 mcg per day
Zinc .... 50 mg per day
Phosphatidyl Choline ....
.... 500 - 1000 mg per day
Phosphatidyl Serine ....
.... 500 mg per day
5–Hydroxy-tryptophan (5-HTP) ....
.... 25 mg per day

Depression

Symptoms of depression include fatigue, insomnia, or frequent sleeping, moodiness, dark negative thoughts, loss of appetite, headaches, colon disorders, and feelings of worthlessness and despair. Depression, especially if serious, should NEVER be self-treated. You need to be under the supervision of a qualified orthomolecular psychiatrist. Depression can be caused by many things and can range from minor to devastating. Nutrients involved in the stress response as well as those affecting brain chemistry are listed below.

Full Spectrum Nutrition

Stress B-Complex .... double the label dosage

Vitamin B12 (sublingual) .... 500 mcg 3 –4 times per day

Magnesium.... 600 mg per day extra

Vitamin B1 .... 100 – 200 mg per day

Vitamin B6 ...... 50 – 100 mg per day

Iron .... 50 mg per day for 1 week

Betaine Hydrochloride .... 300 mg with each meal

5-Hydroxy-Tryptophan (5-HTP) .... 500 mg per day

St. John's Wort .... 100 – 200 mg per day

Acetyl L-Carnitine .... 500 – 1000 mg per day

Phosphatidylserine .... 300 – 600 mg per day

Phenylalanine* .... 1000 mg at bed time

*Note: do not take if you suffer from uncontrolled high blood pressure.

Dermatitis

An allergic reaction of the skin, which manifests as scaling, flaking, and itching. Dermatitis is caused by the skin's exposure to an offending substance such as poison ivy and other plants, certain creams, ointments, rubber, metals, and cosmetics. Avoidance of the offending substance is essential or the condition will worsen and spread.

Full Spectrum Nutrition
High Potency B-Complex...............
.... As indicated on product label
Kelp.............. 5 – 10 tablets per day
Essential Fatty Acids ....
.... 1000 mg per day
Zinc Gluconate ....
.... 100 mg per day for 1 week

Diabetes Mellitus (Type-II diabetes)

The fastest growing epidemic in industrialized nations, adult-onset diabetes accounts for 90 percent of all diabetes worldwide and is the product of over-consumption of refined carbohydrates and sugars. (See Chapter 6 for a complete discussion of this disease.)

Full Spectrum Nutrition (Encapsulated version)
Take the following nutrients with each meal:
Aspartic Acid .... 500 mg
Chromium........................ 200 mcg
Vanadium .... 300 mcg
Bilberry Extract .... 20 mg

Bitter Melon .... 200 mg
Alpha Lipoic Acid .... 50 mg

Consider also taking a high potency antioxidant formula to prevent damage from free radicals generated by this disease.

Diarrhea

This condition can have many causes ranging from nothing more than the rapid elimination of a toxic substance to the result of a chronic chemical imbalance in the digestive system. Loss of fluids can lead to dehydration so extra care must be given to adequate fluid replacement. If the condition persists, even after following the steps below, or if there is blood in the stool, see a qualified medical doctor immediately.

Full Spectrum Nutrition
Fasting ....
.... Eat nothing for 24 – 48 hours
Fluids ....
.............8-10 glasses of water daily

Multi-Acidophilus ....
.... 10 capsules daily
Folic Acid.................... 1 mg per day
Essential Fatty Acids ....
.... 1000 mg per day

Multi-Enzymes with Hydrochloric acid
.... 2 –6 per meal
Herbs such as Carob Pod Powder
and Citrus Seed Extract are also helpful.

Diverticulitis – See Colitis

Drug Addiction (Substance Abuse)

This is a growing problem worldwide. While the single greatest factor is abusive behavior is society, it is believed to be, in part, a gross deficiency of the B-Complex nutrients. The following nutrient program can help reduce the cravings and speed along recovery.

Full Spectrum Nutrition
High potency B-Complex ....
.... 2 –3 times the label dosage
B12 Injections............... 1cc per day
Calcium .... 1500 mg per day
Magnesium............ 750 mg per day
Antioxidant Compound with
Coenzyme Q10, Milk Thistle,
Quercetin, N-Acetyl Cysteine,
Bilberry Extract and Grape Seed.....
.... 400 mg 2 –3 times per day
If diet is poor...
High protein Liquid Meals ....
.... 50 grams protein per day

GABA (gamma-amino butyric acid) .
.... As directed on product label
L-Phenylalanine* ....
.... 1000 mg in the morning
*Note: do not use this if you have
uncontrolled high blood pressure.

Dumping Syndrome – See Inflamatory Bowel Disease

Dysmenorrehea

An all too common condition, dysmenorrehea is the cause of more sick days among menstrual-age women than any other single factor. It is signified by excessive pain during menstruation. While the exact cause in unknown, increased prostaglandins are thought to be part of the principle mechanism.

Full Spectrum Nutrition
Bilberry Extract .... 200 mg per day
Dong Quai ....
.... 100 mg 3 times per day
Papain ....
..........2 –3 capsules with each meal
Bromelain ....
.... 1-2 capsules with each meal
Feverfew ....
.... As indicated on product label

Dyspepsia – See Indigestion

Ear Infection/Ache

The most common cause for a doctor visit, ear infections send more children to the doctor than any other cause. Most ear infections will pass in a few days providing that the child's immune system is functioning properly. If not, then attention to the immune system must be primary.

> ### Full Spectrum Nutrition
> Liquid Oxygen.................................
> 1 ounce twice daily – depending upon age
> Vitamin C ....To bowel tolerance
> Vitamin A......................................
> 5,000 to 25,000 IU – depending upon age
> Consider the protocol under Immunodepression if there are repeated infections.

Ecchymoses – See Vasculitis

Eczema (Atopic Dermatitis)

This skin condition may be closely related to a fatty acid deficiency and/or specific food and airborne allergies. If control is difficult, it is essential to rule out all allergies.

> ### *Full Spectrum Nutrition*
> Vitamin C .... 3-5 grams
> Zinc .... 100 mg for two weeks
> Copper .... 2 mg for two weeks
> Essential Fatty Acids ..... 2 –3 grams
> Vitamin A (from fish liver oil) ....
> .... 25,000 – 100,000 IU
>
> If food allergies are present add:
>   Betaine Hydrochloride ....
> .... 100-400 mg per meal

Edema

This is a general term used for the accumulation of fluid in the body. Also called dropsy, edema may be caused by many underlying conditions. The best treatment for this problem is to address the causes behind it. The fluid is most often retained in the feet and ankles. Ongoing edema may be a sign of kidney, bladder, heart, or liver problems. Another major reason for edema is hypersensitivity to certain foods, especially intolerance to carbohydrates. If all other reasons are eliminated without finding the cause consider an allergy test and/or reduce the amount of carbohydrates in the body. A high protein diet, together with fresh fruits and vegetables, is very helpful. Exercise is also an important part of overall management.

Full Spectrum Nutrition
Protein...................... 80-100 grams
Vitamin B6... 50 mg 3 times per day
L- Carnitine.....................................
.... 500 mg 2 times per day
L- Taurine... 500 mg 2 times per day
Calcium/ Magnesium/ Potassium ...
..... (Lost during diuresis) As needed

Emesis (See Motion Sickness)

Emphysema

An overall deterioration of the lungs and their ability to intake oxygen and exhale carbon dioxide, emphysema is primarily caused by cigarette smoking. Other causes can include related lung disorders, repeated lung infections, and even long-term protein deficiency.

Full Spectrum Nutrition
Multi-purpose Enzyme ....
.... 2-4 with each meal
Coenzyme Q10 ....
.......................50 mg twice per day
Germanium............ 200 mg per day
L-Cysteine/ L Methionine ....
.... 500 –1000 mg twice per day

Protein........ 80 –100 grams per day
Vitamin A (from fish liver oil) ....
.... 25,000-50,000 IU per day
Vitamin C .... 5-10 grams per day
Liquid Oxygen................................
..................1 ounce 3 times per day
on an empty stomach

Endometriosis

This is a disorder results in the growth of cells normally lining the uterus to also grow elsewhere. This condition produces many symptoms and complications including severe pain in the uterus, lower back, and pelvic region. Excessive bleeding together with large clots and shreds of tissue are also common symptoms. Nausea, vomiting, and constipation are common during the menses, and these individuals are frequently infertile. There are many theories, but few facts, as to the actual cause of this condition. Research, being conducted at several centers around the world, is 'shedding new light' on the cause of this condition.

Full Spectrum Nutrition
Vitamin E ...... 800 –1200 IU per day
Chelated Iron .... 12-24 mg per day
Essential Fatty Acids ....
.... 2-4 grams per day
Anti-Stress Nutrient Formula ....
.... As directed

Calcium (citrate/malate) ... 1500 mg
Magnesium .... 1000 mg
Potassium .... 100 – 400 mg per day
Lipotropics:
Choline/Inostitol/Methionine
.... 1000 mg twice per day
Vitamin B6 ....
.. 100 – 200 mg per day for 6 weeks

Environmental Toxicity

There are tens of thousands of foreign chemicals present in our immediate environment. They are in the water, food, air, and virtually everything found in our home and work environments. Detoxification of these chemical residues from the body is essential. (See chapter on cleansing.) Antioxidants are essential to prevent the massive free radical formation, which occurs when these toxins enter the internal environment of the body.

Full Spectrum Nutrition
Coenzyme Q10 .... 30 –50 mg
Milk Thistle .... 100-200 mg
N-Acetyl Cysteine .... 200-400 mg
Garlic .... 2-4 capsules per meal
Vitamin A (from fish liver oil) ....
.........................50,000-100,000 IU
Vitamin E .... 400-800 IU

Liquid Oxygen ....
1 ounce two or three times per day
on empty stomach

Epilepsy

Caused by mild to massive electrical disturbances in the nerve impulses of the brain, epilepsy can result in seizures ranging from petit mal (mild) to grand mal (severe and extremely debilitating). While epilepsy is thought to be hereditary, it can also be suddenly induced by an infection, meningitis, malnutrition, hypoglycemia, head injuries, fever, or severe allergies. For this reason a diagnosis as to the type of epilepsy and probable cause is essential in building a specific support program

Full Spectrum Nutrition
Low Carbohydrate (Ketogenic) Diet
Niacin ....
.1-3 grams per day (work up slowly)
Vitamin B 6 .... 100 mg per day
Copper chelate .... 2 mg per day
Magnesium ....
.... 1000 mg on empty stomach
Note: if magnesium causes diarrhea, take either apple cider vinegar or Betaine hydrochloride with it.
Vitamin B 12 ....
200 mcg sublingual 3 times per day

L-Taurine... 500 mg 3 times per day
L- Tyrosine ....
.... 500 mg 3 times per day
High Potency B-Complex...... 50 mg
combination, 3 times per day

Epstein Barr Virus – See Chronic Fatigue Syndrome

Esophagitis – See Heartburn & Digestive Disorders

Flatulence

Lower intestinal gas is formed when fermented carbohydrates enter the small and large intestines, forming methane gases. This condition can also occur when there is a lack of natural bacterial in the colon.

Full Spectrum Nutrition
Multi-purpose Enzyme ....
.... 2-4 capsules per meal
Betaine Hyrochloride ....
.... 100-200 mg per meal
Acidophilus ....
..... 5-10 capsules per day on empty stomach

Fatigue – See also Chronic Fatigue Syndrome

The biggest cause of fatigue is either a lack of adequate sleep or a diet high in fat and carbohydrates and low in protein. Drug abuse, including alcohol, caffeine, and tobacco, can steal precious energy and cause us to sleep less soundly at night. If the fatigue is severe, a medical examination is in order to expose the underlying cause, which may be another disease or the presence of a virus or bacterial infection. General lack of energy may be remedied with the following program.

Full Spectrum Nutrition
Extra Liquid Organic Source Minerals .... 1-2 ounces per day
High potency B-Complex ....50 mg twice per day
Protein....... 80 – 100 grams per day
Iron .... as needed
Zinc .... 50 mg per day
Folic Acid.............. 400 mcg per day
Ginseng............ per label indication
Vitamin B12 injections .... per your physician

Fatty Liver

Like most problems with the liver, the lipotropic

nutrients work the best in restoring function and fixing the problem.

> ### *Full Spectrum Nutrition*
> Lipotropics
> Choline
> Inositol
> Methionine ....
> .... 1000 mg 2 times per day
> Lecithin Granules.............................
> .... 1-2 tablespoons per day
> Multi Antioxidants ....
> .... 400-800 mg per day

Fever

Fever is always caused by the presence of some pathogen, usually viral or bacterial. Fever, to a point, is beneficial and should be allowed to run its course providing it doesn't go too high. Fever is one of the body's best weapons against infection. Support by boosting the immune response is very helpful.

> ### *Full Spectrum Nutrition as soon as the crisis period is over.*
> Colostrum extract............................
> ..... 200-500mg 4 to 6 times per day
> Mushroom extract mix ....
> .... 100-200 mg 4 to 6 times per day
> Astragallis....... 50 – 100 mg per day

Echinacea .... 100-300 mg per day
1-beta D Glucan ....
.... 50 –200 mg per day

Fibrocystic Disease of the Breast – See Fatty Liver

Fibroid Tumor – See Fatty Liver

Fibromyalgia

This condition is relatively new, yet is appearing in epidemic numbers. There are many theories behind the cause of this, including a virus, although that has never been proven. My work with persons suffering from this condition has shown me that they are all very toxic. When their systems have been properly detoxified their symptoms all but disappear. My personal feeling is that this is a condition of hyper-toxicity and it manifests in persons who are unable to physically cope with the overload of toxins in the system.

Full Spectrum Nutrition
Detoxifying Herbal Combinations....
.... per label instructions
Liquid Oxygen.................................
.... 1 ounce 3 times per day
Glucosamine Sulfate ....
.... 400 mg per day

Chondroitin Sulfate ....
.... 400 mg per day
Vitamin B-6 .... 25 mg per day
Vitamin C .... Bowel Tolerance
5-hydroxy Tryptophan (5-HTP) ....
.... 100 mg 3 times per day
Kava Kava ...... per label instructions

Fibrositis – See Rheumatism

Flu – (Immunodepression)

Food and Chemical Sensitivities – See Allergies

Fractures

A fracture is a break in the bone and may be simple or compound. Once the acute situation has been handled by medical personnel, the following protocol will help accelerate healing.

Full Spectrum Nutrition
Liquid Organic-Source Trace Minerals .... 2-4 oz per day
Liquid Oxygen ....
.... 1 ounce 2 times per day
On an empty stomach
Calcium ..... 1000 –2000 mg per day
Magnesium .... 1000 mg per day

Fungus

Fungus can take many forms both externally, such as under nails, or internally, such as yeast infections or candidiasis. Common sites for yeast infections are the mouth, skin, vagina, nails, or between the toes. While there are many causes of yeast and fungus infections, a depressed immune system, usually through stress, is the main cause. While using topical preparations, the following will help to kill the parasite off from the inside, while boosting the immune system.

Full Spectrum Nutrition

Liquid Oxygen.................................
...... 1 oz 3 times per day for 1 week
2 oz 3 times per day for 4 – 6 weeks
Multi-Acidophilus ....
..... 10 capsules per day for 10 days
on an empty stomach
Colostrum ....
.... 200 –400 mg 3 times per day
Mushroom Extract ....
.... 100-400 mg 3 times per day
Echinacea Extract .... per label
Antiseptic Hydrogen Peroxide.........
.... topically to infected area

Gallbladder Disease/Disorder

Located directly under the liver, the gallbladder serves as a storage site for bile, needed in the digestion of fat. A congested gallbladder can inflame and even infect. This can be a serious condition and should be addressed medically as soon as possible. Another condition of the gallbladder occurs when stones of calcium form in the organ and block the flow of bile. (See Gallstones.) The following nutrients have been shown to assist the gallbladder in both maintenance and function.

Full Spectrum Nutrition
Vitamin C .... 2-4 grams per day
Vitamin E .... 400 IU
Choline .... 500 mg
Essential Fatty Acids ....
.... 2-3 grams per day
Multi Digestive Enzyme ....
.... 2-4 with each meal
Ox Bile .... 50-100 mg per meal
Curcumin .... per label
Milk Thistle .... 100 mg per day

Gallstones

Stones, made up of calcium and other minerals, can form in various sites around the body such as the kidneys, bladder, and the gallbladder. This usually occurs when the overall pH of the body is alkaline too much of the time. Emphasis must therefore be placed upon increasing minerals while adjusting the pH of the body towards greater acidity at the same time.

Full Spectrum Nutrition

Calcium .... 1000-1500 mg per day
Magnesium .... 750-1000 mg per day
Boron .... 2 mg per day
Liquid Organic Trace Minerals ....
.... 1 oz 2 times per day
Betaine Hydrochloride ....
.... 100-400 mg per meal
Apple Cider Vinegar ....
2 tabl 2 or 3 times per day mixed with water
Lecithin Granules .... 2 tabl per day
Dietary Fiber ... 10-15 grams per day
Taurine .... 500 mg 2 times per day

Gingivitis

An advanced disease condition of the gums, gingivitis involves bone loss through infection caused by the buildup of oral plaque. While nothing replaces regular cleaning and maintenance by your dentist, the following will help control the problem.

> ## Full Spectrum Nutrition
> Calcium/ Magnesium........ 2000 mg
> Vitamin C .... to Bowel Tolerance
> Vitamin A (from fish liver oil) ....
> .... 25,000 –50,000 IU per day
> Mouthwash & Toothpaste containing
> hydrogen peroxide
> Licorice Root .... per label
> Bloodroot .... per label

Glaucoma

There are approximately eight million diagnosed cases of glaucoma and it is the second leading cause of blindness worldwide. The condition usually affects people over the age of forty or fifty and is more common in women than in men. This condition results from an increase in the pressure of the fluids within the eyeball. While the condition can have many causes including heredity, the most common causes are nutritional deficiencies and excess stress.

> ## Full Spectrum Nutrition
> Choline .... 1000 mg per day
> Stress B-Complex .... per label
> Vitamin C .... 2000-8000 mg per day
> Rutin........... 50 mg 3 times per day
> Vitamin A (from fish liver oil) ....
> .... 25,000 IU per day
> Beta Carotene .... 10,000 IU per day

Gout

This genetic condition occurs primarily in males and is the result of excess uric acid forming in the blood. The uric acid forms crystals and settles in the joints of the body, most often the feet, creating extremely intense pain and inflammation. Since uric acid is the by-product of certain foods these must be limited at all times and complete eliminated during an outbreak. Further, increasing urine output is also helpful in excreting the excess uric acid.

Avoid purine foods including anchovies, asparagus, herring, meat gravies, mushrooms, mussels, organ meats, sardines, cauliflower, lentils, peas, and spinach. Reduce your overall intake of alcohol and never consume alcohol with purine foods as this greatly increases the production of uric acid.

Full Spectrum Nutrition

Vitamin C .... To Bowel Tolerance
High Potency B-Complex................
.... 50 mg 2 times per day
Pantothenic Acid .. 1000 mg per day
Vitamin E .... 400 IU per day
Multi-Purpose Enzyme ....
...................................2-4 per meal

Folic Acid .... 5-10 mg per day
L-Cysteine .... 1 –2 grams per day
Essential Fatty Acids ....
.... 3-5 grams per day

Avoid taking more than 10,000 IU of vitamin A during an attack and increase the consumption of water as much as possible.

Gum Disease – See Periodontal Disease & Gingivitis

Hair Loss

There are almost as many reasons for hair loss as there are people experiencing the problem. Nutrient deficiencies, stress, and hormone imbalances lead the list. Factors that also affect hair loss include acute illness, surgery, radiation, skin diseases, crash diets, diabetes, thyroid disorders, and many pharmaceuticals. In treating severe hair loss, it is important to uncover the exact underlying cause. The following program will help to meet nutritional needs and eliminate obvious hair loss related deficiencies.

Full Spectrum Nutrition
Liquid Organic –Source Trace Minerals .... 1oz 2 times per day
Biotin .... per label

Essential Fatty Acids ....
.... 2-4 grams per day
High B-Complex ....
.... 50 mg 2 times per day
MSM (organic sulfur) ....
.... 100 mg 2 –3 times per day
Horsetail ... 2 tablets 2 times per day

Hay Fever – See also Allergies

Hay fever or allergic rhinitis, is an allergic response, usually to airborne offenders such as dust, pollen, grasses and flowering plants. It affects the mucous membranes of the nose, eyes, and throat. While treating the underlying allergy is essential the following nutrients will prevent infection by protecting the mucosal lining of the sinuses and throat.

Full Spectrum Nutrition
Vitamin A (from fish liver oil) ....
.... 25,000 – 100,000+ IU per day
Coenzyme Q10 ....
.... 30 mg 2 –3 times per day
Vitamin C .... to Bowel Tolerance
Liquid Oxygen ....
.... 1 oz 2 –3 times per day
Vitamin E .... 400 – 800 IU per day

Headache

Headaches may be caused by dozens of situations and conditions from benign to acutely serious. If you have repeated headaches, I would recommend that you find out the cause behind the condition as this would make management much easier. If you suffer from the occasional headache, it is most often due to stress or allergies. Typical offending foods and food substances that produce headaches include wheat, chocolate, MSG (monosodium glutamate), sulfites, sugar, processed meats, cold cuts, cheeses, sour cream, yogurt, alcohol, vinegar, or other marinated foods. Many airborne allergies can contribute to headache by inflaming the sinuses and related tissues. If you have poor vertebral alignment, headaches can be a regular occurrence and you need to see a chiropractor. Stress still remains the number one cause of headaches and efforts to manage and channel stress effectively are essential.

Full Spectrum Nutrition

Calcium .... 1500 mg per day
Magnesium .... 1000 mg per day
Acidophilus bacteria ...... 1 tsp. daily
Stress B-Complex ....
.........2 –4 capsules 2 times per day
Vitamin C .... 1-3 grams
Essential Fatty Acids ...... 1-2 grams

Gingko biloba extract ....
.... 250-400 mg per day
Cayanne Pepper .... as per label
Ginger .... as per label
Lithium (organic) .... 20 mcg
Feverfew .... as per label
Lavender .... as per label

Hearing Impairment

While there are many causes for a loss of hearing, the following nutrients have proven to be very helpful in both restoring hearing and preventing further loss.

Full Spectrum Nutrition

Ginger .... per label
Gingko Biloba .... 100-300 mg
Vitamin A (fish liver oil) ....
.... 10,000 – 25,000 IU
Calcium .... 1000 mg
Fluoride .... 10-50 mg
Zinc sulfate.................. 100-300 mg
Coenzyme Q10 ....
.... 30 mg 3 times per day
Essential Fatty Acids ....
.... 1-2 grams per day

Rule out aluminum, lead and food poisoning.

Heartburn

This is one of the most misunderstood conditions of modern times. We are repeatedly told that heartburn is the result of excess stomach acid, when in fact, the exact opposite is most often the case. The stomach is a naturally acidic organ. Hydrochloric acid is produced in the stomach in the presence of protein foods. In truth, it is alkalinity that burns the stomach, not acidity. Heartburn is most often the result of too little stomach acid, causing food to ferment and form gases, resulting in further alkaline conditions.

Full Spectrum Nutrition
Multi-purpose enzymes .... 2-4 with each meal
Betaine Hydrochloride .... 100-400 mg with each meal
Licorice Root .... 1-2 capsules per meal

Heart Disease

The majority of all heart disease is caused by a condition known as atherosclerosis (see Chapter 5). The following nutrients will help strengthen the heart muscle while assisting to regulate the heartbeat. Additionally, there are nutrients that assist the body in removing the fat and calcium buildup within the arteries.

```
Oral Chelation Formula ...................
.............................. as per label
Folic Acid ........................... 2-5 mg
Niacin ... 1000 mg 2-3 times per day
work up slowly
Essential Fatty Acids .....................
.......................... 2-3 grams per day
Vitamin B-6 ......... 25-50 mg per day
Pantethine 300 mg 2-4 times per day
Vitamin E ......... 400-800 IU per day
L-Carnitine ......................................
............. 1000 mg 2-3 times per day
Coenzyme Q10 ..............................
................ 30 mg 2-3 times per day
```

Heavy Metal Poisoning

When base elements of potentially toxic nature enter the body they can build up within the soft tissues because our chemistry does not recognize them as readily as if they were present in naturally occurring organic compounds. In fact, many of the so-called 'toxic minerals' are actually of benefit to the body, but they must be ingested in the form of organic compounds and not simply base heavy metals. Regardless of the offending element, be it lead, cadmium, mercury, arsenic, or aluminum, when you ingest organic trace mineral compounds they effectively chelate, or remove these heavy metal counterparts, from your body. This process can take anywhere from three to six months.

> ### *Full Spectrum Nutrition*
> Liquid Organic-Source Trace Minerals .... 2-4 oz per day (Continue to take until diarrhea develops, then back off slowly)
>
> Liquid Oxygen .... 1 oz 2 times per day

Heel or Bone Spurs

A bone spur occurs in the same manner an organ stone, such as a kidney or gallstone, does. When calcium and magnesium are deficient in the body, these minerals are leached from the bone. This bone calcium is very alkaline and easily forms heel or bone spurs when the chemistry of the body is also over alkaline. This alkalinity can occur from eating a diet of dead, lifeless foods for years or it may be rapidly induced through gross calcium deficiency or conditions that product alkalosis. It is very common for people with arthritis to have these conditions as well, since the cause of both disorders is essentially the same.

> ### *Full Spectrum Nutrition*
> Liquid Organic-Source Minerals .... 1-2 oz extra

Calcium .... 1500 mg
Magnesium......................... 750 mg
Multi purpose enzymes..................
.... 2-4 with each meal
Betaine Hydrochloride ....
.... 100-300 mg per meal

Hemophilia

Hemophilia is an obscure blood disorder found only in males. The disease prevents blood from clotting, and the individual is in constant threat of bleeding to death, even from a small cut. Internal bleeding is the biggest threat. There is no known cure for hemophilia. The following nutrient program will assist in managing this difficult condition.

Full Spectrum Nutrition
Calcium .... 1500 mg
Magnesium...................... 1000 mg
Raw Liver Nucleoprotein ....
.... 5-10 tablets per day
Extra B-Complex....... 50 mg per day
Vitamin C .... 3 grams per day
Vitamin K............. 300 mcg per day

Hemorrhoids

Characterized by swollen tissues around the anus, which may protrude out of the rectum, hemorrhoids can be both annoying and uncomfortable.

Full Spectrum Nutrition

Calcium malate/citrate ...... 1000 mg
Magnesium .... 750 mg
Vitamin C .... 3 grams per day
Bioflavonoids .... 2 grams per day
Vitamin E .... 400 IU
Coenzyme Q10 ...... 100 mg per day
Increase natural fiber ....
........,.................... 4-8 grams per day
Colon Cleanse Product ....
.... as per label
Vitamin A (fish liver oil) ....
.... 25,000 IU per day

Soaking in a bath of warm water and Witch Hazel may be helpful.

Hepatitis

There are several types of hepatitis. The most common form is Type A, which is spread through person to person contact. Type B is transmitted via serum or blood through contaminated syringes, needles, insects, and blood transfusions. Another strain, hepatitis C, is often the most dangerous as it frequently becomes chronic and destroys the quality of life for the sufferer.

Full Spectrum Nutrition

High potency Stress B-Complex .....
.... as per label
Milk Thistle (Silymarin) ....
.... 100-500 mg
N-Acetyl Cysteine .... 100-500 mg
Licorice Rood .... as per label
Folic Acid................... 2 mg per day
Coenzyme Q10 ....
.... 30 mg 3 times per day
Lipotropics
Choline
Inositol
Methionine ....
.... 1000 mg 3 times per day
Multi-enzyme formula ....
.... 2-4 with each meal
Betaine Hydrochloride ....
.... 100-300 mg per meal
Vitamin C .... 3-5 grams per day
High Protein Diet ....
.... 80 –100 grams per day

Herpes

There are two basic strains of the herpes virus. Type I (herpes simplex) and is most often acquired during birth from the mother. Type II is genital herpes and is most often transmitted sexually from one person to another. Like most viruses, once herpes enters the body, it never leaves. It can become dormant but will usually surface again during periods of stress or immune suppression.

Full Spectrum Nutrition

L-Lysine ....
1000-3000 mg per day during an outbreak
Vitamin A (fish liver oil) ....
.... 25,000 IU per day
Vitamin C .... to bowel tolerance
Zinc Gluconate ....
  50-100 mg daily during an outbreak
Essential Fatty Acids ....
.... 1-3 grams extra
Multi Acidophilus ....
.... 5-8 capsules per day
Vitamin E oil...................... topically

Herpes Zoster

Also known as shingles, this often painful disorder is caused by the same virus that causes chicken pox and it affects the endings of the nerve lines in the skin. Like most viruses, risk of an outbreak of shingles is greatest when you are under severe stress or have an immune compromise.

Full Spectrum Nutrition

L-Lysine .... 2-4 grams per day
Bilberry extract ....
......................200-400 mg per day
Vitamin C ....
.... 2-4 grams extra per day
Adensoine Monophsphate ....
.... as per label
Vitamin B12 ....
.... 100 mg 3 times per day
Cayenne Pepper .... as per label

High Blood Pressure

A very common occurrence, high blood pressure or hypertension is a result of modern stressful living and electrolyte nutrient imbalance. Efforts to control hypertension must revolve around stress management and electrolyte nutrient intake.

Full Spectrum Nutrition

Calcium ..... 1500 –3000 mg per day
Magnesium .... 1000 mg per day
Potassium .... 100-300 mg per day
L-Carnitine ....
.... 500 mg 2-3 times per day
Essential Fatty Acids ...... 2-3 grams
Garlic Concentrate .... as per label
Selenium .... 200 mcg per day

Coenzyme Q10 ....
.... 30 mg 2 times per day
Taurine............... 1-3 grams per day
Eliminate heavy metal toxicity and
possible allergies.

High Cholesterol

While cholesterol has never actually caused a single case of heart disease in medical history, elevated cholesterol and other fats in the blood are not necessarily healthy. Dietary intake of cholesterol affects the overall cholesterol levels in the blood only marginally in most people. This is because the body produces far more cholesterol than we can possibly consume from our diet. The problems with cholesterol level regulation begin in the liver and must be managed by cleansing and nourishing this organ.

Full Spectrum Nutrition
Lipotropics
Choline
Inositol
Methionine .... 1-2 grams per day
Lecithin Granules ....
.................1-3 tablespoons per day
Multi Antioxidants .... 400mg per day
Increase Fiber ..... 4-8 grams per day
Garlic Capsules ....
.... 2 capsules 3 times per day

Pantethine ..... 500-1000 mg per day
Essential Fatty Acids ....
.... 1-3 grams per day extra
Guggulipids .... 100-300 mg
Gamma-oryzanol .... 250-500 mg

HIV – See AIDS

Hot Flashes – See Menopause (Also Chapter 8)

Hyperactivity (See also ADD)

Hyperactivity usually occurs in children and teenagers, although, if left untreated, can carry on into adulthood. It is characterized by excessive nervousness and irritable behavior. Since the central nervous system is involved, our focus will be on nutrients governing this area.

Full Spectrum Nutrition
Niacin ....
500 mg to 2000 mg depending upon weight
High potency Stress B-Complex .....
.... 2-8 capsules per day
Organic Liquid Trace Minerals ....
.... to bowel tolerance
Calcium .... 100-2000 mg per day

> Magnesium ....
> 10-750 mg per day (depending upon
> weight)
> Rule out food allergies
> Rule out heavy metal poisoning

Hypertension – See High Blood Pressure

Hyperthyroid

An over-active thyroid gland produces excessive amounts of hormone, causing an overactive metabolic environment within the body. Often the body's digestion can speed up, causing mal-absorption. Symptoms of this disorder include nervousness, irritability, increased perspiration, fatigue, weakness, hair and weight loss, insomnia, brittle nails, low tolerance to heat, rapid heartbeat, and hand trembling.

> **Full Spectrum Nutrition**
> High potency Stress B-Complex .....
> ...... 2-4 capsules 2-3 times per day
> Vitamin C .... to bowel tolerance

Hypoglycemia

One of the three phases of carbohydrate intolerance, technically known as hyperinsulinemia, hypoglycemia is characterized by low blood sugar levels, caused by an overproduction of insulin from the pancreas.

Hypoglycemics can be either overweight or underweight, depending upon a variety of factors. Like all disorders involving insulin, hypoglycemia also involves the adrenal glands, which frequently over-secrete adrenaline as a result of low blood sugar levels. Symptoms of hypoglycemia include fatigue, dizziness, headache, irritability, indigestion, obesity, and impaired memory. While proper diet is the key to managing this chronic condition, the following protocol will assist the body in normalizing blood sugar levels and improving insulin regulation.

Full Spectrum Nutrition

High Protein Diet .... 100 grams per day
Low Carbohydrate Diet .... 60 grams per day or less
Vitamin C .... 2 – 4 grams
Pantothenic Acid .... 2000 – 3000 mg per day
Adrenal Glandulars .... 6-10 tablets per day
Vitamin E .... 400 IU extra
Chromium .... 500 mcg per day
Vanadium .... 200 –400 mcg per day
Aspartic Acid ... 100-300 mg per day

Hypothyroid

When the thyroid gland under-produces hormone, a variety of symptoms can arise. These include fatigue, loss of appetite, obesity, painful menstrual periods, weakness, dry/scaly skin, yellow bumps on the eyelids, frequent infections, depression, hair loss, and intolerance to the cold. You can easily test your thyroid with a regular fever thermometer. Before you go to bed at night, shake down a thermometer and place it by your bed. When you first wake up in the morning, before moving about at all, place the thermometer under your arm for 10 minutes. You must remain still and quiet. If the temperature is consistently at 97.6 degrees farenheit or lower, it is a good indication that your thyroid is not producing enough hormone. If it is low on a regular basis you may need Armour Thyroid Extract, which is available only by prescription from your doctor. The following protocol will help support thyroid function and may even adjust thyroid production if it is not too low.

Be sure to avoid anything with chlorine or fluoride, since these substances are not only carcinogenic, but block the action of iodine, necessary for proper thyroid function.

Full Spectrum Nutrition
Kelp (seaweed) . 10-15 Tablets daily
L-Tyrosine .... 500-1000 mg daily

> Raw Thyroid Glandular ....
> .... 4-8 tablet per day
> High Potency Stress B-Complex ....
> .... 30 –100 mg per day

Hysterectomy - See Chapter 8

Immunodepression

Our immune system is really the army of the body, providing protection against invading pathogens, which can cause harm to our health and well being. For years, medical science simply took for granted that the immune system did its job. Through the prominence of such conditions as AIDS and cancer, we can see just how devastating it can be when the immune system fails or is prevented from functioning. Through the tens of thousands of toxins in our environment, our immune system is constantly on overload, having to build antibodies to the many thousands of byproducts produced when these poisons are broken down internally.

> ### Full Spectrum Nutrition
> Colostrum Concentrate
> Mycelium Mushroom Extracts
> .... 1 beta – 1 D Glucan
> Take this combination together according to your health care professional

Echinacea .... as per label
Astragallus membranaceus Extract
.... as per label
Panax Ginseng .... as per label
Garlic Extract .... 4-8 capsules
Multi Antioxidants ....
.... 400-800 mg per day
Dimethylglycine ....
.... 100-400 mg per day
Selenium .... 200 mcg extra
L-Ornithine ....
.... 500 mg 2 times per day
Zinc .... 50-100 mg per day
Beta Carotene ....
.... 10,000 – 25,000 IU per day
Olive Leaf Extract ....
....
.... 500 –1000 mg per day
Glycerol monolaurate ....
.... 1000 mg per day
Goldenseal .... 1-4 capsule per day
Pantethine ..... 500-1000 mg per day

To help prevent infections

Vitamin A .... 25,000 – 100,000 IU
Coenzyme Q10 .... 30 mg

Be sure and rule out heavy metal toxicity. If heavy metal toxicity exists, it will be necessary to chelate or remove these offending substances. (See Heavy Metal Poisoning.)

Impotence

Difficulty in obtaining or maintaining an erection is becoming an increasing problem, even among younger men. There are some organic, physical reasons for this problem such as peripheral vascular disease and low sperm count, but for the vast majority of men it is a nutrient deficiency. I suggest the following protocol, but if it doesn't produce results within 30 days, see your physician and explore other possible causes.

Full Spectrum Nutrition

Yohimbine	100-400 mg
Gingko biloba	50- 100 mg
L-Arginine	500 mg 3 times per day
Zinc	50 mg extra
Octacosanol	per label
Raw Orchic Glandular	4-8 tablets per day
Ginseng	per label
Tribulus terrestris	750 mg 1 or 2 times per day

Indigestion (Dyspepsia)

Most symptoms of indigestion, which include feelings of fullness after a meal, bloating, belching, gas, and heartburn are caused by a lack of natural hydrochloric acid in the stomach. This lack of acids prevents the proper breakdown of protein foods leading to protein and mineral deficiencies. Further, the lack of hydrochloric acid prevents the production of specific enzymes, involved in further digestion of foods. Taking antacids, while often producing relief, does nothing to improve digestion or assimilation of food. The following program will not only bring relief, but solve the problem as well by increasing the absorption of both foods and nutrients.

Full Spectrum Nutrition

Betaine Hydrochloride ....
.... 100-300 mg per meal
Multi-Purpose Enzyme Precursor
Containing
Pancreatin
Papain
Bromelain
Ox Bile .... 100-300 mg per meal

In severe cases of over alkalinity, apple cider vinegar (2 Tbl) and water, taken two or three times per day is often helpful.

Infections – (See also Immunodepression)

Infections are a normal part of living. In fact, an occasional bout with an invading bug actually stimulates the immune system into greater function. However, when infections are prolonged and/or occur often, it is a sign of immune weakness and the immune system needs to be both stimulated and nourished. Follow the protocol under Immunodepression. For topical infections follow the treatment suggestions below.

Full Spectrum Nutrition
Liquid Oxygen ....
.1 ounce two or three times per day
On an empty stomach

Use 3% on skin infections but not on open wounds. Wash infected area with antibacterial soap containing food grade hydrogen peroxide.

Infertility (Men) – See Impotence

Infertility (Women)

The inability to become pregnant after a long period of regular sexual activity usually signals hormonal problems. Some of the more frequent causes in women include pelvic disease, chlamydia infection (untreated), and allergic reactions to their partner's sperm. Since there are so many possible causes, it is wise to seek the advice of a qualified physician. If all the physical causes have been eliminated, the following program will support the woman's body nutritionally and put her in the best possible hormonal position to conceive.

Full Spectrum Nutrition

Folic Acid	400 mcg extra
Vitamin B6	50 mg extra
Zinc	50 –100 mg per day
Vitamin E	400 – 800 IU extra
Ovarian Glandular Extract	4-8 tablets per day
L-Arginine	4 grams per day
Iron	10-20 mg per day
Vitamin B12	100-300 mcg per day

Since stress is often involved in hormone imbalance, a high potency Stress B-complex formula, taken two or three times per day is often helpful.

Inflammation

When the body reacts to trauma or infection, swelling and pain is often the result. Inflammation may be either internal or external and involve almost any organ or other tissue.

> **Full Spectrum Nutrition**
> Vitamin C .... To Bowel Tolerance
> Bioflavonoids .... 3 –6 grams per day
>
> Antioxidant Combination ....
> 400-800 mg per day during inflammation period
> Bromelain ....
> 200-500 mg 3 times per day on empty stomach
> Organic Source Trace Minerals ....
> 1 –3 ounces extra during inflammation
> Horsetail Extract .... per label

Inflammatory Bowel Disease (Irritable Bowel Syndrome)

This condition, which is directly tied into unmanageable stress, is becoming more and more common. Twice as many women suffer from this problem as men. IBD involves the muscular contraction of intestines and when these contractions are not smooth, it affects the movement of waste material to the bowel. Symptoms include constipation alternating with rapid onset diarrhea, abdominal pain and cramping, and an excess production of mucus in the stool. Food allergies are also often at the heart of this problem so it is important to eliminate all offending foods. Stress, the cardinal player in this condition, interferes with the acid/alkaline balance often causing spontaneous dumping of the contents of the colon by flooding it with water.

Full Spectrum Nutrition
Essential Fatty Acids ....
.... 3-6 grams extra
Fiber .... 3-6 grams
Peppermint Extract ....
.... 2 capsules per day
Ginger Root Extract ....
.... 3 capsules with each meal
Multi-Purpose Enzymes ....
.... 2 –6 or more with each meal
High Potency Stress B-Complex ....
... 2-4 capsules 2 or 3 times per day
L-Glutamine .... 3-5 grams per day
Cascara sagrada................ per label
Chamomile .... per label

Eliminate all food allergens.
It is also important to learn to manage and reduce the stress your life.

Influenza – See Immunodepression

Insect Bite

Localized insect bites can be soothed and healed by applying 3 percent hydrogen peroxide to the affected area several times per day. A paste made from baking soda and applied to the skin is often helpful as well.

Insomnia

Sleeplessness is occasionally experienced by everyone and is little cause for concern. If, however, this condition occurs night after night, the underlying cause should be sought. Since there are many causes for this condition, you should seek the advice of a qualified health care practitioner. Poor nutritional habits and excess stress can also contribute to this condition.

Full Spectrum Nutrition
Calcium Lactate............................
.... 1000 mg before bed
Magnesium..... 1000 mg before bed
Valerian Root Capsules ....
.......2-6 capsules 1 hour before bed

If stress is the underlying cause:

Kava Kava Extract..........................
.... 2-4 capsules 2 times per day
High Potency B-Complex................
...... 3 capsules 2 or 3 times per day

Melatonin .... per label
Passion Flower Extract ...... per label

Intermittent Claudication

This condition, often associated with atherosclerosis and other heart and circulatory disorders, is characterized by a weakness in the legs. This weakness occurs most often during exercise and may be accompanied by cramps or spasms in the calves. Intermittent Claudication occurs only at certain times, usually after an extended period of walking. (See also for Atherosclerosis.)

Full Spectrum Nutrition
Bilberry Extract ....
.... 4-8 capsules per day
Bromelain .... 300-500 mg per day
Gingko biloba .... 100 mg per day
Vitamin E .... 400 –800 IU extra
Inositol.................... 500 – 1000 mg
Essential Fatty Acids ....
.... 3-5 grams per day
Centella asiatica .... per label
Hawthorn Berry .... per label
Horsechestnut .... per label
Ruscus aculeatus .... per label

Irritable Bowel Syndrome – See Inflammatory Bowel Disease

Jaundice

Jaundice is caused by an obstruction of the flow of bile from the liver. This can be a sign of serious liver disease and should be addressed by a qualified physician. Nutrients to support the liver are as follows.

Full Spectrum Nutrition
Milk Thistle .... 100 – 400 mg per day
N-acetyl Cysteine .... 200-600 mg per day
Lipotropics
Choline
Inositol
Methionine ....
1000 mg of combination 3 times per day

Kidney & Bladder Problems

Since the kidneys and bladder are responsible for elimination of waste fluids from the body, they must be kept in good health to avoid infections. There are several types of infections of the kidneys, many of them serious and require immediate medical attention. To avoid most of these situations, it is important to keep the bladder healthy and free from pathogens since many kidney problems result from previous bladder infections. The following nutrients will help strengthen both the kidneys and bladder and assist with proper function.

Full Spectrum Nutrition

Water ....
. 6-8 ounce glass every waking hour
Acidophilus capsules ....
.... 5 capsules daily
Vitamin B6 ....
  50 mg 3 times per day during infection
Vitamin C .... to bowel tolerance
Dandelion Root .... per label
Calcium .... 1000 mg extra
L-Arginine .. 500 mg 3 times per day
Vitamin A (natural only) ....
.... 25,000 – 50,000 IU per day
Zinc .... 50 mg per day
Choline & Inositol .. 1000 mg per day

For men: Saw palmetto & Pygeum africanum
For women: Black cohosh & Mexican yam

Kidney Stones

Stones in the kidneys and bladder as well as other deposits, such as heel spurs, are caused by minerals (especially calcium) dropping out of solution and forming crystals. There are two main causes for this problem. Firstly, an over alkaline digestive system, which cannot properly acidify these minerals. Secondly, the over-consumption of sugar foods. When insulin is present in the blood stream in large amounts, it accelerates the excretion of calcium.

Full Spectrum Nutrition

To Acidify:
Betaine Hydrochloride ....
.... 200-400 mg per meal
Apple Cider Vinegar ....
.... 1Tbl 3 times per day in water

Nutritional Support:

Calcium Citrate/Malate only ....
.... 1000 mg total per day
Magnesium chelate ....
.... 300 mg 3 times per day
Vitamin B6 ....
.... 50 mg 2 times per day during problems
Vitamin A .... 25,000 IU per day
Vitamin C .... to bowel tolerance

> Potassium .... 100 mg per day
> L-Lysine ..... 300 mg 2 times per day
> Ginkgo biloba extract .... per label
> Goldenrod .... per label
> Rose hips .... per label
> Cranberry Juice or Capsules ....
> .... 8 oz 4 times per day or
> Label dose 4 times per day

Lead Poisoning – See Heavy Metal Poisoning

Learning Disabilities – See Attention Deficit Disorders

Leg Ulcers

Wounds that do not heal, primarily due to poor circulation, develop an erosion and ulceration is often the result. Diabetes and other diseases, which destroy circulation, are often at the cause of ulcers that will not heal.

> ### Full Spectrum Nutrition
> Liquid oxygen ....
> .... 1 oz 3 –4 times per day on empty stomach
> Hyperbaric Oxygen Treatments... as needed
> Coenzyme Q 10 ....
> .... 30 mg 2- 3 times per day

DMG (Dimethylglycine) ....
.... 100 mg 3 times per day
Vitamin C .... to bowel tolerance
Vitamin E .... 400 – 800 IU extra
Garlic Extract ....
.... 4 capsules 3 times per day

Leukemia – See Cancer

Leukorrhea

This is a vaginal discharge resulting from either an infection, likely chlamydia, or a yeast infection, such as Candida albicans. Other causes can include nutrient deficiencies, especially the B-complex group.

Full Spectrum Nutrition
High Potency B-Complex... per label
Garlic Extract ....
...... 2 capsules 3 or 4 times per day
Essential Fatty Acids ....
.... 4-5 grams per day
Acidophilus ....
.........3 capsules 3 –4 times per day
Vitamin C .... to bowel tolerance
Vitamin A (natural only)...................
.... 25,000 – 50,000 IU per day
Liquid Oxygen Flush ....
.... See Chapter on detoxification

Lupus

This disease belongs to a group of illnesses called autoimmune disorders. This means that the immune system of the patient is actually attacking itself. Since the immune system is already over-active, it is essential that these individuals DO NOT take any supplements that heavily stimulate the immune system, as this can make the condition much worse. There are two types of lupus, Systemic lupus erythematosus, which affects organs and joints, and Discord lupus erythematosus, which is a skin disease. Various theories exist as to the cause of this autoimmune problem.

Full Spectrum Nutrition

Vitamin C .... to bowel tolerance
Essential Fatty Acids ....
.... 4-6 grams per day
Selenium .... 500 mcg
Multi-enzymes ... 2-4 with each meal
Alfalfa Capsules .... per label
Niacin .... 25 mg 2 times per day

Pantothenic Acid ....
.... 500 mg 2 times per day
Vitamin A (Fish liver oil) ....
25,000 IU per day
L-Cysteine . 500 mg 3 times per day
Zinc .... 50 – 100 mg per day
Organic Sulfur .... per label

Lyme Disease – See Immunodepression

Macular Degeneration

This disorder of the eye tissues has taken on almost epidemic expansion in the last 20 years. The result of this condition, if left untreated, is blindness. I have used the following protocol for several years, with excellent results.

Full Spectrum Nutrition

Bilberry Extract ....
.... 250 –500 mg per day
Multi Antioxidant Formula ....
.... 400 – 1200 mg per day
Lutein .... 10 – 20 mg per day
Zinc .... 50 mg per day
Beta Carotene ..... 25,000-50,000 IU
Gingko biloba ....
.... 250- 400 mg per day
Taurine...... 1,500 –3000 mg per day
Vitamin A........................ 25,000 IU
Vitamin C .... 2-4 grams per day

Manic-Depressive Disorder

This disorder of brain chemistry is characterized by extreme mood swings, from excitement and elation to the depths of depression. It is important to understand that no disorder involving brain chemistry imbalances should be self-treated. The chemistry of the brain is very tricky and ignorant experimentation can lead to a much worse condition. We have done considerable work in this area of psycho nutrition, but I have decided not to publish our protocols due to the risk that attempts at self-management. If you suffer from this or any brain chemistry disorder, it is essential that you be under the care of a health care practitioner that understands both the disorder and the alternative methods of management involved. If you have a health care practitioner, I am happy to share my experiences and the results of my work directly with them.

Melanoma – See Cancer

Memory Improvement

We all experience a temporary loss of memory from time to time. The most common cause of short term and brief memory loss is fatigue and excess stress. When memory recall becomes a more regular occurrence this is often a sign of underlying nutritional deficiencies, which are leading to an altered biochemistry. The following protocol represents the latest research into substances that have been shown to improve the memory response.

Full Spectrum Nutrition
L-Carnitine .... 100-300 mg

DMAE .... 150-300 mg
Gotu Kola .... 50 mg
Pantothenic Acid .... 150 mg
Phosphatidyl Serine ..... 200-400 mg
Phosphatidyl Choline ... 200-400 mg
Vitamin B6 .... 10-20 mg
Vitamin B12 .... 100-300 mcg
Choline Bitartrite .... 200-400 mg
1-Pyroglutamic Acid ..... 150-300 mg

Meniere's Syndrome

This condition of the inner ear can have many causes such as allergies, clogged arteries, poor circulation, and spasms. Symptoms of Meniere's included ringing in the ears, loss of hearing, nausea, and loss of balance. The following program represents a combination of the latest nutritional research on managing this annoying condition.

Full Spectrum Nutrition
Manganese .... 5 mg per day
Coenzyme Q10 ...... 100 mg per day
Vitamin A (natural) ....
.... 25,000 IU per day
Vitamin D .... 200 IU extra
Calcium .... 1000 mg
Essential Fatty Acids ....
.... 2-4 grams per day
Fluoride .... per label

Zinc .... 100 mg per day
Valerian Root .... per label
Kava Kava .... per label

Meningitis – See Immunodepression

Menopause – See Chapter 8

Menstrual Cramps

In addition to many of the nutrients found in Chapter 8, the following are especially helpful for the cramping often experienced during menstruation.

Full Spectrum Nutrition

Niacin .... 100 mg total per day
100 mg every 3 hours during cramp-ing
Vitamin E .... 400 IU extra
Iron .... 18 mg
Magnesium...................................
.... 100 mg 4 times per day
Bilberry extract ....
.... 100 mg 3 times per day

Menorrhagia

Characterized by long and excessive menstrual periods, this condition can be very debilitating, causing excessive iron deficiency and other nutrient loss.

This condition often is a complication of uterine fibromyomata and other uterine disorders.

> **Full Spectrum Nutrition**
> Vitamin A (from fish liver oil) ....
> .... 25,000 IU 2 times per day
> Iron .... 100 mg daily for 15 days
> Manganese .... 5 mg per day
> Bioflavonoids ....
> .... 1000 mg 3 times per day
> Vitamin C .... to bowel tolerance

Mercury Toxicity – See Heavy Metal Poisoning

Migraine Headaches

A headache of extreme severity, migraines are usually caused by either a chemical imbalance in brain chemistry or stress, which constricts the arteries of the brain putting pressure on nerves. Allergies are also a common cause of migraine and other headaches and therefore should be either ruled out or managed accordingly. The majority of migraine headache sufferers are women (75%). Migraine headaches may be distinguished from other types of headache by vomiting, blurred vision, tingling and numbness in the limbs, seeing stars, sparks, or flashes, and sometimes speech disorders.

Full Spectrum Nutrition
Liquid Oxygen..................................
..............1 ounce 2-3 times per day
DMG (Dimethylglycine) ..... per label
Magnesium... 200 – 400 mg per day
Essential Fatty Acids ....
.... 2 grams per day
Feverfew .... 25-75 mg per day
Niacin ....
take enough to flush just as headache
begins

Mitral Valve Prolapse

A common heart valve problem often involving lesions on the surface of the valves themselves. The following program is helpful in supporting the heart muscle with many types of valve disturbances.

Full Spectrum Nutrition
Magnesium.....................................
.... 600 –1000 mg per day extra
L-Carnitine......... 2-4 grams per day
Selenium .... 200-400 mcg
Coenzyme Q10 .... 100-200 mg
Potassium ..... 300 –800 mg per day
Hawthorn berry........... 250-500 mg
Taurine................ 2-3 grams per day
Vitamin C .... 1-2 grams per day

Mononucleosis – See Immunodepression

Motion Sickness

Motion sickness can occur while in a car, airplane, or boat. Severe sufferers can experience motion sickness while riding in an elevator or watching a turning object. Symptoms of motion sickness include cold sweats, nausea, vomiting, and dizziness.

Full Spectrum Nutrition
Charcoal Tablets ....
.... 5 tablets 1 hour before travel
Ginger Root Capsules ....
2-4 capsules every 2 hours during travel
Magnesium ..... 500 mg before travel
Vitamin B6 .... 50 mg before travel
Liquid Oxygen ....
2 ounces before travel and as needed
Take on an empty stomach

Mouth and Gum Disorders – See Periodontal Disease

Multiple Sclerosis

This disease affects the central nervous system and is a progressive autoimmune condition. There are many causes for this disease such as allergies, environmental exposure, and many others that have not yet been identified. Since it is an autoimmune condition, sufferers should avoid immune stimulants of all kinds. Currently there is no cure for MS. The late Dr. Hans Neiper of Germany discovered the best treatment methods for control of this condition. His work continues through his foundation. (See Resource section.)

Full Spectrum Nutrition

Liquid Organic Source Trace Minerals .... 2-4 ounces per day
Essential Fatty Acids ....
.... 4-10 grams per day
Multi-Antioxidants ....
.... 400-1200 mg per day
Multi Enzymes with Hydrochloric Acid
.... 3-6 capsules per meal
AEP Salts:
Calcium, Magnesium
Potassium ...... 3-6 capsules per day
Octacosanol .... 25-50 mg
Vitamin B12 (as methylcobalamin) ..
.... 10-30 mg per day
Gingko biloba .... 100 mg per day
High potency B-Complex Stress .....
.... per label
Liquid Oxygen ....
.... 1 oz 3 times per day
on an empty stomach
Kelp .... 10-15 tablets per day

Muscle Cramps

The most common cause of muscle cramping is an imbalance or deficiency of the electrolyte minerals, calcium, magnesium, and, to some extent, potassium. Another cause of this phenomenon is a vitamin E deficiency. Most muscle cramps occur at night and this variety is almost exclusively caused by a calcium/magnesium deficit.

Full Spectrum Nutrition
Calcium .... 1500 mg per day
                    500 mg a bedtime
Magnesium .... 1000 mg per day
Potassium ....
.... 100 mg 2 or 3 times per day
High Potency Stress B-Complex ....
.... per label
Vitamin E .... 200-400 IU extra

Check if sodium levels are low. If so, salt tablets may be helpful, especially during warm weather.

Muscular Dystrophy (see also Myopathy)

This genetic condition involves the destruction and atrophy of skeletal muscles. Symptoms include loss of strength and deformity. While the exact cause is still unknown, errors in metabolism are involved.

> ### Full Spectrum Nutrition
> Selenium .. 200 – 1000 mcg per day
> Vitamin E .... 200-400 IU extra
> Free Form Amino Acids ..... per label
> Choline ....
> .... 3,000 – 10,000 mg per day
> Liquid Organic Trace Minerals ....
> .... 2-4 oz per day

Myasthenia Gravis – See Myopathy

Myocardial Infarction – See Chapter 5

Myopathy

A wasting away of skeletal muscle associated with many diseases such as muscular dystrophies.

> ### Full Spectrum Nutrition
> Riboflavin (B2) ....
> .... 100-200 mg per day
> Vitamin A (natural) ....
> .... 25,000 IU per day
> Vitamin E .... 400-800 IU per day
> Magnesium ....
> .... 200 mg 3 times per day
> Selenium .... 500 mcg
> Phosphatidyl Choline ....
> .... 1000 mg per day
> Vitamin B6 ... 50 mg 2 times per day

Coenzyme Q10 ....
.... 50 mg 3 times per day
Vitamin C .... 2-4 grams per day

Nail Problems

The fingernails have often been called a mirror to the inside of the body. Many problems with fingernails often stem from a lack of quality protein in the diet. Deficiencies of vitamin A or calcium can cause the nail to become dry and brittle. Ridges in the nail can either be caused from damage to the nail bed or a lack of B-complex nutrients. White marks on the nails are a sign of zinc deficiency. Low protein consumption and/or vitamin C deficiencies can lead to hangnails. Insufficient amounts of natural stomach acid can cause fingernails to split or peel.

Full Spectrum Nutrition
Protein................ 80 grams per day
Vitamin A........................25,000 IU
Gelatin/ Chondroitin sulfate...........
.... 400 mg per day
Zinc .... 25- 50 mg per day
B-Complex .... 25 mg per day
Horsetail .... per label
Vitamin C .... 2-3 grams per day

Nausea (During Pregnancy) – See Motion Sickness

Nausea (w/ Vomiting) – See Motion Sickness

Neuritis

This painful condition is the result of an inflammation of the nerves in a particular grouping. Prolonged neuritis can lead to nerve deterioration. Symptoms include pain, tingling, loss of sensation, swelling, and redness of the affected area(s). There are many causes for this condition, which include nutritional deficiencies, but may also be a side effect from a bone fracture, nerve infection, or diseases such as diabetes or gout. Toxic metals, such as mercury, lead, or cadmium, in the body can also cause this condition and should be eliminated through chelation.

Full Spectrum Nutrition
Lecithin Granules ....
.... 1 tbl 2 or 3 times per day
Vitamin B1 ....
100 mg 2 times per day during flair up
High potency Stress B-Complex .....
.... per label
Calcium .... 2000 mg daily
Magnesium .... 500 mg daily

Increase fluid intake and avoid caffeine

Neuromuscular Degeneration

When the impulses from the nerves have difficulty signaling muscle response, a variety of neuromuscular conditions are suspected. The following program will support nerve impulse and strengthen function.

Full Spectrum Nutrition
Folic Acid................. 800-1200 mcg
Vitamin B6... 50 mg 3 times per day

Vitamin B12.....................................
.... 500 mcg 3 or 4 times per day
Calcium .... 2000 mg
Magnesium........................ 750 mg
Free Form Amino Acids ..... per label
L-Carnitine.......................................
.... 500 mg 3 times per day
Coenzyme Q10 ....
.... 50 mg 2 times per day

Be sure and rule out allergies such as gluten as well as heavy metal poisoning.

Nickel Toxicity – See Heavy Metal Poisoning

Night Blindness

If your vision is normally stable, with or without glasses, during the daylight hours but you have difficulty seeing well at night, due to the reflection and glare of bright lights, this condition is referred to as 'night blindness'. This condition can be a signal of more serious eye trouble but generally it is a symptom of vitamin A deficiency.

> **Full Spectrum Nutrition**
> Vitamin A (from fish liver oil) ....
> ....25,000 – 100,000+ per day
> Leutin .... per label

Obesity

It is important to determine the cause of your weight gain and then to plan a proper eating program based on the way your body handles food. (I have written a book covering this subject – contact the Institute for availability.) Once you understand the right type of diet for your body chemistry, the following nutrients are often helpful.

Full Spectrum Nutrition

Essential Fatty Acids .... 1-2 grams per day

L-Carnitine .... 1000-2000 mg per day

Phenylalanine* .... 500-1000 mg at bedtime

*Note: Do not take if you have un-controlled high blood pressure.

Choline .... 1000 mg

Inositol .... 1500 mg

Methionine .... 400-800 mg

Conjugated Linoleic Acid 2-4 grams per day

Ma Huang* (Ephedrine) .... 10 – 20 mg per day

*Note: Do not take if you suffer from heart disease, diabetes, hypoglyce-mia, or are over 50 years old and more than 50 pounds overweight.

Osteoarthritis – See Chapter 7

Osteoporosis – (See also Chapter 7)

Osteoporosis is a condition which results in the thinning of bone tissue and a loss of bone density. The leaching or depletion of calcium and other minerals from the bone tissue results in osteoporosis. Although osteoporosis primarily affects women, men do suffer from this condition as well. We previously thought that estrogen depletion was the chief causes of this condition. While hormone imbalance during and after menopause certainly does play a part, we now know that micro trace mineral deficiencies are at the root of the problem.

Full Spectrum Nutrition

Multi-Enzymes with Hydrochloric Acid .... 4-6 capsules with each meal

Calcium (citrate/malate) .... 1000-1500 mg per day
Magnesium .... 750 mg per day
Manganese .... per label
Copper .... 2 mg
Zinc .... 10 mg
Boron .... 2-4 mg
Vitamin D .... 400-600 mg
Strontium .... per label
Horsetail .... per label

Otosclerosis – See Ear Dysfunction

Overweight – See Obesity

Pain

Pain is nature's way of telling us that there is something wrong with the body. All too frequently we take drugs designed to elevate the pain but we do not look to find the cause of the discomfort. Neglect and continued abuse can lead to the problem worsening. Once the cause of the pain has been determined and properly addressed, the following nutrients may help you naturally manage the pain until the underlying cause has an opportunity to correct itself.

Full Spectrum Nutrition
dl- Phenylalanine* ....
.... 500 mg 3 times per day
*Note: do not take if you have uncontrolled high blood pressure
Curcumin .... per label

Topical Pain Relief
Capsaicin Cream .... as needed

Pancreatitis

An inflammation or infection of the pancreas, which is often caused by pancreatic stones, scarring, or even cancer. This condition can either be acute or become chronic.

Full Spectrum Nutrition
Chromium .... 300-400 mcg
Pancreas Glandular Extract ....
.....................................4-10 tablets
Stress B-Complex .... per label

> If infection is present, use protocol under Immunodepression.

Parasites/Amebas

The biggest reason parasites and other similar organisms take up residence within the human body is due to a deficiency of hydrochloric acid in the stomach as well as a lack of available oxygen within the body. This oxygen deficiency is caused by lack of exercise, lung disorders, advanced age, or other disease. Fortunately, regardless of the invading parasitic organism, most all of them are anaerobic in nature and are effectively destroyed with a liquid oxygen flush.

Full Spectrum Nutrition
Liquid Oxygen* ....
.... 1 ounce 3 times per day
Then 2 ounces 3 times per day after 1 week
Stay at a total of 6 ounces per day for a period of 4 to 6 weeks.
*Note: Liquid oxygen must be taken on an empty stomach, 30 minutes before, or three hours after a meal.
Acidophilus ....
10 capsules per day on empty stomach for ten days after the liquid oxygen flush.

Consider also using a short duration of immune boosting nutrients as discussed under Immunodepression.

Parkinson's Disease

This degenerative disease affects the nervous system. While the exact cause is still not fully understood, we do know that there is an imbalance between two chemicals, dopamine and acetylcholine. Symptoms of this condition include shaking, drooling, loss of appetite, shuffling gait, tremors, and impaired speech. The most common pharmaceutical for the management of this disease is Levodopa. If you are taking this drug be sure NOT take vitamin B6 as they interact, causing an elevation of dopamine in the brain. Levodopa must be carefully administered, since it can produce serious side effects. Evidence has shown that taking vitamin B6 alone, in mega doses, is often as effective as levodopa and much safer.

Full Spectrum Nutrition (with low B6 if taking levodopa)

Calcium .... 1500 mg
Magnesium...................... 1000 mg
Lecithin Granules...........................
.... 1 tbsp. 3 times per day
Folic Acid................. 400 –800 mcg
Vitamin B6 ..... 300-1000 mg per day

Note: Do not take B6 if you are taking the medication Levodopa.
Vitamin C .... 2-4 grams
Vitamin E .... up to 3,000 IU
Essential Fatty Acids ...... 4-8 grams
Stress B-Complex ....
.... 100 mg 3 times per day

Rule out the possibility of heavy metal poisoning by taking a hair mineral test.

Pellagra

This is a vitamin disease caused by prolonged and severe deficiency of the B-complex nutrients. Full Spectrum Nutrition and B-complex vitamins will completely cure the disorder.

Full Spectrum Nutrition
B-complex

Peptic Ulcers

The stomach lining ulcerates primarily when the natural stomach pH is disturbed for long periods of time. We often think that ulcers are caused by stomach acid, but this is not true. Stomach acid can irritate an open ulcer, once it has developed, but it is actually a lack of stomach acids combined with an infection that produces this disorder. Emphasis must be placed upon healing the open ulceration then re-establishing the proper pH of the stomach with enzymes and betaine hydrochloride.

Full Spectrum Nutrition
Multi – Enzymes ....
.... 3-4 with each meal
Bilberry Extract .... 200-500 mg
Licorice Root Extract .... per label
Rhubarb .... per label
Fatty Acids .... 2-4 grams
Vitamin A (natural only) ....
.... 50,000 – 100,000 IU
Vitamin C .... 2-4 grams
Organic Aluminum (from plant sources) .... 1-3 ounces per day
Bismuth ..... 150 mg 4 times per day
Zinc . 25-50 mg 2 or 3 times per day

Periodontal Disease

This is a general term for infections and other disease pathology of the gums and supporting tissues around the teeth. When addressing these conditions, we must place emphasis upon both the infection, usually present, as well as the rebuilding of bone, which holds teeth in place. The Standard American Diet (SAD Diet) provides so many soft foods that plaque, which builds up on the teeth, never gets cleaned off. This leads to infection and inflammation, which can result in one of two major gum problems, gingivitis and eventually, pyorrhea (periodontitis).

Full Spectrum Nutrition

Coenzyme Q10 .... 50 mg 2 or 3 times per day
Vitamin C .... 4 – 10 grams
Calcium .... 1000 – 1500 mg
Magnesium .... 800 mg
Phosphorus .... as per label
Folic Acid .... 1 mg per day
Vitamin A (natural only) .... 10,000 – 20,000 IU
Zinc .... 50 mg
Centella asiatica .... 2-4 capsule per day
Licorice Root .... per label
Bloodroot .... per label
Chlorella .... 1 tsp. per day

Ensure you have adequate Hydrochloric Acid production in the stomach Rule out leaking dental fillings, which can lead to mercury poisoning, by taking a hair mineral test.

Peripheral Vascular Disease

This deterioration of the vascular system can lead to inflammation and infection of the vascular system.

When this condition exists, you may also have athero-sclerosis and varicose veins.

Full Spectrum Nutrition

Bilberry Extract ....
.... 100 mg 4 times per day
Hawthorn Berry .... 250-500 mg
Gingko biloba ....
.... 50 mg 3 times per day
Horsechestnut ....
.... 50 mg 3 times per day
Bromelain ....
.... 250 – 500 mg 3 times per day
on empty stomach
Zinc .... 50 mg
Magnesium.....................................
...... 200 mg extra 2-3 times per day
Essential Fatty Acids ......2-4 Grams
Inositol....... 500 mg 2 times per day
Vitamin E .... 400-1400 IU extra
Vitamin A (natural only)....25,000 IU

Phlebitis

This condition is caused by an inflammation of the veins, often causing blood clots. It occurs, mostly, as a result of a trauma to the blood vessel wall, an infection, prolonged sitting, standing, or inactivity.

Full Spectrum Nutrition

Vitamin E .... 800 – 1200 IU
High Potency B-Complex ....
.... 50 mg 2 times per day
Vitamin C w/bioflavonoids ....
.... to bowel tolerance
Essential Fatty Acids ....
.... 3-6 grams per day
Increase Fiber .... 10-20 grams
Water .... 64 oz per day

Pneumonia

This condition of the lungs may be caused by a variety of viruses, bacteria or even fungi. When the body is compromised with other infections, or during the presence of chronic diseases or prolonged inactivity, pneumonia is more likely to occur. Age is also a factor. Since there is most often an infection of some sort at the root of pneumonia, immune-boosting supplements should be considered. (See Immunodepression.)

Full Spectrum Nutrition

Immune building protocol
Vitamin A .... 25,000- 100,000 IU
Vitamin C .... 3-10 grams
Acidophilus if taking antibiotics 10 capsules per day on empty stomach

> Raw thymus extract ....
> .... 500 mg 3 times per day
> Zinc .... 50 mg
> Antioxidant Mix ....
> .... 400 mg 2-3 times per day

Polyps

Polyps are non-cancerous growths, which may grow on any mucous lining such as bladder, cervix, large intestine, and the sinuses. Since those with polyps are much more likely to develop cancer, attention to the management and surgical removal, if necessary, is of paramount importance. (See Immunodepression.)

> ### Full Spectrum Nutrition
> Beta Carotene ....
> 25,000 IU
> Vitamin A (natural only) .... 25,000 IU
> Vitamin C ....
> .... 5-10 grams
> Vitamin E ....
> .... 400 IU extra
> Multi-Antioxidant Mix 400 mg 2 or 3 times per day

Pregnancy

The period of pregnancy lasts about 280 days, and

for most women, this is a happy time with very little complication. The most common problems during pregnancy are morning sickness, indigestion, hemorrhoids, edema and hemorrhage. These are addressed in the following protocol.

Full Spectrum Nutrition

Ginger Root (morning sickness) .... 3-5 capsules 3or 4 times per day
Increase Fiber ...... 10 grams per day
Exercise (walking) ..... 1 mile per day
Essential Fatty Acids ....
.... 2 grams extra
Vitamin K .... 100 mg per day
Folic Acid ..... 400 mcg extra per day
Potassium ....
.... 100 mg 2 times per day
Iron .... 10-14 mg extra
Protein ....
.... 100 grams per day minimum

Note: a lack of protein is the main cause of toxemia of pregnancy, especially during the last trimester.

Pregnancy Toxemia – (See also Pregnancy)

Usually occurring during the last trimester, this is almost often caused by a lack of protein in the diet. The typical symptom is edema of the hands and feet.

> **Full Spectrum Nutrition**
> Protein........ 100-150 grams per day
> Liquid Amino Acids .... per label
> Vitamin B6.......................................
> 25 –50 mg per day (stop after birth)
> Water .... 64 or more oz per day

Premenstrual Syndrome

PMS is another disorder of the hormone balance of the body and, oddly enough, is related to and shares many of the same causes as symptoms of the menopause. Typical effects of PMS include headaches, bloating, backache, breast swelling, fatigue, irritability, and emotional outbursts, which can be severe enough to produce anger, violence, and even thoughts of suicide. In the past, doctors thought that women with these symptoms were psychotic and recommended either psychopharmacology or that they be institutionalized. Thankfully, today we realize that these symptoms are not only very real but they have a biochemical origin as well. This means that they can be effectively treated with diet and nutritional supplements.

> **Full Spectrum Nutrition**
> Progesterone Cream .... per label
> Calcium .... 1500 mg
> Magnesium....................... 1000 mg

Vitamin B 6 ....
.... 50 mg 3 times per day
Essential Fatty Acids ....
.... 4-6 grams per day
High potency Stress B-Complex .....
.... 4 capsules 2 times per day
Corn silk ....
.... 2 capsules 3 times per day
Gingko biloba .... 150 mg per day
Vitamin A (natural only) ....
.... 100,000 to 200,000 IU per day
Tyrosine ....
.... 3-6 grams per day in the morning
Choline .... 200 mg
Inositol .... 1000 – 1500 mg
GABA .... 500 – 2000 mg per day
Black cohosh ....
.... 25 mg 2 times per day
DHEA .... 20 mg per day

Prostatitis – See Chapter 9

Prostate Enlargement – See Chapter 9
Psoriasis

This condition, often hereditary, is the result of an over replication of the cells in the outer layer of the skin. Most often it is a lack of fats and fatty acids in the diet. For example, a prolonged very low fat diet can induce this condition.

Full Spectrum Nutrition

Essential Fatty Acids ....
.... 2-6 grams per day
Multi-Enzymes ....
.... as needed per meal
Vitamin A (from fish liver oil) ....
.... 50,000 –100,000 IU
Vitamin B12 .... 500 –1000 mcg
Selenium .... 200 mcg extra
Hypoallergenic cream with selenium
apply topically 2or 3 times per day
Capsaicin .... per label
Sarsaparilla .... per label
Milk Thistle .... 200 mg
Lecithin Capsules ....
.... 2 capsules with each meal

Rule out the possibility of food allergies by taking a RAST blood test.
Also, test for a lack of hydrochloric
acid in the stomach by taking a pH
test.

Puppura – See Peripheral Vascular Disease

Raynaud's Disease – See Peripheral Vascular Disease

Restless Leg Syndrome

This is a symptom of nervousness or inner stress that is not managed. See recommendations under stress management as well.

Full Spectrum Nutrition
Folic Acid... 50 mcg 3 times per day
Calcium .... 1500 mg
Magnesium .... 800 mg
Vitamin E .... 400 IU extra
Iron .... 10 mg
L-Tryptophan (if you can find it) or 5-hydroxy Tryptophan (5-HTP) per label
High Potency Stress B-Complex ....
...... 4 capsules 2 or 3 times per day

Retinopathy – See Macular Degeneration

Rheumatic Fever – See Immunodepression

Rheumatism – See also Arthritis

An inflammatory disorder of joints and connective tissue, rheumatism can be very painful and debilitating.

Full Spectrum Nutrition
Vitamin B1 .... 200 mg per day

Vitamin B6... 50 mg 3 times per day
Vitamin E ....400-800 IU
Copper ....2-3 mg per day
5-hydroxy Tryptophan .... per label
Selenium .... 200 mcg extra
Magnesium........................ 800 mg

Be sure to rule out the possibility of food allergies by taking a RAST blood test.

Rheumatoid Arthritis – See Also Arthritis

This is an autoimmune disease, which results in the destruction of cartilage and connective tissues due to over-activity of the immune system. As with all autoimmune conditions, do not use any immune stimulants of any kind.

Full Spectrum Nutrition
Chicken Cartilage ....
.... Double the label suggestion
Bromelain ....
1000 mg for 60 days then 500 mg thereafter
Liquid Oxygen........... 2-3 oz per day
Take on an empty stomach
MSM (organic sulfur)........ per label
Follow arthritis protocol listed under Arthritis

Capsaicin .... per label
Devils claw .... per label
Feverfew .... per label
Ginger Root extract .... per label
Pantothenic Acid ....
.... 500 mg 4 times per day
Vitamin A .... 25,000 IU
Vitamin C .... to bowel tolerance
Copper salicylate ....
.... 1-3 tablets per day
For 10 days only
Colloidal Gold .... per label
L-Histidine ....
.... 1000 mg 2 or 3 times per day
Essential Fatty Acids ...... 2-6 grams
Quercitin .... 200 mg per day
Bromelain ....
...... 2 capsules 3 or 4 times per day
Rule out the possibility of food allergies by taking a RAST allergy test. Also, ensure adequate hydrochloric acid in stomach. To check your acid/alkaline levels take a pH test.

Scleroderma

A rare autoimmune disease affecting the blood vessels and connective tissue of the body. The disease produces fibrous degeneration of the connective tissue of the skin, lungs, and internal organs. Most of the cases of scleroderma occur in middle aged females.

Full Spectrum Nutrition

Bromelain .... 150 –500 mg 3 times per day

Gotu kola ..... twice label suggestion

Vitamin E ...... 800 IU with each meal Decrease to a total of 1600 IU after a week

Then down to 800 IU after two weeks

Essential Fatty Acids .... 4-6 grams per day

Para-amino Benzoic Acid .... 4 grams 2 or 3 times per day

Bovine Cartilage .... 6-12 capsules per day

Seborrhea – See Seborrheic Dermatitis

Seborrheic Dermatitis

This condition is caused by a malfunction of the sebaceous glands, which secrete oil. The most likely spots for flair ups to occur are on the scalp, face, or chest, but can occur anywhere on the skin. This condition is frequently caused by a combination of vitamin A and essential fatty acid deficiencies.

Full Spectrum Nutrition

Essential Fatty Acids .... 4-8 grams per day

Vitamin A (from fish liver oil) .... 50,000 IU

Vitamin E .... 400-800 IU extra

Folic Acid.................... 2 mg per day

Vitamin B12 ....500 mcg 3 times per day under tongue

Selenium .... 200 mcg extra

Lithium .... per physicians instruction

Be sure and rule out the possibility of a hydrochloric acid deficiency in the stomach. Take a pH test to determine your acid/alkaline levels.

Senility (Senile Dementia)

Senility is really a very rare disorder, most often affecting the elderly. Many times this condition is misdiagnosed and really turns out to be something else such as nutrient deficiencies due to mal-absorption, drug overdose, depression, thyroid deficiency, and liver or kidney disorders.

Full Spectrum Nutrition

Multi Enzymes with HCl .... 2-4 with each meal

Protein.....at least 60 grams per day
High Potency B-Complex...............
.... 100 mg 3 times per day
Vitamin B12............2,000 mcg daily
Choline..
.... 1000 mg 2 or 3 times per day
Niacin ..... 25-50 mg 3 times per day
Antioxidant Multi Formula ....
.... 400 –1200 mg per day

Shingles – See Herpes Zoster

Sinusitis

An inflammation and infection of the sinuses, sinusitis is most often the result of either a respiratory infection or repeated irritation from airborne allergies. Symptoms of this condition include loss of the sense of smell, pain and tenderness in the face, fever, headache, earache, and toothache. If the cause is another infection, treatment of both is essential. (Use the Immunodepression program.)

Full Spectrum Nutrition
Vitamin A (from fish liver oil) ....
.... 25,000 –100,000 + IU per day
Vitamin C .... 2-4 grams

Skin Cancer – See also Cancer

Over-exposure to radiation, primarily from the sun, is the biggest single cause of most skin cancers. The lighter your skin, the more likely you will develop skin cancer due to over-exposure to sunlight. It is essential to use a sun screen and limit your exposure to the sun if you are fair skinned, since you have minimal protective pigmentation.

Full Spectrum Nutrition
Multi Anti-oxidants .... 400 –1600 mg per day
DMG .... per label

Liquid Oxygen................................. 1 oz 3 or 4 times per day on empty stomach
Essential Fatty Acids .... 2 grams with each meal
Germanium............. 200 mg per day
Coenzyme Q10 ...... 100 mg per day
Selenium .... 200 mcg extra
Vitamin A (from fish liver oil) .... 50,000 –100,000 IU per day
Vitamin E .... 800 –1000 IU

Sore Throat – See Immunodepression

Spasmodic Colon – See Colitis

Sports Injuries

Most sports related injuries involve soft tissues, bones and connective tissue, or both. Healing of these types of injuries may be accelerated by aggressive nutrition with an emphasis upon liquid organic mineral compounds.

Full Spectrum Nutrition

Liquid Organic Source Trace Minerals .... 3-5 oz per day
Vitamin C .... 3-6 grams
Bioflavonoids .... 2-4 grams
Coenzyme Q10 ...... 100 mg per day
Glucosamine Sulfate ....
.... 400 mg 2 times per day
Bromelain ....
.... 200-400 mg 3 times per day
On an empty stomach

Stress and Anxiety

Excess stress is almost a given in today's society. Each of us is trying to cram 90 minutes into every hour, resulting in stress related illnesses including anxiety, mood swings, aggressive behavior, and depression. Nutrition can play an important role in managing stress from the physical angle but stress management from the mental or emotional side is also essential.

Full Spectrum Nutrition
Vitamin C .... to bowel tolerance
Vitamin B12 ....
.... 500 mcg 3 times per day
Pantothenic Acid ....
.... 1000-2000 mg per day
Adrenal Glandular Extract ....
..............2-4 tablets 3 times per day
Calcium .... 1500-2000 mg per day
Magnesium.... 800-1000 mg per day

Stroke

A stroke, or cerebral hemorrhage, is caused by the rupturing of a blood vessel in the brain and is a common source of debilitation and death. The most common cause of this condition is elevated blood pressure. The best treatment for stroke is prevention by keeping blood pressure down and managing stress effectively. If you have had a stroke, it is essential that you get the right treatment as soon as possible. Hyperbaric oxygen treatments are one of the best methods of helping restore brain function.

Full Spectrum Nutrition
Vitamin E ....400-1200 IU
Essential Fatty Acids ...... 3-6 grams
Multi-Antioxidant Mix ....
.... 800 –1200 mg per day

Liquid Oxygen ....
. 1 oz 3 or 4 times per day on empty
stomach

Sunburn

Overexposure to the sun can lead to painful burning of the upper layers of the skin. If you are fair skinned, it is important to limit your exposure to the sun and stay completely out of the sun during peek radiation periods, which are from 10 AM until 2 PM.

Full Spectrum Nutrition
Liquid Organic Source Trace Minerals .... 1 oz 2 or 3 times per day
Apply liquid trace minerals topically to burned area 2 or 3 times per day
Vitamin C .... 3-4 grams
Vitamin A .... 25,000 IU
Vitamin E .... 400 IU extra
Apply vitamin E directly on skin once or twice per day
Aloe Vera Gel ....
.... apply as needed to skin

Temperomandibular Joint Syndrome (TMJ)

This common condition affects over 20 million people worldwide. The causes of TMJ are poor bite, grinding of teeth, and stress. If you are under more stress than you can manage, you must consider dealing with this issue independently of the following protocol.

> ## Full Spectrum Nutrition
> Calcium .... 2000 mg
> Magnesium.....................................
> .... 1500 mg in divided doses
> Stress B-Complex ....
> .... 2-4 capsules 2or 3 times per day
> Co Enzyme Q10 ....
> .... 30 mg 3 times per day
> L-Tyrosine......................................
> .... 500-1000 mg on empty stomach
> 1 hour before bed
> Vitamin C ....1000 mg extra
> Vitamin B6.....................................
> ....25 mg taken with the Tyrosine

Tendon Problems – See Sports Injuries

Tendinitis – See Inflammation

Thrombophlebitis – See Peripheral Vascular Disease

Thrush – See Candidiasis

Thyroid – See either Hyperthyroid (over-active) or Hypothyroid (underactive)

Tinnitus

This condition of the middle ear causes a ringing in the ears, which may be anything from barely noticeable to almost deafening. It can be caused by repeated or prolonged acoustic trauma, Meniere's disease, otosclerosis, or some physiological blockage to the ear passages.

Full Spectrum Nutrition

Essential Fatty Acids .... 2-4 grams per day
Vitamin A (natural only).... 25,000 IU
Zinc .... 50 mg
Calcium .... 1500 mg
Magnesium......................... 700 mg
Potassium .... 100 mg

It is important to reduce refined carbohydrates and sugars from the diet. Also, rule out the possibility of any allergies by taking a RAST blood test.

Tonsillitis – See Immunodepression

Toxicity – See Heavy Metal Poisoning

Triglycerides Elevated

Excess triglycerides, unlike cholesterol, are caused by a combination of the over-consumption of sugar and refined carbohydrates and a lack of activity or exercise. Reduce sugar and sugar forming foods in the diet and exercise at least three times per week for 30 minutes each time.

Full Spectrum Nutrition
Essential Fatty Acids ....
.... 2-4 grams per day
Chromium.................. 200-400 mcg
Vanadium .... 500+ mcg per day
Aspartic Acid .... 300 mg per day
Selenium .... 500 mcg
Vitamin C .... to bowel tolerance

Tuberculosis – See Immunodepression

Ulcers, Stomach & Duodenal (See also Indigestion)

Ulcers of the stomach and duodenum are caused by an imbalance in the pH of the organ. When the pH of the stomach becomes alkaline, it compromises the integrity of the stomach lining. When bacteria are present in an alkaline stomach environment, the tissues of that organ are highly susceptible to infection since the bacteria cannot be effectively killed off. Once an ulcer has formed, even the smallest amount of naturally occurring stomach acid will irritate the open sore.

Full Spectrum Nutrition

Vitamin A (from fish liver oil) ....
.... 100,000 – 200,000 IU
Bioflavonoids .... 2 –3 grams per day
Multi-enzyme without HCl ....
.... 2- 4 with each meal
Vitamin B6 ....
.... 100 mg per day during healing
Zinc .... 50 mg per day
Vitamin B12 ....
.......500 mcg per day during healing
Gamma oryzanol.............................
.....................500-1000 mg per day
Glutamine .... 1000-3000 mg
Pantethine .... 500-1000 mg
Licorice Root ....
.... 1-2 caps with each meal
Cat's claw extract ....
.... 1-2 caps with each meal

Rule out the possibility of food allergies by taking a RAST blood test.

Urinary Tract Infections – See Kidney and Bladder Infections

Urticaria – See also allergies

Also known as hives, this is a serious skin rash caused by an allergic reaction to a variety of substances, but most often foods are responsible. The best treatment is identifying and avoiding the offending substances. The use of antihistamines is frequently required.

Full Spectrum Nutrition
Beta Carotene .... 20,000 IU
Niacin ... 25 mg 2 or 3 times per day
Vitamin B12 ....
 200 mcg sublingual 3 times per day
Magnesium .... 500 mg extra

Rule out the possibility of food allergies by taking a RAST blood test.

Vaginitis

This condition is most often caused by a bacteria or yeast infection. Other causes may be excessive douching or a nutrient deficiency. Symptoms include burning and itching along with a vaginal discharge. Antibiotic abuse can also lead to this condition.

Full Spectrum Nutrition
Multi-Acidophilus ....
10 capsules per day for 10 days on

empty stomach
Liquid Oxygen.....................................
.. 1 ounce 3 times per day on empty
stomach
Garlic Capsules ....
.... 2 capsules with each meal
Essential Fatty Acids ....
.... 2-4 grams per day
High Potency B-Complex... 50 mg 2
times per day

Varicose Veins – See Peripheral Vascular Disease

Vasculitis – See Peripheral Vascular Disease

Venous Insufficiency – See Peripheral Vascular Disease

Vericose Veins – See Peripheral Vascular Disease

Vertigo – See Inner Ear Dysfunction

Extreme dizziness, vertigo is usually the result of an inner ear dysfunction.

Viral Infections – See Immunodepression

Vitiligo

This is a skin condition, identified by white patches, which is caused by a loss of melanin or skin pigment in the area. Sometimes thyroid problems can be at the heart of this problem and should be considered.

Full Spectrum Nutrition
Para-amino Benzoic Acid (PABA)....
.... 100-200 mg 3 times per day
Pantothenic Acid ....
.... 200 mg 2 times per day
Essential Fatty Acids ...... 2-4 grams
Copper .... 2 mg per day
L-Phenylalanine* ....
.... 500 mg 2 times per day
*Note: Do not use if you have uncontrolled high blood pressure.
Vitamin C .... 2-4 grams per day
High Potency Stress B-Complex ....
.... 2 capsules 2 times per day

Weakened Immune System – See Immunodepression

Worms

These are a variety of parasites that live in the gastrointestinal tract. They are most common in children.

Full Spectrum Nutrition
Garlic Capsules ....
2 capsules 3 times per day with meals
Liquid Oxygen................................
.... _ to 1 oz 3 or 4 times per day
on an empty stomach
Pumpkin Extract................ per label

Wound Healing

Slow wound healing can be the result of a deficient immune system or the side effect of chronic diseases such as diabetes. If the immune system is depressed, follow the protocol under Immunodepression as well as the following.

Full Spectrum Nutrition
Aloe Vera .... apply topically
Bromelain .. 100 mg 3 times per day
Gotu kola .... per label
Vitamin A..
.... 10,000 – 25, 000 IU per day
Vitamin C .... 2-3 grams
Zinc .... 50 mg
Essential Fatty Acids ...... 2-4 grams

Yeast Infection – See Candidiasis

Conclusion

The field of nutrition, like few other areas of science, is changing almost by the day. What we know today can change the course of human health and longevity, yet it will be dwarfed by how much we will know in just a few years from now.

One of the truly final frontiers here on Earth is the vast complex chemical laboratory known as the human body. Its ability to adapt and change is phenomenal, its wisdom immense. Yet in spite of this adaptability, we have pushed the internal body rhythms so far out of balance that disease and deterioration has been the result.

We now hold in our hands, the ability to dramatically extend the human life span. Those born today will have a better than 70 percent chance of living well past 100 years of age, but at what price?

In order to enjoy the extended years, we must also have the quality of life as well. What value is living an extra 20 or 30 years if they will be spent in compromised health? What value is aging if we must spend that extra time at doctor's offices, therapy sessions, or in repeated convalescence? If I invented a magic pill that could automatically and assuredly extend everyone's life by an extra ten years, would everyone want it? Suppose I took my discovery to the local convalescent home where the majority of residents have lost 90 percent of their body functions. Do you think that they would be thrilled at the idea of taking my magic pill so that they could spend another decade in that miserable state? Surely they would not be.

Quality and quantity must go hand in hand. The threshold of genetic understanding at which science currently stands will provide the quantity, but nutrition and a greater responsibility for our own lifestyle will provide the quality – or lack thereof.

When we buy a new car or the latest piece of electronic wizardry almost invariably we also buy a maintenance plan to go with it. We would never think of paying $30,000 for a new car and then simply driving it into the ground. No, we have the maintenance schedule clearly posted on the inside of the car door and we know when the oil must be changed and the tires rotated. Yet the most prized possession that each of us has is this human body of ours, and we rarely look after it half as much as we do our new car. We have come to believe that the body will just run and run no matter what we do to it. We seem to think that we can feed it junk food, work two or more jobs, get less sleep than we need, and pile insurmountable stress on top of everything else with no ill effect. In fact, we are often amazed and shocked when we finally develop a chronic degenerative disease. We ask, "Why me?" A better question would be to ask and marvel as to how the body was able to somehow prevent these illnesses for so long. When we finally develop a chronic degenerative disease we have probably been working on its development for years or even decades of time.

Life is about choices. We must make them every-day and these choices affect our lives in countless ways. The choices we make about our health can either add or detract from the quality of our remaining life.

The late George Bernard Shaw once said, to the effect, that a human life could be divided into three parts. The first third of our life is made up of what we were born with, our genetics, our families, etc. The second third of our life is what we have made of it, our education, our jobs, whether we have a family of our own, etc. The last third of our life is what we deserve! This last third will be determined by how we have lived the first two thirds of our life.

What does the future hold for humanity? The answer to that question is vast. We do know that our knowledge of genetics will eliminate many devastating diseases. Illnesses like cancer, heart disease, and many others will likely be history within the next 50 years, but they will likely be replaced by other health challenges we haven't yet realized.

Regardless of how advanced science becomes, we as individuals will always have to take responsibility for our own lives and our own health through the choices we make. Wise choices can only be made through knowledge. Even though our knowledge will grow with each passing year, we owe it to ourselves to utilize what we have today. Live, love, and be happy. Enjoy your life, it's everyone's birthright. Provide yourself with true health insurance, not merely disease insurance. Ensure that the chemicals of life, called nutrients, are available to the master chemical laboratory of your body on a daily basis, and you will be in the best possible position to both heal and maintain your wellbeing.

This book represents much of the body of knowledge that I have learned and taught for the last 27 years. Now that you have read it, use it wisely and let it enrich your life.

References

Chapter 1

1. Study finds NSAIDS often prescribed unnecessarily for elderly patients. Annals of Internal Medicine, Sept. 1997
2. Wicox, S., et al. Inappropriate drug prescribing for the community-dwelling elderly JAMA July 1994
3. Avorn, J., et al. Scientific versus commercial sources of influence on the prescribing behavior of physicians. American Journal of Medicine 73:4, 1982.
4. Heart Facts, Dallas Texas, American Heart Association 1985.
5. Chipponi. J. et al. Total parenteral nutrition often causes nutrient deficiencies. Am. J. Clin Nutr. May 1982 1112-1116.
6. Beecher, HK. Surgery as a placebo. JAMA 176:1102, 1961.
7. Steffee, W. Malnutrition in hospitalized patients JAMA 244:2630-2635, 1980.
8. Trubo, R. The Achilles' heel of medicine. Medical World News. January 1985, 127-135.
9. Presont, T. Bypass surgery: A placebo? MD Feb. 1985, 30-38.
10. Jacobs, Paul. Prescribing drugs: The hard sell. Los Angeles times December 29th, 1982.
11. Stamler J. Primary prevention of coronary heart disease: The last 20 years. Am J Cardiology. 47:722-735, 1981.
12. Williams, Roger J. Nutrition Against Disease, New York, Pitman Publishing Co. 1971.
13. Talley, R and Laventurier, MF., Drug-induced illness. JAMA 244: 2630-2635, 1980.

Chapter 2

1. Hertog M, et al. Dietary antioxidant flavonoids and risk of coronary heart disease: the Zutphen Elderly Study. Lancet 1993; 342: 1007-1011
2. Hertog M and Hollman PCH. Potential health effects of the dietary flavonol quercetin. Eur J Clin Nutr. 1996;50: 63-71
3. Agullo G, et al. Quercetin exerts a preferential cytotoxic effect on active dividing colon carcinoma HT29 and Caco-2 cells. Cancer Letters. 1994;87: 55-63
4. Singhal R, et al. Quercetin down-regulates signal transduction in human breast carcinoma cells. Biochemical and Biophysical Research Communications. 1995 208;1: 425 - 431
5. Hertog M, et al. Antioxidant flavonols and ischemic heart disease in a Welsh population of men: the Caerphilly Study. Am J Clin Nutr.

1997; 65: 1489-1494

6. Huk I, et al. Bioflavonoid quercetin scavenges superoxide and increases nitric oxide concentration in ischaemia-reperfusion injury: an experimental study. British Journal of Surgery 1998; 85:1080-1085

7. Muldoon MF and Kritchevsky SB. Editorial: Flavonoids and heart disease. BMJ. 1996; 312: 458-459

8. Fischer S, Mills G, and Slaga T. Inhibition of mouse skin tumor promotion by several inhibitors of arachidonic acid metabolism. Carcinogenesis 1982;3(11):1243-1245

9. Virgili F, Kobuchi H, and Packer L. Procyanidins extracted from pinus Maritima (Pycnogenol() Scavengers of free radical species and modulators of nitrogen monoxide metabolism in activated murine raw 264.7 macrophages. Free Rad Biol Med 1998;24(7/8): 1120-1129

10. Bagchi D, et al. Protective effects of grape seed proanthocyanidins and selected antioxidants against TPA-induced hepatic and brain lipid peroxidation and DNA fragmentation, and peritoneal Macrophage activation in mice. Gen. Pharmac. 1998;30(5): 771-776

11. Howard D, et al. Oxidative stress induced by environmental tobacco smoke in the workplace is mitigated by antioxidant supplementation. Ca Epidem Bio Prev 1998;7: 981-988

12. Pastori M, et al. Lycopene in association with a-Tocopherol inhibits at physiological concentrations proliferation of prostate carcinoma cells. Biochemical and Biophysical Research Communications 1998;250:582-585

13. De Flora S, Grassi C, and Carati L. Attenuation of influenza-like symptomatology and improvement of cell-mediated immunity with long-term N-acetylcysteine treatment. Eur Respir J. 1997;10:1535-1541

14. De Vries N, et al. N-Acetyl-l-Cysteine. Journal of Cellular Biochemistry 1993;Suppl 17F: 270-277

15. De Flora S, et al. Adducts to nuclear DNA and mitochondrial DNA as biomarkers in chemoprevention. Principles of Chemoprevention 1996;139: 291-301

16. Harrison PM, et al. Improved outcome of paracetamol-induced fulminant hepatic failure by late administration of acetylcysteine. Lancet 1990;335:1572-1573

17. Ruan E, et al. Glutathione levels in chronic inflammatory disorders of the human colon. Nutrition Research 1997; 17(3): 463-473

18. Izzotti A, et al. Chemoprevention of carcinogen-DNA adducts and chronic degenerative diseases. Cancer Research 1994 Suppl;54: 1994-1998

19. Millman M, et al. Use of Acetylcysteine in bronchial asthma- another look. Annals of Allergy 1985 54: 294-296.

20. De Mattia G, et al. Reduction of oxidative stress by oral N-acetyl-l-

cysteine treatment decreases plasma soluble vascular cell adhesion molecule-1 concentrations in non-obese, non-dyslipidaemic, normotensive, patients with non-insulin-dependent diabetes. Diabetologia 1998;41:1392-1396.

21. Shutenko Z, et al. Influence of the antioxidant quercetin in vivo on the level of nitric oxide determined by electron paramagnetic resonance in rat brain during global ischemia and reperfusion. Biochem Pharmocol. Jan, 1999;57(2):199-208

22. Laplaud PM, et al. Antioxidant action of Vaccinium myrtillus [Bilberry] extract on human low density lipoprotein in vitro: initial observations. Fundam Clin Pharmacol. 1997;11(1):35-40

23. Harman D. Role of free radicals in mutation, cancer, aging, and the maintenance of life. Radiation Res. 1962;16:753-763

24. Bomser J, In vitro anticancer activity of fruit extracts from Vaccinium species. Planta Med. Jun, 1996;62(3):212-6

25. Flora K, et al. Milk thistle (Silybum marianum) for the therapy of liver disease. Am J Gastroenterol. Feb, 1998;93(2):139-43

26. Katiyar SK, et al. Protective effects of silymarin against photocarcinogenesis in a mouse skin model. J Natl Cancer Inst. Apr 16, 1997;89(8):556-66

27. Basaga H, et al. Free radical scavenging and antioxidant properties of 'silibin' complexes on microsomal lipid peroxidation. Cell Biochem Funct. Mar 1997;15(1):27-33

28. Dehmlow C, et al. Scavenging of reactive oxygen species and inhibition of arachidonic acid metabolism by silibin in human cells. Life Sci. 1996;58(18):1591-600

29. Matthews RT, et al. Coenzyme Q10 administration increases brain mitochondrial concentrations and exerts neuroprotective effects. Proc Natl Acad Sci USA. Jul 1998;95(21):8892-7

30. Aejmelaeus R, et al. Ubiquinol-10 and total peroxyl radical trapping capacity of LDL lipoproteins during aging: the effects of Q-10 supplementation. Mol Aspects Med. 1997;18 Suppl:S113-20

31. Sinatra ST and DeMarco J. Free radicals, oxidative stress, oxidized low density lipoprotein (LDL), and the heart; antioxidants and other strategies to limit cardiovascular damage. Conn Med. Oct, 1995;59(10):579-88

32. Emonet-Piccardi N, et al. Protective effects of antioxidants against UVA-induced DNA damage in human skin fibroblasts in culture. Free Radic Res. Oct, 1998;29(4):307-13

33. Bagchi D, et al. Oxygen free radical scavenging abilities of vitamin C and E, and a grape seed proanthocyanidin extract in vitro. Res Commun Mol Pathol Pharmacol. Feb, 1997;95(2):179-89

34. Hussain S, et al. Role of metallothionein and other antioxidants in scavenging superoxide radicals and their possible role in neuroprotection. Neurochem Int. Aug, 1996;29(2):145-52

35. Lizard G, et al. Glutathione is implied in the control of 7-ketocholesterol-induced apoptosis, which is associated with radical oxygen species. FASEB J. Dec, 1998;12(15):1651-63

36. Obrador E, et al. Regulation of tumor cell sensitivity to TNF-induced oxidative stress and cytotoxicity:role of glutathione. Biofactors. 1998;8(1-2):23-6

37. Matsumoto K, N-acetylcysteine inhibits IL-1 alpha-induced IL-8 secretion by bronchial epithelial cells. Respir Med. Mar, 1998;92(3):512-5

38. Erkkila K, N-acetyl-L-cysteine inhibits apoptosis in human male germ cells in vitro. J Clin Endocrinol Metab. Jul, 1998;83(7):2523-31

39. Gillissen A and Nowak D. Characterization of N-acetylcysteine and ambroxol in anti-oxidant therapy. Respir Med. Apr, 1998;92(4):609-23

40. Kelly GS. Clinical applications of N-acetylcysteine. Altern Med Rev. Apr, 1998;3(2):114-27

41. Murray Michael. 5-HTP: The natural way to overcome depression, obesity, and insomnia. Bantam Books:New York;1998

42. Kohlmeier L, et al. Lycopene and myocardial infarction risk in the EURAMIC Study. Am J Epidemiol. Oct, 1997;146(8):618-26

43. Flatt A, et al. Reduced selenium in asthmatic subjects in New Zealand. Thorax. 1990;45:95-99

44. Scheef W. Combined Tumor Therapy:Basic Possibilities and Related Adjunctive Therapeutic Methods, 1995, Heinrich Wrba, ed,; Stuttgart:Hippocrates

45. Pastorino U, et al. Adjuvant treatment of stage I lung cancer with high-dose vitamin A. J Clin Oncol. Jul 1993;11(7):1204-7

46. Gensini GF, et al. Changes in fatty acid composition of the single platelet phospholipid induced by pantethine treatment. Int J Clin Pharmacol Res. 1985;5(5):309-18

47. Redman C, et al. Inhibitory effect of selenomethionine on the growth of three selected human tumor cell lines. Cancer Lett Mar 13, 1998;125(1-2):103-10

48. Rodier M, et al. Relationship between serum lipids, platelet membrane fatty acid composition and platelet aggregation in type 2 diabetes mellitus. Diabete Metab Nov-Dec, 1993;19(6):560-5

49. Melichar B, et al. Urinary zinc excretion and acute phase response in cancer patients. Clin Investig Dec 1994;72(12):1012-4

50. Combs GF, Clark LC, Turnbull BW. Reduction of cancer mortality and incidence by selenium supplementation. Med Klin Sep 15 1997;92Suppl(3): 42-5

51. Wood RJ and Zheng JJ. High dietary calcium intakes reduce zinc absorption and balance in humans. Am J Clin Nutr. Jun 1997;65(6):1803-9

52. Verhoef P, et al. Homocysteine metabolism and risk of myocardial

infarction: relation with vitamins B6, B12, and folate. Am J Epidemiol May 1996;143(9):845-59

53. Peretz AM, Neve JD, Famaey JP. Selenium in rheumatic diseases. Semin Arthritis Rheum Apr 1991;20(5):305-16

54. Prisco D, et al. Effect of oral treatment with pantethine in platelet and plasma phospholipids in Iia hyperlipoprotienemia. Angiology Mar 1987;38(3):241-7

55. Cohen M and Bhagavan HN. Ascorbic acid and gastrointestinal cancer. J Am Coll Nutr. Dec 1995;14(6):565-78

56. Kritchevsky SB, et al. Dietary antioxidants and carotid artery wall thickness. The ARIC Study. Atherosclerosis Risk in Communities Study. Circulation Oct 15 1995; 92(8):2142-50

57. Stephens NG. Randomized controlled trial of vitamin E in patients with coronary disease: Cambridge Antioxidant Study. Lancet Mar 23 996; 347(9004):781-6

58. Prasad AS, et al. Zinc status and serum testosterone levels of healthy adults. Nutrition May 1996;12(5):344-8

59. Paiva SA, et al. Assessment of vitamin A status in chronic obstructive pulmonary disease patients and healthy smokers. Am J Clin Nutr Dec 1996;64(6):928-34

60. Honnorat J, et al. Effects of diabetes type and treatment on zinc status in diabetes mellitus. Biol Trace Elem Res Jan-Mar 1992;32:311-6

61. Clark LC, et al. Effects of selenium supplementation for cancer prevention in patients with carcinoma of the skin. A randomized controlled trial. Nutritional Prevention of Cancer Study Group. JAMA Dec 25 1996; 276(24):1957-63

62. Gomot MJ, et al. Effect of acute zinc deficiency on insulin receptor binding in rat adipocytes. Biol Trace Elem Res Jan-Mar 1992;32:331-5

63. Boers GH. Hyperhomocysteinaemia: a newly recognized risk factor for vascular disease. Neth J Med Jul 1994;45(1):34-41

64. Solomons NW. Mild human zinc deficiency produces an imbalance between cell-mediated and humoral immunity. Nutr Rev Jan 1998;56(1 Pt 1):27-8

65. Beharka A, et al. Vitamin E status and immune function. Methods Enzymol 1997;282:247-63

66. Meydani SN, et al. Vitamin E supplementation and in vivo immune response in healthy elderly subjects. A randomized controlled trial. JAMA May 7 1997;277(17):1380-6

67. Noroozi M, Angerson WJ, Lean ME. Effects of flavonoids and vitamin C on oxidative DNA damage to human lymphocytes. Am J Clin Nutr Jun 1998;67(6):1210-8

68. De Whalley CV, et al. Flavonoids inhibit the oxidative modification of low density lipoproteins by macrophages. Biochem Pharmacol. 1990;39(11):1743-1750

69. Bohm F, et al. Beta-carotene with vitamins E and C offers synergistic cell protection against NOx. FEBS Letters. 1998;436:387-389

70. De la Fuente M, et al. Immune function in aged women is improved by ingestion of vitamins C and E. Can J Physiol Pharmacol. 1998;76:373-380

71. Heinonen OP, et al. Prostate cancer and supplementation with alpha-tocopherol and beta-carotene: incidence and mortality in a controlled trial. J Natl Cancer Inst. Mar 1998;18;90(6):440-6

72. Norozi M, et al. Effects of flavonoids and vitamin C on oxidative DNA damage to human lymphocytes. Am J Clin Nutr. 1998;67:1210-8

73. Siow RC, et al. Vitamin C protects human arterial smooth muscle cells against atherogenic lipoproteins: effects of antioxidant vitamins C and E on oxidized LDL-induced adaptive increases in cystine transport and glutathione. Arterioscler Thromb Vasc Biol. Oct 1998;18(10):1662-70

74. Campbell NR, et al. Effect of cysteine on the survival of mice with transplanted malignant thyoma. Nature Sep 13,1974;251:158

75. Bjorksten J. The crosslinkage theory of aging. J Am Geri Soc 1968;16(4):408-427

Chapter 3

1. Dortch S. American Weighs In. American Demographics. June 1997; 19-6

2. Obesity Research Center. A review of long-term studies evaluating the efficacy of weight loss in ameliorating disorders associated with obesity. Clin Ther. 1996 Nov-Dec. 18:6.

3. Reigler, E. Weight reduction by a high protein, low carbohydrate diet. Med Klin. Jun 1976: 71:24.

4. Burton, BJ, Foster WR. Human Nutrition. 4th Ed. McGraw Hill, 1988.

5. Kasper H. Dietetic treatment of obesity with low and high carbohydrate diets: Comparative studies and clinical results. Int J Obes. 1979; 3:3.

6. Manton, KG, et al. Estimates of change in chronic disability and institutionalization, incidence and prevalence rates in the United States elderly population from the 1992, 1984 and 1989 National Long-Term Care Surveys. Jour. Of Gerontology 48:S153.

7. Hermanson, B., et al. Beneficial six-year outcome of smoking cessation in older men and women with coronary artery disease. New England Journal of Medicine 319: 1365. 1988.

8. Higgins, MW., et al. Smoking and lung function in elderly men and women. JAMA, 269: 2741, 1993.

9. Seeman, T., et al. Predicting changes in physical functioning in a high-functioning elderly cohort: MacArthur studies of successful aging.

Journal of Gerontology. 49: M97, 1994.

10. Blair, SN., et al. How much physical activity is good for health? Annual Review of Public Health 13:99, 1992.

11. Breslow, L., and Belloc, N. Relationship of Physical Health Status and health practices. Preventive Medicine, 1, 1972; 409-421.

12. Cheraskin, E., et al. Eating habits of smokers and nonsmokers. Journal of the International Acadamy of Preventive Medicine, 2; 9-18, 1975.

13. Russell, MA and Feyerabend, C. Nicotine from other smokers. Lancet, Jan 1975.

14. Montagu, Ashley, The Endangered Environment. New York; mason and Lipscomb, 1974.

15. Brady, Edwards and Cluff. Drugs and the Elderly. In Drugs and the Elderly. Los Angeles: Ethel Percy Andrus Gerontlogy Center. (University of Southern California), 1973.

16. Iber, F. In alcoholism, the liver sets the pace. Nutrition Tody 6, 2-9, 1971.

17. DeVries, H. Exercise intensity threshold for improvement of cardiovascular-respiratory function in older men. Geriatrics, 26: 94-101, 1971.

Chapter 4

1. Diabetes In America 2nd ed. 1995.

2. American Diabetes Association "Diabetes Facts", 1997.

3. Decisions Resource, Inc. Waltham, MA; 1998.

4. The Arthritis Foundation 1998

5. The National Centers for Health Statistics: 1998

6. "Impact of CVD", National Center for Health Statistics 1998

7. Osteoporosis. NIH Consens Dev Conf. Consens Statement Online 1984, April 2-4; 5(3): 1-6, 1997.

8. National Osteoporosis Foundation, Washington DC, State by State Report 1997.

Chapter 5

1. Benditt, EP, University of Washington, School of Medicine. American Journal of Pathology 1974.

2. McGill, HC, The Geographic Pathology of Atherosclerosis. Laboratory Investigation. Vol 18, 5, May 1968

3. The Pathogenesis of Atherosclerosis. Edited by RW Wissler and JC Geer. The Williams & Wilkins Company, 1972.

4. Benditt, EP and Benditt, JM, Evidence For A MonoClonal Origin of Human Atherosclerotic Plaques. Proceedings of the National Academy of Sciences of the United States of America. Vol 70: (6) 1753-1756; June 1993.

5. Benditt, EP, Implications of the MonoClonal Character of Human Atherosclerotic Plaques. Beitrage zur Pathologie, Vol 158: (4) 405-416; 1976.

6. Yudkin, J Dietary Fat and Dietary Sugar in Relation to Ischemic Heart Disease and Diabetes. Lancet, 4-5; 1964.

7. Yudkin, J, Levels of Dietary Sucrose in Patients with Occlusive Atherosclerotic Disease. Lancet 6-8; 1964.

8. Yudkin, J, Diet and Coronary Thrombosis. Lancet 155-62, 1957.

9. Blankenhorn, DH, et al. The Influence of Diet on the appearance of New Lesions in Human Coronary Arteries. JAMA, 1990; 263: 1646-1652.

10. Witztum, JL, The Oxidation Hypothesis of Atherosclerosis. Lancet, 344: 793-5; 1994.

11. Scharts, CJ, et al. The Pathogenesis of Atherosclerosis: An Overview. Clin Cardiol 14(1): 1-16; 1991.

12. Ross, R. The Pathogenesis of Atherosclerosis - An Update. NEJM 314(8): 488-500; 1986.

13. Steinberg, D, et al. Beyond Cholesterol. NEJM, 320(14); 915-24; 1989.

14. Goodnight, SH, et al. Polyunsaturated Fatty Acids, Hyperlipidemia and Thrombosis. Arteriosclerosis. 2: 87-113; 1982.

15. Newbold, HL, Reducing the Serum Cholesterol Level With a Diet High in Animal Fat. Southern Med J. 81(1); 61-63; 1988.

16. Gorringe, JAL, Why Blame Butter?: A Discussion Paper. J Royal Soc Med, 79: 661-663; 1986.

17. Klurfeld, DM and Kritchevsky, D, The Western Diet: An Examination of its Relationship with Chronic Disease. J Am Coll Nutr, 5: 477-485; 1986.

18. Eaton, SB, et al. Stone Agers in the Fast Lane: Chronic Degenerative Diseases in Evolutionary Perspective. Am J Med, 84: 739-49; 1988.

19. Mensink, RP and Katan, MB, Effect of Monounsaturated Fatty Acids verses Complex Carbohydrates on High-Density Lipoprotein in Healthy Men and Women. Lancet, 122-5; 1987.

20. Ginsberg, H, et al. Induction of Hypertriglyceridemia by a Low-Fat Diet. J Clin Endocrinol Metab, 42: 729-35; 1976.

21. Leaf, DA, Omega-3 Fatty Acids and Coronary Artery Disease. Postgrad Med, 85(8); 237-42; 1989.

22. Mann, GV, et al. Journal of Atherosclerosis Research, 1964.

23. Ball, KP, et al. Lancet 1965.

24. Rose, GA. British Journal of Medicine 1965.

25. Malhorta, SL. American Journal of Atherosclerosis Research, 1964.

26. Hunter, JD. Atiu and Mitiaro Natives of Polynesia. Federation Proceedings, 21:36; 1962.

27. Cohen, AM. Jews Living in Yemen. American Heart Journal, 1963.

Chapter 6

1. Lowenstein & Preger. *Diabetes - New Look At An Old Problem*. Harper & Row

2. West & Kalbfleisch. Influence of Nutritional factors on Prevalence of Diabetes. *Diabetes*. 1971;20: 99-108

3. Yudkin, J. Dietary Fat and dietary sugar in relation to ischemic heart-disease and diabetes. Lancet. 1964; 4-5

4. Durrington, PN. Is insulin atherogenic? *Diabetic Medicine*. 1992; 9: 597-600

5. Yudkin, J. Medical problems from modern diet. *J Royal Coll of Physicians of London*. 1975; 9(2): 161-164

6. Allred, JB. Too Much of A Good Thing? *J Amer Dietetic Assoc*. 1995; 95(4): 417-418

7. Cohen, MP, et al. High Prevalence of Diabetes in Young Adult Ethiopian Immigrants to Israel. *Diabetes*. 1988; 37: 824-828

8. Paolisso, G. et al. Pharmacologic Doses of Vitamin E Improve Insulin Action in Healthy Subjects and Non-insulin-dependent Diabetic Patients. *Am J Clin Nutr*. 1993; 57: 650-656

9. Urberg, M. And Zemel, MB. Evidence for Synergism Between Chromium and Nicotinic Acid in the Control of Glucose Tolerance in Elderly Humans. *Metabolism*.1987; 36(9): 896-899

10. Moan, A, et al. Mental Stress Increases Glucose Uptake During Hyperinsulinemia: Associations with Sympathetic and Cardiovascular Responsiveness. *Metabolism*. 1995; 44(10): 1303-1307

11. Nicholson, AL, and Yudkin, J. The Nutritional Value of the Low-Carbohydrate Diet Used in the Treatment of Obesity. *Proc Nutr Soc*. 1968; 28(1):13 A

12. Klurfeld, DM and Kritchevsky, D. The Western Diet: An Examination of its Relationship With Chronic Disease. *J Am Coll Nutr*. 1986; 5: 477-485

13. Mouratoff, GJ and Scott, EM. Diabetes Mellitus in Eskimos After a Decade. *JAMA*. 1973; 226(11): 1345-1346

14. O'Dea, K. Westernisation, Insulin Resistance and Diabetes in Australian Aborigines. *Med J Aust*. 1991; 155: 258-264

15. Yudkin, J. Evolutionary and Historical Changes in Dietary Carbohydrates. *Am J Clin Nutr*. 1967; 20(2): 108-115

16. Garg, A, et al. Effects of Varying Carbohydrate Content of Diet in Patients with Non-insulin-dependent Diabetes Mellitus. *JAMA*. 1994; 271(18): 1421-1428

17. Cahill, GF and Boston, MD. Physiology of Insulin in Man. *Diabetes*. 1971; 20(12): 785-799

18. Hollenbeck, CB and Coulston, AM. Effects of Dietary Carbohydrate and Fat Intake on Glucose and Lipoprotein Metabolism in Individuals with Diabetes Mellitus. *Diabetes Care*. 1991; 14: 744-785

19. Chen, YD, et al. Why do Low-fat High-carbohydrate Diets Accentuate Postprandial Lipemia in Patients with NIDDM? *Diabetes Care.*1995; 18(1): 10-16

20. Farquhar, JW, et al. Glucose Insulin and Triglyceride Responses to High and Low Carbohydrate Diets in Man. *J Clin Invest.* 1966; 45(10): 1648-1656

21. Zimmet, PZ. Hyperinsulinemia - How Innocent a Bystander. *Diabetes Care.* 1993;16(3): 56-70

Chapter 7

1.Sperling, RI et al. Arthritis and Rheumatism 25: 133 (1983)

2. Lee, TH, et al. New Eng. J Med 312 (19) 1217-24, May 1985.

3. Kremer, J et al, Clin Res. 33: A778, 1985.

4. McCormick, JN et al, Lancet 2:508, 1977

5. Aaseth, J, et al, Selenium In Biology and Medicine May 1980.

6. McKenzie, LS, et al, Osteoarthrosis: Uncertain Rationale for Anti-inflammatory Drug Therapy. Lancet 1:908-909, 1976.

7. Vidal y Plana, RR, et al, Articular Cartilage Pharmacology: In Vitro Studies on Glucosamine and Non-steroidal Anti-inflammatory Drugs. Pharmacological Research Communications. 10(6): 557-569, 1978.

8. Arthritis Information: Osteoarthritis. Atlanta, GA. The Arthritis Foundation, Brochure No. 4040, May 1995.

9. Liang MH and Fortin, P, Management of Osteoarthritis of the Hip and Knee. JAMA 325(2): 125-127, 1991.

10. Mueller-Fabbender, H, et al. Glucosamine Sulfate Compared to Ibuprofen in Osteoarthritis of the Knee. Osteoarthritis andCartilage 2:61 - 69, 1994.

11. Crolle, G and D'Este, E. Glucosamine Sulphate for the Management ofarthosis: A Controlled Clinical Investigation. Current Medical Research and Opinion 7(2): 104-109, 1980.

12. Tapadinhas, MJ, et al, Oral Glucosamine Sulphate in the Management of Arthosis: Report on a Multi-centre Open Investigation in Portugal. Pharmatherapeutica. 3(3): 157-168, 1982.

13. Piptone, VR, Chondroprotection with Chondroitin Sulfate. Drugs in Experimental and Clinical Research 17(1): 3-7, 1991.

14.Mazieres, B, et al. Le Chondroitin Sulfate Dayns le Traitement de la Gonarthrose et de la Coxarthrose. Rev. Rheum Mal Osteoartic 59(7-8): 466-472, 1992.

15.Kerzberg, EM, et al. Combination of Glycosaminoglycans and Acetylsalicylic Acid in Knee Osteoarthrosis. Scandinavian Journal of Rheumatology.

16. Gay, G. Another Side Effect of NSAIDs. JAMA 264(20): 2677-2678, Nov. 1990.

17. Sandler, DP. Analgesic Use and Chronic Renal Disease. New Eng. J. Med. 320: 1238-1243, 1989.
18. Fredericks, Carlton; Arthritis: Don't Learn to Live With It, Grosset & Dunlap, New York. 1981.
19. Charnot, A, et al, Ann. Endocrinol. 32:397, 1971.

Chapter 8

1. Adlercreutz, H., et al. Soybean phytoestrogen intake and cancer risk. J. Nutrition 125:757-770.
2. Adlercreutz H., Mazur W. Phytoestrogens and western diseases. Annuals Med 29: 95-120 1997.
3. Blatt MHG., et al. Vitamin E and climacteric syndrome: Failure of effective control as measured by menopausal index. Arch Intern Med 91:792-9, 1953.
4. Finkler, RS. The effect of vitamin E in the menopause. J Clin Endocrinol Metab 9: 89-94, 1949.
5. Clemetson, CAB, et al. Capillary strength and the menstrual cycle. Ann N Y Acad Sci 93: 277-300, 1962.
6. Smith, CJ. Non-hormonal control of vaso-motor flushing in menopausal patients. Chic Med 67(5): 193-5, 1964.
7. Miksicek RJ. Interaction of naturally occurring nonsteroidal estrogens with expressed recombinant human estrogen receptor. Journal of Steroid Biochemistry and Molecular Biology. 49: 153-160, 1994.
8. Joannou, GE., et al. A urinary profile study of dietary phytoestrogens. The identification and mode of metabolism of new isoflavonoids. J Steroid Bio and Molecular Biology, 54: 167-184, 1995.
9. Ingram D., et al. Case control study of phyto-oestrogens an breast cancer. Lancet, 350: 990-994, 1997.
10. Cassidy, A., et al. Biological effects of a diet of soy protein rich in isoflavones on the menstrual cycle of premenopausal women. Am J Clin Nutr. 60: 333-340, 1994.
11. Horoschak, A., Nocturnal leg cramps, easy bruisability and epistaxis in menopausal patients: Treated with hesperidin and ascorbic acid. Del State Med J. January 1959, pp. 19-22.
12. Wilcox G., et al. Oestrogenic effects of plant foods in postmenopausal women. Br Med J 301:905-6, 1990.
13. Thompson J. et al. Relationship between nocturnal plasma oestrogen concentration and free plasma tryptophan in perimenopausal women. J Endocrinol 72(3): 395-6, 1977.
14. Duker EM, et al. Effects of extracts from Cimicifuga racemosa on gonadotropin release in menopause women and ovariectomized rats. Plant Med 57(5): 420-4, 1991.
15. Zhy DPQ. Dong quai. Am J Chin Med 15(3-4): 117-25, 1987.

16. Costello CH, Lynn, EV. Estrogenic substances from plants: I. Glycyrrhiza. J Am Pharm Soc 39: 177-80, 1950.
17. Kumagai, A. et al. Effect of glycyrrhizin on estrogen action. Endocrinol Japan 14: 34-8, 1967.
18. Kaldas Rs, Hughes, CL. Reproductive and general metabolic effects of phytoestrogens in mammals. Reprod Toxicol 3: 81-9, 1989.
19. Rose, DP. Dietary fiber, phytoestrogens, and breast cancer. Nutrition 8: 47-51, 1992.
20. Messina, M., Barnes, S. The roles of soy products in reducing risk of cancer. J Natl Cancer Inst. 83: 541-6, 1991.

Chapter 9

1.Braeckman, J, The extract of Serenoa Repens in the Treatment of Benign Prostatic Hyperplasia: a Multi center Open Study. Current Therapeutic Research, July 1994; 55: 776-85.
2. Carroll, KK and Khor, HT, Dietary Fat in Relation to Tumorigeneses. Prog. Biochem Pharmacol., 1975; 10: 308-53.
3. Carrilla E, et al, Binding of Permixon, a new treatment for prostatic benign hyperplasia, to the cytosolic androgen receptor in the rat prostate. J Steroid Biochem 1984; 20: 521-23.
4. Champault, G, et al, A Double-Blind Trial of an Extract of the Plant Serenoa Repens in benign Prostatic Hyperplasia. British Journal of Clinical Pharmacology, 1984; 18: 461-62.
5. Wynder EL, et al. Nutrition and prostate cancer: a proposal for dietary intervention. Natr Cancer. 1994; 22: 1-10.
6. Pusateri, DJ et al. Dietary and Hormonal Evaluation of Men at Different Risks for Prostate Cancer, Plasma and Fecal Hormone - Nutrient Interrelationships. Am J Clin Nutr. 1990; 51: 371-77.
7. Vitramo J, and Huttunen, J. Vitamin A and Prostatic Cancer. Ann Med. 1992; 24: 143-44.
8. Marchand L, et al. Vegetable and Fruit Consumption in Relation to Prostate Cancer Risk in Hawaii: a Reevaluation of the Effect of Dietary Beta-Carotene. Am J Epidemiol. 1991; 133: 215-19.
9. Oshi K, et al. A Case-Control Study of Prostatic Cancer with Reference to Dietary Habits. Prostate 12: 179-90. 1988.
10. Carter JP, et al. Hypothesis: Dietary Management May Improve Survival from Nutritional Linked Cancers Based on Analysis of Representative Cases. J Am Coll Nutr. 3: 209-29. 1993.
11. Dumrau, F., Benign Prostatic Hyperplasia: Amino Acid Therapy for Symptomatic Relief. American Journal of Geriatrics, 1962; 10: 426-30.
12. Lu-Yao, GL, et al. An Assessment of Radical Prostatectomy. JAMA, 1993; 269 (20) 2633 - 36.
13. Tripoli, V. Et al. Treatment of Prostatic Hypertrophy with Serenoa

Repens Extract. Med Praxis, 1983; 4: 41-46.

14. Rhodes, L et al. Comparison of Finasteride (Proscar), a 5-alpha-reductase Inhibitor and Various Commercial Plant Extracts in Vitro and in Vivo 5-Alpha-reductase Inhibition. The Prostate 1993; 22: 43-51.

15. Johansson, JE, et al. Natural History of Localized Prostatic Cancer. Lancet, 1989; 799-803.

16. Flemming , C, et al. A Decision Analysis of Alternative Treatment Strategies for Clinically Localized Prostate Cancer. JAMA 1993; 269 (20): 2650-58

17. Tasca A, et al. Treatment of Obstructive Symptomology Caused by Prostatic Adenoma with an Extract of Serenoa repens. Double-blind Clinical Study vs Placebo. Minerva Urol Nefrol 1985; 37: 87-97.

18. Mattei FM, et al. Serenoa repens extract in the Medical Treatment of Benign Prostatic Hypertrophy. Urologia 1988; 55: 547-52.

19. Hart JP, and Cooper, WL: Vitamin F in the Treatment of Prostatic Hyperplasia (No.1) Lee Foundation for Nutritional Research, Milwaukee, WI 1941.

20. Scott WW. The Lipids of the Prostatic Fluid, Seminal Plasma and Enlarged Prostate Gland of Man. J Urol. 1945; 53: 712-8.

21. Fahim M, et al. Zinc Treatment for the Reduction of Hyperplasia of the Prostate. Fed Proc 1976; 35: 361.

22. Judd AM, et al. Zinc Acutely, Selectively and Reversibly Inhibits Pituitary Prolactin Secretion. Brain Res 1984; 294: 190-2.

23. Vescovi PP, et al. Pyridoxine (vitamin B-6) Decreases Opiods-Induced Hyperprolactinemia. Horm Metab Res 1985; 17: 46-7.

24. Pansadoro V and Benincasa, A. Prostatic Hypertrophy: Results Obtained with Pygeum africanum extract. Minerva Med 1972; 11: 119-44.

25. Carani C, et al. Urological and Sexual Evaluation of Treatment of Benign Prostatic Disease Using Pygeum africanum at High Dose. Arch Ital Urol Nefrol Androl 1991; 63: 341-5.

26. Netter A, et al. Effect of Zinc Administration on Plasma Testosterone, Dihydrotestosterone and Sperm Count. Arch Androl 1981; 7: 69-73.

27. Prodromos PN, et al. Cranberry Juice in the Treatment of Urinary Tract Infections. Southwest Med 1968; 47: 17.

28. Kahn, DH, et al. Effect of Cranberry Juice on Urine. J Am Dietetic Assoc 1967; 51: 251.

29. Frohne V. Untersuchungen zur Frage der Harndesifizierenden Wirkungen von Barentraubenblatt-extracten. Planta Medical 1970-18: 1-25.

30. Wynder, D, et al. Nutrition and Prostate Cancer: A Proposal for Dietary Intervention. Nutrition and Cancer 1994; 22: 4-10.

Chapter 10

1. Crook, T., et al., Neurology, 1991; 41: 644-649.
2. Someya, H., Journal of Tokyo Medical College. 1985; 43: 815-826.
3. Appa, M., et al., Indian Journal of Psychiatry, 1977; 19: 54-58.
4. Funfgeld, E., et al. Progress in Clinical Biological Research, 1989; 317: 1235-1246.
5. Monteleone, P., et al., European Journal of Clinical Pharmacology, 1992; 41: 385-388.
6. Bjorksten, J. Chemical causes of the aging process. Proceedures of the Scientific Section of the Toilet Goods Association 41: 32-34, 1964.
7. Bjorksten, J. The crosslinkage theory of aging. Journal of the American Geriatrics Society. 16:408-427, 1968.
8. Pauling, L and Rath M. An orthomolecular theory of human health and disease, Journal of Orthomolecular Medicine, Vol 6, 3, 4: 135-138, 1991.
9. Dhalla, KS., et al. Measurement of adrenolutin as an oxidation product of catecholemines in plasma. Molecular and Cellular Biochemistry 87: 85-92, 1989.
10. Bjorksten, J., The crosslinkage theory of aging. Journal of the American Geriatrics Society. 16:408-427, 1968.
11. Otani, M. et al. Effect of an extract of ginkgo biloba on triethyltin-induced cerebral edema, Acta Neuropathol, 69(1-2), 1986, 54-65.
12. Allard, M. Treatment of the disorders of aging with ginkgo biloba extract. Presse Med, 15(31) Sept 25, 1986, 1540-1545.
13. Huguet, F., et al. Decreased cerebral 5-HT1A receptors during aging: Reversal by ginkgo biloba extract. Journal of Pharm Pharmacol, 46(4), April 1994, 316-318.

Chapter 11

1. 1. Lamminpaa, A., et al. Human Experimental Toxicology 1993; 12 (1): 29-32.
2. Pizzorno, J., and Murray, M., Textbook of Natural Medicine. 1993; Bothell, Wash: Bastyr University Press.
3. Lechago, J., et al., Gastroenterology, 1993; 105: 1591-1592.
4. Bray, G. Quarterly Journal of Medicine, 1931; 24: 181-197.
5. Recker, R. New England Journal of Medicine 1985; 313 (2): 70-73.
6. Howitz, J., et al., Lancet 1971; 1: 1331-1335.
7. Giannella, R A., et al., Annals of Internal Medicine 1973; 78: 271-276.
9. Oral Enzymes: Basic information and clinical studies, 1992, Geretsried, Germany, Mucos Pharma Co.

Chapter 12

1. MRCA Information Services, Eating In America, Edition II (Eat II), Chicago: National Livestock and Meat Board, 1994.

2. Westerterp, KR, Food Quotient, respiratory quotient, and energy balance. Am J Clin Nutr. 57 (1993).
3. Glore, SR, et al. Soluble fiber and serum lipids: A literature review. Journal of the American Dietetic Association 94. 1994.
4. Eastwood, MA The physiological effects of dietary fiber: An update. Annual Review of Nutrition. 12, 1992, 19-35.
5. Wolever, TM, et al. The glycemic index: Methodology and clinical implications. Am J Clin Nutr. 54: 846-854, 1991.
6. Mariani, JF, Dictionary of American Food and Drink. New York: Hearst Books, 1994.
7. Campbell, TC., & Chen, J., Diet and chronic degenerative diseases: A summary of result from an ecologic study in rural China. Western Diseases. Totowa, NJ: Humana Press, 1994.
8. Nestle, M. Mediterranean diets: Historical and research overview. Am J Clin Nutr. 61: 1313S-1320S, 1995.
9. Kittler, PG, & Sucher, K., Food and Culture in America. New York: Van Nostrand Reinhold, 1989.
10. Carroll, KK., Biological effects of fish oil in relation to chronic diseases. Lipids, 21: 731-732, 1986.
11. Willett, WC., et al. Intake of trans fatty acids and risk of coronary heart disease among women. The Lancet. 341: 581-585, 1993.
12. Shils, ME, et al. Modern Nutrition in Health and Disease, 6th ed. Philadelphia: Lea and Febiger, 1994.
13. Rasch, PJ., et al. Protein dietary supplementation and physical performance. Medicine and Science in Sports 1: 195-199, 1969.
14. Zemel, MB., Calcium utilization: Effect of varying level and source of dietary protein. Am J Clin Nutr. 48: 880-883, 1988.

Chapter 14

1. Hill, R. et al. The discovery of vitamins, in The Chemistry of Life. Cambridge: Cambridge University Press, 1970.
2. Mertz, W. A balanced approach to nutrition for health: the need for biologically essential minerals and vitamins, Journal of the American Dietetic Association 94: 1259-1262, 1994.
3. McCarthy, MA., & Matthews, RH., Conserving Nutrients in Foods. Administrative report No 384. Hyattsville, MD: Nutrition Monitoring Division, Human Nutrition Information Service, U.S. Dept. of Agriculture. 1988.
4. National Research Council, Recommended Dietary Allowances, 10th Ed. Washington DC, National Academy Press. 1989.
5. Goodhart RS & Shils, ME., Modern Nutrition in Health and Disease, Philadelphia: Lea & Febiger, 1980.
6. Orten, JM., & Neuhaus, OW., Human Biochemistry. St. Louis: The CV Mosby Co. 1994.

1. Bone, RA, et al. Distribution of lutein and zeaxanthin stereoisomers in the human retina. Exp Eye Res 64 (2): 658-62, 1997.

2. Hammond BR., et al. Cigarette smoking and retinal carotenoids: Implications for age-related macular degeneration. Vision Res 36 (18): 3003-3009, 1996

3. Landrum JT, et al. A one-years study of the macular pigment: The effect of 140 days of a lutein supplement. Exp Eye Res 65 (1): 57-62, 1997.

4. Snodderly, DM, Evidence for protection against age-related macular degeneration by carotenoids and antioxidant vitamins. Am J Clin Nutr 62 (6): 1448S-1416S, 1995.

5. Martin, KR, et al. Beta-carotene and lutein protect HepG2 human liver cells against oxidant-induced damage. J Nutr. 126 (9): 2098-2106, 1996.

6. Middleton, E. and Drzwiecki, G. Flavonoid inhibition of human basophil histamine release stimulated by various agents. Biochem Pharmacol 33 (21): 3333-3338, 1984.

7. Baumann, J., et al. Flavonoids and related compounds and inhibitors of arachidonic acid peroxidation. Prostaglandins 20: 627-639, 1980.

8. Bronner, C., and Landry, Y., Kinetics of the inhibitory effect of flavonoids on histamine secretion from mast cells. Agents Actions 16 (3-4): 147-151, 1985.

9. Alschuler, L, Kava root: Herbal treatment for anxiety conditions. Am J Nat Med 4 (10): 22, 1997.

10. Kinzler, E., et al. Effect of a special kava extract in patients with anxiety, tension, and excitation state of non-psychotic genesis: double blind study with placebos over four weeks. Arzneimittel-forschung 41 (6): 584-588, 1991.

11. Balderer, G, Borbely, AA., Effect of valerian on human sleep. Psychopharmacology. 87 (4): 406-409, 1985.

12. Eagon, CL., et al. Estrogenicity of traditonal Chinese and Western herbal remedies. Proc Annu Meet Am Assoc Cancer Res 37: A 1937, 1996.

13. Jarry, H., et al. Studies on the endocrine efficacy of the constituents of Cimicifuga racemose II. In vitro binding of compounds to estrogen receptors. Planta Med 4: 316-319, 1985.

14. Ruiz-Larrerea, MB., Mohan, AR., et al. Antioxidant activity of phytoestrogenic isoflavones. Free Radic Res 26: (1): 63-70, 1997.

15. Liske, E., Therapeutic efficacy and safety of Cimicifuga racemosa for gynecologic disorders. Adv Ther 15 (1): 45-53, 1998.

16. Champhault, G., et al. A double-blind trial of an extract of the plant Serenoa repens in benign prostatic hyperplasia. Br J Clin Pharm 18: 461-462, 1984.

17. Carbin, BE., et al. Treatment of benign prostatic hyperplasia with phytosterols. Br J Urol 66 (6): 639-641, 1990.
18. Berges, jRR., et al. Randomized, placebo-controlled, double-blind clinical trial of betw-sitosterol in patients with benign prostatic hyperplasia: beta-sitosterol Study Group. Lancet 345: 1529-1532, 1995.
19. Shimade, H., et al. Biologically active acylglycerides from the berries of saw-palmetto (Serenoa repens). J Nat Prod 60 (4): 417-418, 1997.
20. Caffarra, P., and Santamaria, jV., The effects of phosphatidylserine in subjects with mild cognitive decline: an open trial. Clin Trials J 24: 109-114, 1987.
21. Delwaide, PJ., et al. Double-blind randomized controlled study of phosphatidylserine in demented subjects. Acta Neurol Scand 73: 136-140, 1986.
22. Monteleone, P., et al. Effects of phosphatidylserine on the neuroendocrine response to physical stress in humans. Neuroendocrinol. 52: 243-248, 1990.
23. Bernard, GR., N-acetylcysteine in experimental and clinical acute lung injury. Am J Med 91 (3C): 54S-59S, 1991.
24. Akerlund, B., et al. Effect of N-acetylcysteine (NAC) treatment on Hiv-1 infection: a double-blind placebo-controlled trial. Eur J Clin Pharmacol 50 (6): 457- 461, 1996.
25. Flanagan, RJ., and Meredith, TJ., Use of N-acetyl-cysteine in clinical toxicology. Am J Med 91 (3C): 131S-139S, 1991.
26. MacNee, W., et al. The effects of N-acetylcysteine and glutathione on smoke-induced changes in lung phagocytes and epithelial cells. Am J Med 91 (3C): 60S-66S, 1991.
27. Kreast, D., et al. Depression of plasma Glutamine concentration after exercise stress and its possible influence on the immune system. Med J Aust 162 (1): 15-18, 1995.
28. Klimber, VS., et al. Oral glutamine accelerates healing of the small intestine and improves outcome after whole abdominal radiation. Arch Surg 125 (8): 1040-1045, 1990.
29. Droge, W., and Holm, E., Role of cysteine and glutathione in HIV infection and other diseases associated with muscle wasting and immunological dysfunction. FASEB J 11 (13): 1077-1089, 1997.
30. Klimber, VS., and Mcclellan, JL., Glutamine, cancer, and its therapy. Am J Surg 172 (5): 418 – 424, 1996.
31. Harward, TR., et al. Glutamine preserves gut glutathione levels during intestinal ischemia/reperfusion. J Surg Res 56 (4): 351-355, 1994.
32. Ames, B., et al. Oxidants, antioxidants, and the degenerative diseases of aging. Proc Natl Acad Sci USA 90: 7918, 1993.
33. Baggio E., et al. Italian multicenter study on the efficcy of coenzyme Q10 as adjunctive therapy in heart failure (interim analysis). Clin Invest 71:S145-149, 1993.

34. Hanaki, Y., Coenzyme Q10 and coronary artery disease. Clin Investig 71: S112-S115, 1993.

35. Kamikawa, T., et al. Effects of Coenzyme Q10 on exercise tolerance in chronic stable angina pectoris. Am J Cardiol 56:247-=251, 1985.

36. Witt, jEH., et al. Exercise, oxidative damage and effects of antioxidant manipulation. J Nutr. 122 (Suppl 3): 766-773, 1992.

37. Folkers, K., et al. Biochemical rationale and the cardiac response of patients with muscle disease to therapy with coenzyme Q10. Proc Natl Acad Sci 82: 4513-4516, 1985.

38. Muriel P., and Mourell, M., Prevention by silymarin of membrane alteration in acute CC14 liver damage. J Appl Toxicol 10 (4): 275-279, 1990.

39. Velussi, M., et al. Long-term (12 months) treatment with an antioxidant drug (silymarin) is effective on hyperinsulinemia, exogenous insulin need and malondialdehyde levels in cirrhotic diabetic patients. J Hepatol 26 (4): 871-872, 1989.

40. Lang, I., et al. Immunomodulatory and hepatoprotective effects of in vivo treatment with free radical scavengers. Ital J Gastroenterol 22:283-287, 1990.

41. Adlercreutz, CH., et al. Soybean phytoestrogen intake and cancer risk. J Nutr 125 (suppl 3) 757-770S, 1995.

42. Wang, TT., et al. Molecular effects of genistein on estrogen receptor mediated pathways. Carcinogenesis 17 (2): 271-275, 1996.

43. Messina, M., Barnes, S., The role of soy products in reducing the risk of cncer. J Natl Cancer Inst 83 (8): 541-546, 1991.

44. Tikkanen, MJ., et al. Effect of soybean phytoestrogen intake on low density lipoprotein oxidation resistance. Proc Natl Acad Sci USA 95 (6): 3106-3110, 1998.

Chapter 17

Note: The following is only a partial list of the references used for this chapter. There were literally hundreds of studies that went into the protocols recommended.

1. Stillians, AW Pyridoxine in treatment of acne vulgaris. J Invest Dermatol 7:150-151, 1946.

2. Plewig G, et al. Action of isotretinoin in acne rosacea and gram-negative folliculitis. J Invest Dermatol 86:390-393, 1986.

3. Bogden JD, et al. Micronutrient status and human immunodeficiency virus (HIV) infection. Ann NY Acad Sci 587: 189-195, 1990.

4. Shambaugh, jGE Jr. Zinc and AIDS. J Appl Nutr 40(20): 138-139, 1989.

5. Baines, M. Detection and incidence of B and C vitamin deficiency in alcohol-related illness. Ann Clin Biochem 15:307-312, 1978.

6. Cleary, JP, Niacinamide and addictions. Letter. J Nutr Med 1: 83-84, 1990.
7. Simon, SW. Vitamin B12 therapy in allergy and chronic dematoses. J Allergy 2: 183-185, 1951.
8. Clemetson, CA Histamine and ascorbic acid in human blood. J Nutr 110(4):662-668, 1980.
9. Reed, JD et al. Nutrition and sickle cell disease. Am J Hematol 24(4): 441-55, 1987.
10. Wray D. A double blind trial of systemic zinc sulfate in recurrent aphthous stomatitis. Oral Surg 53(5): 559-561, 1977.
11. Meyer, EC et al. Vitamin E and benign breast disease. Surgery 107(%): 549-551, 1990.
12. Gately, CA, Mansel RE. Managemetn of the painful and nodular breast. Br Med Bull 47(2):284-294, 1991.
13. Schwartz J, Weiss ST. Dietary factors and their relation to respiratory symptoms. The Second National Health and Nutrition Examination Survey. Am J Epidemiol 132(1): 67-76, 1990.
14. Truss CO. Metabolic abnormalities in patients with chronic candidiasis: The acetaldehyde hypothesis. J Orthomol Psychiatry 13: 66-93, 1984.
15. Fujii T. The clinical effects of vitamin E on purpuras due to vascular defects. J Vitaminology 18: 125-130, 1972.
16. Cox BD, Butterfield WJ. Vitamin C supplements and diabetic cutaneious capillary fragility. Br Med J 3:205, 1975.
17. Roden DM. Magnesium treatment of ventricular arrhythmias. Am J Cardiol 63(14):43G-46G, 1989.
18. Fujioka T, et al. Antiarrhythmic action of coenzyme Q10 in diabetics. Tohoku J Exp Med. 141 (suppl): 453-463, 1983.
19. Driskell JA et al. Effectiveness of pyridoxine hydrochloride treatment on carpal tunnel patients. Nutr Rep Int 34: 1031-1040, 1986.
20. Devamanoharan, P, et al. Prevention of selenite cataract by vitamin C. Exp Eye Res 52: 563-568.
21. Bhat KS. Plasma calcium and trace minerals in human subject with mature cataract. Nutr Rep Int 37:157-163, 1988.
22. Butterworth CE. Et al. Improvement in cervical dysplasia associated with folic acid therapy in usuers of oral contraceptives. Am J Clin Nutr 35: 73-82, 1982.
23. Palan PR et al. Plasma levels of antioxidant beta-carotene and alpha-tocopherol in uterine cervix dysplasias and cancer. Nutr Cancer 15:13-20, 1991.
24. Altura, BM, Altura BT. Biochemistry and pathophysiology of congestive heart failure: Is there a role for magnesium? Magnesium 5(3): 134-143, 1986. Azuma J et al. Double-blind randomized crossover trial of taurine in congestive heart failure. Curr Ther Res 34(4): 543-557, 1983.

672

25. Gorbach SL. Bismuth therapy in gastrointestinal diseases. Gastroenterology 99(3):863-875, 1990.

26. Morse PF et al. Meta-analysis of placebo-controlled studies of the efficacy of Epogram in the treatment of atopic exzema: relationship between plasma essential fatty changes and treatment response. Br J Dermatol 121:75-90, 1989

27. Asregadoo ER. Blood levels of thiamine and ascorbic acid in chronic open-angle glaucoma. Ann Ophthalmol 11(7): 1095-1100, 1979.

28. Campbell RE, Pruitt FW. The effect of vitamin B12 and folic acid in the treatment of viral hepatitis. Am J Med Sci 229:8-15, 1955.

29. McCune MA et al. Treatment of recurrent herpes simplex infections with L-lysine monohydrochloride Cutis 34(4): 366-373, 1984.

30. Zureick M. Treatment of shingles and herpes with vitamin C intravenously. J de Praticiens 64:586-, 1950.

31. Digiese V, et al. Effect of coenzyme Q10 on essential arterial hypertension Curr Ther Res 47:841-845, 1990.

32. Shansky, A. Vitamin B3 in the alleviation of hypglycemia. Drug Cosmetic Industry 129(4):68, 1981.

33. Gugliano D, Torella R. Prostaglandin E1 inhibits glucose-induced insulin secretion in man. Prostaglandins Med 48:302, 1979.

34. Bernstein J et al. Depression of lymphocyte transformation following oral glucose ingestion. Am J Clin Nutr. 30:613, 1977.

35. Cohen B, et al. Revesal of postoperative immunosuppresion in man by vitamin A. Surg Gynecol Obstet 149: 658-662, 1979.

36. Anderson R. The immunostimulatory, anti-inflammatory and anti-allergic properties of ascorbate. Adv Nutr Res 6:19-45, 1984.

37. Chandra RK. Trace element regulation of immunity and infection. J Am Coll Nutr 4 (1): 5-16, 1985.

38. Reynolds JV, et al. Immunomodulary mechanisms of arginine. Surgery 104(2): 142-151, 1988.

39. Pinnock CB et al. Vitamin A status in children who are prone to respiratory tract infections. Aust Paediatr J 22(2): 95-99, 1986.

40. Carr AB et al. Vitamin C and the common cold: Using identical twins as controls. Med J Aust 2: 411-412, 1981.

41. Baer MT et al. Nitrogen utilization, enzyme activity, glucose intolerance and leukocyte chemataxis in human experimental zinc depletion. Am J Clin Nutr 41(6): 1220-1235, 1985.

42. Roberts P. et al. Vitamin C and inflammation. Med Biol 62:88, 1984.

43. Cichoke AJ, Marty L. The use of proteolytic enzymes with soft tissue athletic injuries. Am Chiropractor, October 1981, P 32.

44. Romeo G.The therapeutic effect of vitamins A and E in neurosensory hearing loss. Acta Vitaminol Enzymol 7 Suppl: 85-92, 1985

45. Moser M et al. A double-blind clinical trial of hydroxyethylrutosides in Meniere's disease. J Laryngol Otol 98(3): 265-272, 1984.

46. Mitwalli A et al. Control of hyperoxaluria with large doses of

pyridoxine in patients with kidney stones. Int Urol Nephrol 20(4): 353-359, 1988.

47. Welsh AL Lupus erythematosus: Treatment by combined use of massive amounts of pantothenic acid and vitamin E. Arch Dermatol Syphilol 70:1810198, 1954.

48. Katz ML et al. Dietary vitamins A and E influence retinyl ester composition and content of the retinal pigment epithelium Biochim Biophys Acta 824(3):432-441, 1987.

49. Newsome DA et al. Oral zinc in macular degeneration. Arch Ophthalmol 106(2):192-198, 1988.

50. Wright JV et al. Improvement of vision in macular degeneration associated with intravenous zinc and selenium therapy: two cases J Nutr Med 1:133-138, 1990.

51. Sotonishi T et al. Treatment of climacteric complaints with gamma oryzanol plus tocopherol. Folha Med (Brazil) 77(2): 235, 1978.

52. Wilcox G et al. Oestrogenic effects of plant foods in postmenopausal women. Br Med J 301: 905-906, 1990

53. Reynolds, EH, Linnell JC. Vitamin B12 deficiency, demyelination and multiple sclerosis. Lancet 2-920, 1987

54. Mai J. et al. High dose antioxidant supplementation to MS patients. Biol Trace Element Res 24:109, 1990.

55. Wolfgram, F et al. Serum linoleic acid in multiple sclerosis. Neurology 25(8): 786-788, 1975.

56. Page EW, Page EP, Leg crams in pregnancy: Etiology and treatment. Obstet Gynecol 1(94):1953.

57. Milhorat AT Bartels WE. The defect in utilization of tocopherol in progressive muscular dystrophy. Science. 101:93-94, 1945

58. Tomasi LG. Reversibility of human myopathy caused by vitamin E deficiency. Neurology 29:1182, 1979.

59. Nurmikko T et al. Attentuation of tourniquet-induced pain in man by D-phenylalanine, a putative inhibitor of enkephalin degradation. Acupunct Electrother Res. 12 (3-4):185-191, 1987.

60. Reilly DK et al. On-off effects in Parkinson's disease: a controlled investigation of ascorbil acid therapy. Adv Neurol 37:51-60, 1983.

61. Snider SR. Octacosanol in parkinsonism. Letter Ann Neurol 16(6):723, 1984.

62. Rubinoff, AB et al. Vitamin C and oral health. J Can Dent Assoc 55(9):705-707, 1989.

63. Khmelevski IuV et al. Effect of vitamins A, E, and K on the indices of the glutathione antiperoxidase system in gingival tissues in periodontosis. Vopr Pitan (4): 54-56, 1985.

64. Piesse JW. Vitamin E and peripheral vascular disease. Int Clin Nutr Rev 4(4):178-182, 1984.

65. Brevetti G et al. Increases in walking distance in patients with peripheral vascular disease treated with L-carnitine: A double-blind,

cross-over study. Circulation 77(4):767-773, 1988.

66. Chuong CJ, et al. Vitamin A levels in premenstrual syndrome. Fertil Steril 54(4):643-647, 1990.

67. Doll H et al. Pyridoxine and the premenstrual syndrome: A randomized crossover trial. JR Coll Gen Pract 39:364-368, 1989.

68. Morimoto S et al. Therapeutic effect of 1,25-dihydroxyvitamin D3 for psoriasis: Report of five cases. Calcif Tissue Inter 38: 119-122, 1986.

69. Dochao A et al. Therapeutic effects of vitamin D and vitamin A in psoriasis: A 20-year experiment. Actas Dermosifiliogr 66(3-4):121-130, 1975.

70. DiGiacomo RA et al. Fish-oil dietary supplementation in patients with Raynaud's phenomenon: da double-blind, controlled, prospective study. Am J Med 86:158-164, 1989.

71. Ellis JM Folkers K. Clinical aspects of treatment of carpal tunnnel syndrome with vitamin B6. Ann NY Acad Sci 585:302-320, 1990.

72. Barton-Wright EC, Elliott WA. The pantothenic acid metabolism of rheumatoid arthritis. Lancet 2: 862-863, 1963.

73. Honkanen V et al. Vitamins A and E, retinol binding protein and zinc in rheumatoid arthritis. Clin Exp Rheumatol 7:465-469, 1989.

74. Block MT. Vitamin E in the treatment of diseases of the skin. Clin Med Jan. 1953.

75. Gey GO, et al. Effect of ascorbic acid on endurance performance and athletic injury. JAMA 211(1):105, 1970.

76. Shimomura Y et al. Protective effect of coenzyme Q10 on exercise-induced muscular injury. Biochem Biophys Res Commun 176:349-355, 1991.

77. Salomon P et al. Treatment of ulcerative colitis with fish oil in n-3-omega fatty acid: an open trial. J Clin Gastroenterol 12(2):157-161, 1990.

Alvarez OM Gilbreath RL, Thiamin influence on collagen during the granulation of skin wounds. J Surg Res 32:24-31, 1982.

RESOURCES

Many of the recommendations in this book may be difficult to find in some areas. The following sources offer mail order on specific products we have used and found to meet our specifications.

How to reach us:

The Institute of Nutritional Science
9528 Miramar Road #180
San Diego, CA 92126
Tel. 858-653-6566
Fax 858-271-0912
Website: www.healthyinformation.com
www.instituteofnutritionalscience.org

In Europe:

The Institute of Nutritional Science
Van Boetzelaerlaan 155
2518 AR Den Haag
The Netherlands

For Full Spectrum Nutrition and specific formulations for arthritis, prostate, heart disease, diabetes and other chronic conditions as described and used by us, contact:

In the United States:

The Institute of Nutritional Science
At the above address

In Europe & Canada:

Vitmin International
UK Freephone: 08000 265 265
NL Bel Gratis: 08000 240 505
Main Office Tel. +31 70 306 3202
Fax +31 70 306 3204
E-mail: info@VitMin.com

Low Carbohydrate Foods – for those who are carbohydrate intolerant

Life Services Supplements Inc
3535 Hwy 66,
Neptune, NJ 07753
1-800-542-3230

European Chicken Cartilage – used with Rheumatoid Arthritis

Personal Health Lifestyles
1-800-943-1123

Referral Organizations and Services

IV Chelation Therapy

Provides a nation-wide listing of participating physicians
American College for the Advancement in Medicine
1-800-532-3688

PO Box 3427
Laguna Hills, CA 92654

Holistic Psychiatry

Provides a listing of participating psychiatrists in Canada and the US
Orthomolecular Psychiatry Association
416-733-2117
www.orthomed.org
16 Florence Avenue
Toronto, Ontario M2M 1E9
Canada

Naturopathic Physicians

Provides a nation-wide referral service for naturopathic physicians
National College of Naturopathic Medicine
503-255-4860
11231 SE Market Street
Portland, Oregon 97216

Hyperbaric Oxygen Therapy

Facility provides actual service
Health Restoration Center
Dr. David Steenblock
949-367-8870 or 1-800-300-1063

Multiple Sclerosis – calcium orotate etc.

Provides the works of the late Dr Hans Neiper, renowned specialist in the natural treatment of MS.

A. Keith Brewer Foundation
International Science Library
325 North Central Avenue
Richland Center, WI 53581
608-647-6513

Index